The Heart of Wisdom: Studies on the Heart Amulet in Ancient Egypt

Rogério Sousa

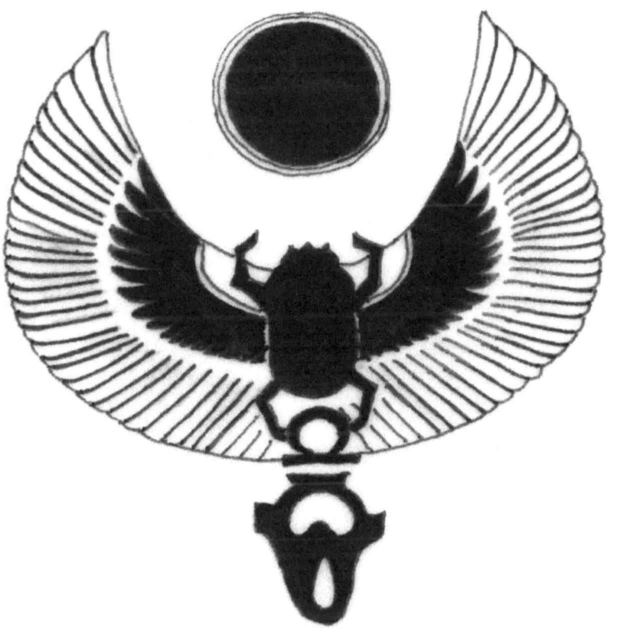

BAR International Series 2211
2011

Published in 2016 by
BAR Publishing, Oxford

BAR International Series 2211

The Heart of Wisdom: Studies on the Heart Amulet in Ancient Egypt

ISBN 978 1 4073 0769 5

BAR Publishing is the trading name of British Archaeological Reports (Oxford) Ltd. British Archaeological Reports was first incorporated in 1974 to publish the BAR Series, International and British. In 1992 Hadrian Books Ltd became part of the BAR group. This volume was originally published by Archaeopress in conjunction with British Archaeological Reports (Oxford) Ltd / Hadrian Books Ltd, the Series principal publisher, in 2011. This present volume is published by BAR Publishing, 2016.

Printed in England

BAR
PUBLISHING

BAR titles are available from:

BAR Publishing
122 Banbury Rd, Oxford, OX2 7BP, UK
EMAIL info@barpublishing.com
PHONE +44 (0)1865 310431
FAX +44 (0)1865 316916
www.barpublishing.com

Can you get through life with a good heart?

That´s been my struggle: to try and get the heart to rebound and bloom again

Joni Mitchel (2003)

To my sister Laura,

and to her quest for truth, strength and beauty

CONTENTS

ACKNOWLEDGEMENTS

Some of the studies presented in this volume have been previously published in egyptological journals. I am deeply in debt to the critical contributions of many of their reviewers and to the colleagues who generously and patiently enriched this work with their knowledge. I would like here to address my especial gratitude to Eugene Cruz-Euribe (*Journal of the American Research Center in Egypt*), Jean-Luc Chappaz (*Bulletin de la Société Egyptologique de Genève*), Carla Balconi (*Aegyptus: Revista Italiana de Egittologia e Papirologia*), Alejandro Serrano (*Boletín de la Associacion Española de Egiptologia*) and most specially to Herman de Meaulenaere (*Chronique d'Égypte*) who provided me the most careful and attentive editorial assistance.

This work was only possible thanks to the active collaboration of the staff from the Egyptian Antiquities Department of the Louvre Museum and of the Cairo Egyptian Museum, who provided full support for our research. For that reason we would like to address our acknowledgement to Sylvie Guichard, Patricia Rigault and Mahmoud Ibrahim. To the curators who kindly sent us museological documentation, we would also like to express our gratitude, namely to Cláudia Monte Farias and Isabel Stuenkel (Metropolitan Museum of Art), Nigel Strudwick (Bristish Museum), Richard Langley (Petrie Museum) and Christian Loeben (August Kestner Museum).

I would like to address a thankful acknowledgement to those that contributed in one way or another to improve my work. To Rune Nyord who read some chapters of this book. A significant contribution has been given to this book by Erik Hornung who carefully reviwed the totality of the text and provided encouragement and precious suggestions to improve it. Kerstin Hoffmeister provided translations of German texts that could not otherwise have been used in my work. As regards the English text, the final outcome of this volume would never be possible without the careful and dedicated revision provided by Maria Macedo, Daniel Miguel and by Marie Bryan who generously and most paciently assisted me in this difficult task.

Some of the drawings published in this book are only possible to present thanks to Andrzej Niwinski who generously allowed me the possibility to explore his extensive photographic resources on the Egyptian coffins of the 21st Dynasty. I also thank him for the authorization to publish in this book some of his own drawings.

I also could not forget the support and encouradgement of my colleagues and students from the Instituto Superior das Ciências da Saúde – Norte and from the CITCEM, the research center from the Faculdade de Letras da Universidade do Porto, especially in what concerns to the endless support provided by their Directors, Jorge Proença and Gaspar Martins, respectively.

I am deeply indebted to all of these contributions but I cannot ignore the primary role undertaken by Luís Manuel de Araújo, from the University of Lisbon, who directed my PhD research and always has been an enduring inspiration to my work.

Last but not the least, I would like to thank to all my family and friends for their constant source of support throughout my life, namely to Daniel, Maria do Carmo, my parents, my sister Laura and my nephews, Tomás e João Pedro, who have been able to join to my work so much love, wisdom and joy.

Porto, June 2010

ROGÉRIO SOUSA

INTRODUCTION

When we started to study heart amulets in ancient Egypt we could not guess that we were about to find one of the most complex sets of images and symbols ever created to express the nature of the human mind. Notwithstanding the richness (both in quality and in quantity) of the material related to the heart amulets, we were surprised to find that few studies have been published on the symbolism of this object.

Nevertheless, studies on the Egyptian concept of the heart are almost as old as Egyptology itself. Numerous archaeological findings certainly helped to direct the attention of early scholars to the prominent role of the heart in ancient Egypt. Particularly intriguing in the eyes of the first explorers would have been the large funerary scarabs that were found over or within the chest of the mummies. Depictions of these funerary items are abundantly documented in the Napoleonic *Description de l'Égypte* as well as the depictions of the judgement of the dead that illustrated the funerary papyri. Thus, even before the decipherment of the hieroglyphs, it was possible to gain insights into the major significance of the heart in the Egyptian afterlife.[1]

Notwithstanding the huge number of depictions and objects related to the heart, in the early days of Egyptian archaeology the decipherment of hieroglyphs overshadowed the study and interpretation of iconography. Throughout the nineteenth century, efforts were focused on Egyptian philology with early scholars working on the translation of hieroglyphic texts. In the mid-nineteenth century, Samuel Birch published important contributions to the identification of the terminology of the 'heart'.[2] By the beginning of the twentieth century the maturity and ongoing security gained in the decipherment of the hieroglyphic writing, along with the increasing number of published documents, allowed the development of the first systematic approaches to the Egyptian sources. The first attempts to study the heart can be found in the pioneering work of Alexander Piankoff. [3] The author inventoried a large repertory of semantic contexts in which the use of the cardiac words can be found in the hieroglyphic writing. It was immediately clear to Piankoff that, although they refer to the anatomical organs, the words used to denote the heart were mainly used to designate the seat of the mind, being strongly connected to the feelings, reasoning and will. It also became evident that the Egyptian notion of the heart was multidimensional, combining anatomical and psychological aspects in a one all-encompassing entity.

It was only after the two world wars that further studies sought to define and detail the subtleties that this anthropological concept achieved in the Egyptian literary texts. Following this line of philological research, Adrian de Buck published several articles that aimed to define various aspects of the Egyptian 'psychology' through the study of the cardiac chapters of the *Book of the Dead*.[4] Another important contribution to estimate the Egyptian definition of the heart was provided by Helmutt Brunner. Several articles, compiling the bulk of his research in this area, still provide the quintessential definition of the multiple aspects of the heart as it was depicted in the wisdom and religious literature.[5] With the work of this author the heart came to be fully understood as the centre of the human being, a pivotal piece that united the body, the *ka* and all the multiple set of elements that were seen as part of the human nature.

Following the heyday of cross-cultural biblical approaches, many studies pointed out to the similarities between Egyptian and biblical wisdom literature. Biblical scholars were able to identify the influence of Egyptian texts on the Jewish tradition, for example the *Teachings of Amenemope* in the *Book of Proverbs*, or even the influence of the *Great Hymn of Aten* in the Psalm 104. At this point it also becomes clear that the Egyptian view of the heart revealed strong affinities with the biblical characterization of the heart.[6] These similarities showcased, for example, that behind the rhetorical contrast of the 'hardened heart' of the Pharaoh (Ex 9,12) and the chosen people who were 'wise of heart' (Ex 36:8), one could clearly identify identical categories of thought in both biblical and Egyptian wisdom literature and therefore recognize the wide cultural influence of Egypt among Israelite sages.

As first attempted on biblical texts, tracing back the genealogy of Egyptian wisdom texts proved to be a fruitful task. In her authoritative study on Egyptian autobiographies, Miriam Lichtheim was also able to demonstrate that interest in the characterization of the heart

[1] See heart amulet in *Description de l'Égypte*, 2002, p. 554 (n° 50), p. 555 (n° 10). Heart scarabs can be seen in *Idem*, p. 550 (n° 8 and n° 11). Also vignettes of the weighing of the heart, in *Idem*, p. 241, and p. 250-251.

[2] See S. BIRCH, 'On formulas relating to the heart', *ZÄS* 4 (1866), pp. 89-92; *Idem*, 'On formulas relating to the heart', *ZÄS* 5 (1867), pp 16-17; *Idem*, 'On formulas of three royal coffins', *ZÄS* 7 (1869), pp. 49-53; *Idem*, 'On formulas relating to the heart', *ZÄS* 8 (1870), pp 30-34.

[3] A. PIANKOFF, *Le 'Coeur' dans les Textes Égyptiens depuis l'Ancien jusqu'à la fin du Nouvel Empire*, 1930.

[4] A. DE BUCK, ‚Een groep dodenboekspreuken betreffende het hart', *JEOL* 9 (1944), pp. 9-24. Also *Idem*, 'Un chapitre de Psychologie Egyptienne', in *Cd'É* 41 (1946), pp. 17-24.

[5] H. BRUNNER, ‚Herz', in Wolfgang Helck e Wolfhart Westendorf (ed.), *Lexikon der Ägyptologie,* II, cols 1158-1168; H. BRUNNER, *Das hörende Herz. Kleine Schriften zur religions und Geitesgeschichte Ägyptens*, 1988.

[6] M. LICHTHEIM, *Moral Values in ancient Egypt*, 1997. Also N. SHUPAK, *Where wisdom can be found? The Sage's Language in the Bible and in Ancient Egyptian Literature*, 1993.

in Egyptian texts was connected to a growing interest in the definition of the character, which was seen as a way to assure a positive outcome for the judgement of the dead.[7] Literary concern in the characterization of the inner man, i.e., the heart, developed as early as the First Intermediate Period. Although expressed in the context of Egyptian wisdom literature, reflection about the heart was clearly the result of the development and democratization of the funerary belief system of the afterlife. The flourishing exploration of the multiple aspects of the heart was thus related both to the wisdom literature and to the Osirian beliefs about the afterlife.

It was, however, Jan Assmann who, in the nineties, first attempted to establish a complete theory to explain the development of the concept of the heart through an innovative approach that consisted in the relation between the heart and the development of the notion of *maet* along in Egyptian civilization. My means of this conceptual approach he was able to define three major phases in the characterization of the heart.[8] Although the heart, as the seat of the mind, was always seen as the crucial 'piece' in assuring the cosmic integration of each individual, i.e., to assure the realization of *maet*, the way that this integration was understood developed according to the changes that affected the problematization of *maet* throughout Egyptian history. To Jan Assmann, the lack of interest that autobiographies from the Old Kingdom display in the description of the subject's hearts is due to the way that *maet* was seen in this period: only the Pharaoh was responsible for the *maetic* order. Thus, in order to be aligned with the Pharaoh's rule, each individual should guide his heart by the command of the king. This was the period of the 'king-guided individual'. Later, after the collapse of the Old Kingdom, the ability of the Pharaoh to keep *maetic* order was 'democratized' and transferred to the private context. From than on, each individual was responsible for assuring the cosmic order in his own sphere of action. This delegation of royal responsibilities did not come without an equal sharing of royal prerogatives: once reserved to the Pharaoh, the possibility of living in the afterlife as a god could then be shared with royal subjects. Still, this 'justification' was only accessible through a judicial process which took place in the court of Osiris, the weighing of the heart. These symbolic features are typical of the second stage of the development of the heart: in order to be accepted among the justified ones, each individual should follow his own heart, i.e., his wisdom, in order to assure the maintenance of *maet*. This was the period of the 'heart-guided individual'. The rise of personal piety, toward the end of the 18th Dynasty, prompted a second transformation in the understanding of the heart. By this time, Assmann postulates what he defines as the absorption of the reflection about *maet* within the context of a personal relationship to god. As a consequence, the notion of the 'god-guided individual' emerges and with it the heart is seen as directly guided by the command of god.

With regard to the study of anatomical concepts related to the heart, multiple attempts were made to distinguish the precise meaning of the terms and *ib* and *haty* in medical texts. Gustave Lefebvre presented views that would remain as important references with which to understand the anatomical use of these words.[9] Also James Walker in indispensable work on Egyptian medical terminology, proposed an anatomical definition of these words.[10] In this particular area Thierry Bardinet made a decisive contribution to shedding light on an issue that, both before and after his work, has often been the subject of heated debate.[11] It is interesting to note that, although he deals with different sources, Rune Nyord also corroborates Bardinet's point of view about the anatomical definition of the cardiac words in his work about the anatomical concepts of the *Coffin Texts*.[12]

Of course, a concept as central as the heart has produced a large quantity of scientific literature and many important contributions to the understanding of this notion came out of the study of other Egyptian anthropological notions. The study of the *ba*, the *ka*, the *akh*, just to list some of the key elements of human nature, provided important clarifications of the relationship of the heart to these ontological dimensions. Following the seminal philological work of Piankoff about the heart, studies developed by Gertie Englund[13] and Louis Zakbar[14] focused on textual evidence. This has been, in our opinion, one of the remaining barriers to a broader view of Egyptian anthropology: the abundance of iconographic sources related to anthropological elements had not yet been systematically approached and integrated with textual sources.

With regard to the notion of the heart, we have found that a study concerned with the extensive iconographical repertoire of the heart was still lacking. This absence clearly contrasts with the overwhelming abundance of the heart related artefacts or representations in museological collections and in archaeological sites. Nevertheless, important studies concerning particular objects or depictions related to the heart have been published over the years. The seminal work of Michel Malaise remains the reference work on the topic of heart scarabs.[15] The author explored the symbolism of these objects, inventoried symbols and inscriptions found among them

[7] M. LICHTHEIM, *Maat in Egyptian Autobiographies and related studies*, 1992

[8] J. ASSMANN, ‚Zur Geschichte des Herzens im alten Ägypten', *Idem* (ed.) *Die Erfindung des inneren Menschen: Studien zur reliogiösen Anthropologie*, 1993, p. 81-113. See also *idem*, *The Mind of Egypt: History and meaning in the time of the pharaohs*, 2002, p. 135-137 and p. 229-230.

[9] G. LEFEBVRE, *Tableau des Parties du Corps Humain mentionées par les Égyptiens*, 1952.

[10] J. WALKER, *Studies in Ancient Egyptian Anatomical Terminology*, 1996

[11] T. BARDINET, *Les papyrus médicaux de l'Égypte pharaonique*, 1995.

[12] R. NYORD, *Breathing Flesh. Conceptions of the Body in the Ancient Egyptian Coffin Texts*, 2009

[13] G. ENGLUND, *Akh - une notion religeuse dans l'Égypte pharaonique*, Boreas 11, 1978.

[14] L. ZABKAR, *A study of the Ba concept in Egyptian texts*, 1968.

[15] M. MALAISE, *Les Scarabées de coeur dans l'Égypte Ancienne*, 1978.

CHAPTER ONE

THE DEPICTION OF THE HEART AMULET IN EGYPTIAN ART

The heart amulet is one of the amulets more often depicted in Egyptian art. Due to the scarcity of archaeological information available about the heart amulet, its artistic depictions represent an important and decisive source for the study of the meaning of these objects. In fact, the artistic rendering of the heart amulet, supplemented with information available in the archaeological context, can offer us a vivid picture of its use through time. We know that the amulet was already in use as early as the 11th Dynasty among the circle of Theban royalty.[1] However, the first known depiction of the heart amulet only occurs at the beginning of the 18th Dynasty, in the Donation Stela, where the object is used by the young prince.[2] It must also be noted that the heart amulet can be found as well in a group sculpture dated from the same period depicting royal children on the knees of a nurse.[3]

However, the most important example of royal use of the amulet is found in Deir-el-Bahari.[4] A solar heart amulet is clearly depicted in the Punt expedition relief of the funerary temple of Hatshepsut.[5] Hatshepsut/Thutmosis III wears the amulet in a ritual where she/he gives to Amun all the incense brought from Punt.

Interestingly enough, in the context of Thebes, the first documents that portray the use of the amulet by non-royalty date only from the reign of Amenhotep II on. For example, Amenhotep, "overseer of the builders of Amun," in the reign of Amenhotep II is portrayed with this amulet on the chest of his coffin.[6] Sennefer, governor of Thebes during the reign of the same king, is also shown with a double heart amulet in the decoration of his tomb (TT 96). Maherpa, "bearer of the fan" and an intimate friend of Thutmose IV, also wears a heart amulet on the chest of one of his precious wooden coffin found in his tomb of the Valley of the Kings (KV 36).[7] Yuia, father of queen Tiye, is depicted with a heart amulet in a vignette of the *Book of the Dead*,[8] on a *shawabty* statuette[9] and on a *ba* bird statuette.[10] Khaemhat, royal scribe of Amenhotep III, is shown with different kinds of heart amulets in his tomb decoration (TT 57).[11] Ramose, governor of the city of Thebes, also uses the object in a purification ceremony depicted in his famous Theban tomb (TT 55).[12] Also the governor of Memphis, Menkheper, was depicted in his Theban tomb wearing the heart amulet.[13]

However important the use of the heart amulet might have been in this period, it seems to have vanished from the depictions of Akhenaten's reign. Curiously enough, it became increasingly popular in the pictorial and sculptural production of the Ramessid Period. In tomb decoration in particular, the heart amulet is frequently depicted in scenes related to funerary ceremonies or to the afterlife of royal subjects, as in the case of Rai, "royal scribe and supervisor of the domains of Horemheb and Amun" (TT 255),[14] Amenemopet "overseer of the domains of Amun" (TT 41) and Userhat, "funerary priest of the royal cult of Tutmose I" (TT 51).[15] At Deir el-Medina, the tombs of Neferabu (TT 5), Nebenmaet (TT 219) and Irinefer (TT 290)[16] also show the deceased portrayed with the amulet in afterlife scenes. Occasionally, funerary sculpture also portrays the deceased with the amulet.[17]

During the 21st Dynasty the object retained much of its magical importance and is frequently depicted on the chest of the anthropoid coffins of the period. Among the coffins found in the royal cache of Deir el-Bahari, some of the most impressive were decorated with depictions of the heart amulet, sometimes associated with images of the solar scarab.[18] It is also among the finest anthropoid

[1] This is the case of the golden object inscribed with the cartouche of Nebhetepre Mentuhotep II (Louvre Museum, N 551). See Fig. 8.

[2] See Fig. 94. See also I. HARARI, "Nature de la Stéle de Donation de Fonction du roi Ahmôsis a la reine Ahmès-Nefertari", *ASAE* 56 (1956), Pl. II. Before the 18th Dynasty the identification of heart amulets in Egyptian art is doubtful. The amulet weared by prince Rahotep in his famous statue (CG 3, Cairo Egyptian Museum), seems more to be a turtle amulet than a heart. Other amulets in use before the Middle Kingdom presenting a resemblance with the heart amulet seem to be amuletic bourses used to keep other objects within. Royal statues from the Middle Kingdom present sometimes a amulet with a strange resemblance with the heart depicted among the vignettes of chapter 28 of the *Book of the Dead* from the Late Period on (see for instance, papyrus N 3081 from the Louvre Museum, Fig. 38)

[3] JE 98831 (Cairo Egyptian Museum). See C. SHEIKHOSLESLAMI, *The Egyptian Museum at the Millenium: a Special Exhibition in honor of the VIIIth International Congress of Egyptologists*, 2000, pl. 22.

[4] Nevertheless, archaeological data show that, early in 18th Dynasty, the amulet was already used among the Theban royal elite. For example, the object was found in the mummies of the king Ahmose and queen Ah-hotep.

[5] See Fig. 70 and Fig. 45.

[6] See ECM 1876 (Eton College): in S. SPURR, N. REEVES, S. QUIRKER, *Egyptian Art at Eton College: Selections from the Myers Museum*, 1999, p. 24.

[7] JE 31378/CG 4219 (Cairo Egyptian Museum). See Fig. 77.

[8] See T. DAVIS, *The Funeral Papyrus of Iouiya. With an Introduction by Édouard Naville*, 1908, pl. I.

[9] SR 95368 (Cairo Egyptian Museum): in J. QUIBELL, *The Tomb of Yuaa and Thuiu*, Cairo, 1908, pl. XVIII

[10] JE 95312 (Cairo Egyptian Museum). See Fig. 64.

[11] See Fig. 72 and Fig. 73.

[12] See Fig. 75.

[13] See Fig. 71.

[14] See Fig. 78.

[15] See Fig. 76.

[16] See Fig. 85.

[17] See group statue of Meriptah, N. Inv. 48 (Kunsthistorisches Museum, Viena). In H. SATSINGER, *Das Kunsthistorisches Museum in Wien*, p. 38.

[18] Both coffins of Pinedjem II (Cairo Egyptian Museum, JE 26197) and the outer coffin of Nesikhonsu (Cairo Egyptian Museum, JE 26199), his wife, have an elaborated iconographic programme where the heart or the heart amulet stands as a central element. See G. DARESSY, *Cercueils des cachettes royales*, 1909, pl. XLII, XLV. See also Fig. 66.

coffins from Bab el-Gasus that we find the most striking depictions of the heart amulet, especially on their chests.[19] Items such as these suggest that complex depictions of the heart amulet were an attribute of high rank. The object is occasionally found on a few women's coffins,[20] but it seems that the depiction of the heart amulet is still more closely related to the male priests. Besides the depiction of the amulet on the lids of the coffins, it was also frequently drawn in the scenes painted on the exterior walls of the cases, most of them alluding to the vignettes of the *Book of the Dead*.[21] Similar depictions are also found in the so-called "mythological papyri" typical of the period.[22]

Latter, in Late Period editions of the *Book of the Dead*, the heart amulet remains an important symbol but, especially in the context of the vignettes of the weighing of the heart, it seems to be more an attribute of the solar child than of the deceased.[23] In fact, after the 21st Dynasty, the amulet is rarely depicted in human contexts and it is used mainly as an iconographical attribute of specific divinities, such as the divine children (Horpakhered, Nefertum or Ihy) or the falcon gods, such as Horus[24] or the Akhet bird.[25] In a few Greco-Roman artefacts, the amulet finds its final use among the iconographic features of Isis-Aphrodite or Nut-Hathor.[26]

Examining the information collected thus far, we can ascertain an important development in the use of the heart amulet from the early New Kingdom until the Late Period. Archaeological and iconographic data suggest that, until the beginning of 18th Dynasty, the object seemed to have a strong connection to Theban royalty and could have been used to indicate "divine" status. From the reign of Amenhotep II on, perhaps reflecting the desire to strengthen the loyalty of the high officers towards the king, it is possible that the amulet started to be used as a very exclusive royal decoration. This is suggested by the fact that it can only be found among individuals more closely connected to the king. Although the depiction of the ceremony of the gold of honour seems to retain all of its political significance in the tombs of Amarna, the depiction of the heart amulet has disappeared from these scenes, which may alert us to some peculiarities of its meaning. Since it could still be viewed as an important sign of the Theban elite, the heart amulet was possibly seen as an unacceptable symbol to the spirit of Amarna's reform, which re-established the king as the sole keeper of *maet*.

Curiously enough, in the Ramessid Period, depictions of the heart amulet were found more and more frequently in the tomb decoration of the Theban necropolis. However, after the Amarna Period the object seems to have been used with a different meaning, since it was not used in a political context but in a religious one, in strong association with the afterlife and the judgement of the dead. It was also used with this same meaning in the iconography of the Theban 21st Dynasty.

From then on, a new change occurred and the object came to be an iconographic attribute of child divinities. Even when the Pharaoh used the amulet, it seems that the intention was to express an identification between the king and a child god (such as Ihy or Horpakhered).

Following this diachronical trend of the use of the heart amulet we have found it useful to group the artistic renderings of this object into four major symbolic contexts in which it seems to be invested with distinct symbolic meaning and perhaps also used in various ritual contexts.[27]

1. The heart of illumination

In this particular and highly exclusive context we group depictions that present the heart amulet adorned with the solar disk. Depictions such as these seem to be an attribute of the avian form of the god Horus. In fact, the object is frequently depicted in later divine statues of the god.[28]

More rarely, the solar amulet is also shown in the context of royal rituals. This is the case with the dedication of

[19] It is usually on the finest coffins that the amulet is represented. See the coffin and mummy cover of Padiamun (Cairo Egyptian Museum, CG 6233/CG 6235) and the mummy cover of Pakharu (Cairo Egyptian Museum, CG 6122, now in Alexandria National Museum). About this coffin see E. HORNUNG & B. BRYAN, *The Quest of Immortality: Treasures of Ancient Egypt*, 2002, p. 158. Depictions of the amulet are also found on CG 6153 and CG 6191. To these coffins see A. NIWINSKI, *The Second Find of Deir el-Bahri (Coffins)*, 1999, fig. 113. Similar depictions can be found in the coffin CG 6028 (Cairo Egyptian Museum) and in many other monuments. Also the coffin AE 10 (Berna Historical Museum): in R. SCHULZ, M. SEIDEL, *Egipto: O Mundo dos Faraós*, 1997, p. 476. Also N 2503533 (Vatican Gregorian Museum): in A. GASSE, *Les Sarcophages de la Troisiéme Periode Intermédiaire du Museo Gregoriano Egizio*, 1996, p. 81, pl.XIII, 2. Coffin AF 9593 (Louvre Museum) – Fig. 46. See also Fig. 49, Fig. 65, Fig. 67 and Fig. 109.

[20] Unet (AF 9593, Louvre Museum), Direpu (CG 6028, Cairo Egyptian Museum,) and Ikhi (N 2503532) were songstresses of Amun. They wear the amulet on the chest of their coffins. Nesitanebetacheru and Unet also show the amulet on the scene of the weighing of the heart displayed on their coffins. However, the coffin of Unet was not made for a lady, but for a male priest: the lid of the coffin depicts a male priest, but the side decoration of the coffin depicts the female songstress. Anyway, we may take as a rule that, when a couple is depicted, it is always the man that wears the amulet. See *Book of the Dead* of the architect Kha and his wife Merit, from Deir el-Medina (TT 8) and the funerary papyrus of Yuya (from KV 46).

[21] Most of these scenes depict the heart amulet in the context of the weighing of the heart (outer coffin of Pakharu, CG 6122/6121, in Alexandria National Museum) but it can also be found among other vignettes such as the deceased before the Tree goddesses (see also outer coffin of Pakharu). See Fig. 81 and Fig. 82.

[22] See Fig. 53 - vignette of the weighing of the heart in the funerary papyrus of Nesipakhashuti, E 17401 (Louvre Museum). In A. PIANKOFF, N. RAMBOVA, *Mythological Papyri*, 1955, Pl. 104.

[23] See Fig. 100 – (OIM 10486, Oriental Institut Museum). In T. ALLEN, *The Egyptian Book of the Dead*, Pl. LXXXII. To the depiction of the heart amulet in the cardiac vignettes (chapters 26-30) of the late versions of the *Book of the Dead* see R. SOUSA, "The cardiac vignettes of the Book of the Dead (Late Period)", *BAEDE* 17 (2007), 39-53.

[24] See Fig. 44 - JE 30335 (Cairo Egyptian Museum): in J.-P. CORTEGGIANI, *L'Égypte des Pharaons au Musée du Caire*, 1986, p. 160. See Fig. 44.

[25] See SR 6850 (Cairo Egyptian Museum).

[26] See Fig.105 and See Fig. 106.

[27] Although these categories may in fact be largely representative of the depictions of the heart amulet in Egyptian art, we can add to these major themes a few exceptional motifs which will be the focus of our analysis in another chapter.

[28] See avian statue of Horus, Fig. 44 - JE 30335 (Cairo Egyptian Museum): J.P. CORTEGGIANI, *L'Égypte des Pharaons au Musée du Caire*, 1986, p. 160. See Fig. 44.

offerings performed by Hatshepsut/Thutmosis III to the god Amun, in Deir el-Bahari. Here, the sovereign wears a pectoral composed of a heart amulet flanked by two sacred serpents. Each figure, including the heart, wears a solar disk on its top. This splendid piece of jewellery was used by the sovereign in a ritual context, probably as an attribute of Horus. As such, the solar heart amulet was probably seen as the symbol of the divine status of the Pharaoh. Topped by the solar disk, the amulet might have been a symbol of the identification of the king's heart with the sun, and may have signalled the illumination of his conscience (i.e., his ability to perform *maet* in the same way that the sun did on the cosmic level). In this way, the solar heart amulet could help to demonstrate that the sovereign successfully performed the royal task of connecting the divine realm and the earthly world, through his "illuminated" mind.

It is also interesting to note that the solar amulet was frequently depicted on the chest of the 21st Dynasty coffins of the Theban priests of Amun.[29] This use seems an appropriation of an object that, in the past, had been invested with a strong royal status and, from the religious point of view, symbolized the illumination of the conscience or, in other words, the identification of the heart with the sun, probably seen as a divine attribute of Horus. However, an important distinction must be drawn between these two uses: in the 18th Dynasty the object was used in earthly life by the king in order to demonstrate the divine status that enabled him to perform the divine cult, while, amongst 21st Dynasty Amun priests, the object was used in the afterlife as a funerary symbol of resurrection. Furthermore, these later representations depict an important mystery of the beyond: instead of being the symbol of the solar heart of Horus, the object now seems to illustrate the solar-Osirian union between the heart (taken as a symbol of Osiris) and the solar disk, which guarantees the perpetual renewal of the world.[30] It is certainly with this funerary meaning that some later solar heart amulets were produced.[31]

2. The heart of wisdom

From the reign of Amenhotep II to the Amarna period, the heart amulet became an object frequently depicted in the Theban necropolis, especially among the highest officials of the king. Most of the time coloured with yellow pigments, the object depicted in these situations is usually of considerable size. Among tomb decoration the object is usually depicted as an attribute of the tomb owner and sometimes of his son,[32] thus being an object used almost exclusively by men. In these early depictions of the heart amulet it is particularly stricking the use of the object among the lustration scenes, a complex ceremonial that fully provided the tomb owner with the dignity of a justified one and simingly intend to identify the deceased with the newborn sun.[33] Particularly in this context, the heart amulet seems to stand as the symbol of the *maetic* heart of the deceased, perhaps mirroring the role of a similar object among royal rituals that could celebrate the "illuminated" heart of the Pharaoh.

Sometimes this type of objects carries a royal cartouche. Such is the case of Sennefer, the governor of the city of Thebes during the reign of Amenhotep II. This important officer was depicted with a double heart amulet in a group statue found in Karnak[34] and in the pictorial decoration of his tomb (TT 96), in Sheikh Abd el-Gurnah. His statue also wears the typical necklace of the "gold of honour," which is an argument frequently presented to defend the function of the double heart amulet as a royal decoration. This interpretation is also supported by the fact that, in his tomb, this amulet is inscribed with the cartouches of Amenhotep II. Although rarely represented elsewhere, the double heart amulet is also depicted in the splendid tomb of Khaemhat (TT 57), royal scribe and inspector of the granaries of Upper and Lower Egypt under the reign of Amenhotep III. Georges Legrain pointed out that the double heart amulet was in fact an iconographical expression of the term *ibwi* that can be translated as a superlative ("heart of hearts") or as "icon" or "image," in the sense of a tangible image of a god.[35] At Karnak, Pharaohs had an "image," *ibui*, that was the object of a special cult. It is possible that the officers invested with this decoration might have been involved in a cult of the king. In that case, these officers were themselves an "image" of the king for those subjects who never saw the Pharaoh directly. In such a context, the amulet became a powerful symbol of wisdom that distinguished the officer as an ally of the Pharaoh in his task of keeping the cosmic order. Given the scarcity of these depictions, such an object was certainly a very exclusive distinction.

[29] See Fig. 46, Unet's coffin (Louvre Museum, AF 9593) but specially the outer coffins of Pinedem II and Nesikhonsu (Cairo Egyptian Museum, JE 26197 and 26199). Also Fig. 49, mummy-cover of Padiamun CG 6235 (Cairo Egyptian Museum).

[30] These depictions follow the iconographic trend of the period that was significantly enriched by motifs that celebrated the duality between the symbols of Osiris and Re. See A. NIWINSKI, "The solar-Osirian unity as principle of the theology of the 'State of Amun' in Thebes in the 21st Dynasty", *JEOL* 30 (1987-1988), 87-106.

[31] See Fig. 41 - CG 5223 (Cairo Egyptian Museum) and Fig. 40 - UC 22526 A (Petrie Museum).

[32] Such is the case of the later stela of Mesu and Api (C 280, Louvre Museum), from the Ramessid Period, where the deceased and his son wear the heart amulet. During the Third Intermediate Period the amulet is already used by women as in the papyrus of the lady Nesitanebitacheru. See J. TAYLOR, *Death and the Afterlife in ancient Egypt*, 2001, p. 20. See also Fig. 80.

[33] Representations of this kind can be seen in some of the most elaborate tombs from Theban necropolis. Tombs of Duauaneheh (TT 125), Sennefer (TT 96) and Ramose (TT 55) provide some of the finest examples of the use of the heart amulet in this context. The tomb of Userhat (TT 51), from the Ramessid Period, also provides a similar depiction of the heart in the context of lustral purification. To the lustral depiction in Userhat tomb see Norman de G. DAVIES, *Two Ramesside Tombs at Thebes*, 1927, pl. XI. See also Fig. 76. To the description of the ritual see J. ASSMANN, *Mort et l'au-delà dans l'Égypte ancienne*, (Monaco, 2003), 468-474. These depictions must be distinguished from the funerary libation which had a distinct meaning. See A. GARDINER, "The Baptism of Pharaoh", *JEA* 36 (1950), 3-12. Also A. BLACKMAN, "Sacramental ideas and usages in Ancient Egypt", *RT* 39 (1920), 45-48 and C. SPIESER, "L'eau et la regeneration des morts d'après les representations des tombes thébaines du Nouvel Empire", *DdÉ* 72 (1997), 221-228.

[34] Cairo Egyptian Museum, JE 36574, see E. HORNUNG, *The Quest for Immortality*, 2002, pp. 95-96

[35] See G. LEGRAIN, "Le mot *ibwy*, image, icone," *RT* 11 (1905), 181.

Without neglecting the political reading of the object, it seems that it became invested with a funerary, thus magical, purpose, as well. Thanks to the virtue and knowledge gained during earthly life, the officer could receive a royal honour that would also be useful in the beyond, since it could be used by the deceased in the court of Osiris as a royal gift to assure eternal life. In fact, once used in the court of Osiris, the object could attest that the Pharaoh regarded the deceased as righteous, a man who performed *maet* during his earthly life. Therefore, the fact that the amulet was given by the king during the lifetime of the officer does not preclude a funerary use: the golden amulet symbolized after all the immortal heart of the officer, literally the 'heart of gold', a conquest by his wisdom and honour. An example of such use can be seen in contemporary representations of the adoration of Osiris.[36] Most often yellow-coloured, the object depicted in these situations certainly is intended to represent the golden heart amulet. In fact, rather than a magical substitute for the cardiac organ, the amulet depicted in this context seems to be the symbol of the virtue and the wisdom required to be accepted before Osiris.

Ultimately important is, as we have seen, the depiction of the heart amulet in lustration ceremonies that, from the reign of Amenhotep II on, became an important feature of tomb decoration in elite funerals of the period. Probably reminiscent of this use of the amulet is the depiction of the object on the chest of the anthropoid coffins produced until the end of 18th Dynasty. In some of these monuments the amulet, painted yellow or even covered in gold leaf, is shown between the hands of the deceased (sometimes holding the signs *djed* and *tjet*) and worn on a heavy necklace.[37] The depiction of the amulet in this context probably follows the general symbolism of the object in this period: it shows that the deceased had already been decorated by the king as a keeper of *maet* and, in this way, he could demonstrate before the gods of the hereafter that he had accomplished the realization of *maet* during his lifetime. The depiction of the amulet on the chest of some funerary statuettes of this period, including *ushebtis*[38] and statuettes of *ba* birds probably had the same meaning.[39] Such examples lead us to believe that, despite being bestowed during earthly life as a decoration (as a symbol of royal acknowledgement), it was also used in the afterlife to promote a positive outcome in the judgement of the dead. In this context, the heart amulet could have been seen as a powerful help in the court of Osiris, where the royal gift would be noted and respected.

Thus, depictions such as these may refer to the golden heart amulet, which has actually been found in archaeological contexts.[40] In fact, rather than a magical substitute for the heart, such an object may have been seen as a distinctive sign of high rank and royal favour due to the virtue and wisdom of the official.

3. The heart of justification

From the Ramessid Period on the depiction of the heart amulet in the funerary context is prevalent.[41] This can mainly be seen among the vignettes of the weighing of the heart (very often painted on tomb walls), where the deceased seems to receive the amulet as the result of a positive outcome obtained on the *maetic* scale. The fact that the deceased raises feathers in his hands in a gesture of joy[42] makes it very clear that, when used in that context, the heart amulet is a reward given by the court of the dead to designate the deceased as an Osiris.[43]

The vignettes that depict the amulet in scenes of adoration of Osiris must also be interpreted in this manner. Curiously enough, the amulet is used as a decoration of justice that allows the deceased to be in the presence of the god.[44]

[36] See *Book of the Dead* of Kha and Merit (TT 8) in Turin Egyptian Museum. In A.M ROVERI, *Museo Egizio*, s/d, p. 32.

[37] The oldest known type of these representations goes back to the reign of Thutmose III and is seen in the coffin ECM 1876 (Eton College) that was elaborated to Amenhotep, the "Overseer of the builders of Amen": see S. SPURR, N. REEVES & S. QUIRKE, *Egyptian Art at Eton College: Selections from the Myers Museum*, 1999, p. 24. Maherpa, "intimate friend" of king Thutmose IV, was another great personality to present one of these amulets depicted on the chest of the anthropoid coffin JE 31378/CG 4219 (Cairo Egyptian Museum) discovered in its tomb from the Valley of the Kings (KV 36) – see Fig. 77. The stone anthropoid sarcophagus of Khai (nº 2686), an high official buried in Nubia, currently conserved in the Elefantine Museum, also presents a depiction of a heart amulet on its chest.

[38] Although, unfortunately, most of these statuettes do not display the titles of the deceased represented, one of them belonged to Yuya, one of the most eminent individuals of the reign of Amenhotep III. See shabti nº SR 95368/CG 51033 (Cairo Egyptian Museum): in J.E QUIBEL, *The tomb of Yuaa and Thuiu*, 1908, pl. XVIII The quality of these objects must alert us to the equally high status of its owners. See also shabti of Tacheri nº 1914.597 (Cleveland Museum of Art): in L. BERMAN, K. BOHAC, *Catalogue of Egyptian Art*, p. 342.

[39] An interesting *ba* statuette from the tomb of Yuya (JE 95312, Cairo Egyptian Museum), also presents a heart amulet on its chest. See Fig. 64.

[40] See AF 9101 (Louvre Museum), UC 38422 (Petrie Museum), UC 58020 (Petrie Museum), CG 5259 (Cairo Egyptian Museum).

[41] The scene of the weighing of the heart is a common theme depicted among the tombs of Theban necropolis. This is the case of the tombs of Amenemuia (TT 178), Nefersekheru and Pabasa (TT 296), Neferenepet (TT 178), Userhat (TT 51), Rai (TT 255), Nakhtamon (TT 341), Amenemopet (TT 41), Khonsu (TT 31) and Simut (TT 409), only to mention a few of them. The depiction of the heart amulet in these early scenes is missing. In the tomb of Rai (TT 255), from the late 18th Dynasty, the deceased present the amulet in this context.

[42] This gesture is especially depicted on mythological papyri produced during the 21st Dynasty. See mythological papyri of Khonsumes (AOS 3859, Kunsthistorisches Museum). About this papyrus see A. PIANKOFF, N. RAMBOVA, *Mythological Papyri*, 1955, pl. 147. See also Fig. 53 and Fig. 79 - papyrus of Nesipakachuti (E 17401, Louvre Museum). About this papyrus see *idem* pl. 104. Papyrus Nesitanebetaui (SR 40017, Cairo Egyptian Museum). The same gesture is also depicted on the 21st Dynasty coffins, where this theme is very common. See coffins of Pakharu (CG 6122/6121, Cairo Egyptian Museum, now in National Museum of Alexandria), Padiamun (CG 6233/6235, Cairo Egyptian Museum), Ankhefenmut (CG 6109, Cairo Egyptian Museum), Chebet (CG 6028, Cairo Egyptian Museum), Paser (N 2570, Louvre Museum) and Amenempermut (CG 6153, Cairo Egyptian Museum).

[43] In the vignettes of the weighing of the heart, the presentation of the deceased to the god Osiris is the natural consequence of a positive outcome of that procedure. Usually the amulet is given to the deceased before the scene of the adoration of Osiris. Although couples can be depicted, men are always the ones that wear the amulet. This is the case of the tomb of Rai and his wife, Nebetaui, (TT 255) where the amulet seems to be connected to the weighing of the heart. Fig. 78.

[44] See *Book of the Dead* of Kha and Merit (TT 8), in Turin Egyptian Museum. This is one of the earliest depictions of the heart amulet in a funerary context. See also *Book of the Dead* of Yuya (KV 46), in T.

This use of the amulet is detected not only among the vignettes of the *Book of the Dead* but also among temple decoration. In the Abidean Cenotaph of Seti I, Merenpat is depicted in the 'burial chamber' before Osiris wearing the amulet cleary as an allusion to the weighing of the heart.[45] Although such a royal context might be seen as exceptional it is certainly paradigmatic of the private use of the object.

The amulet is always depicted with this meaning on the chests of anthropoid coffins produced in the 21st Dynasty. They are completely surrounded by a plethora of other funerary symbols: the *benu* bird, a dog-like figure of Anubis, the solar winged scarab, many winged goddesses, sacred objects like the Tawer totem and hieroglyphs such as *wedjat*, *nefer* and *neb*.[46] Instead of the yellow pigments or the golden leaf used to colour the amulet in earlier periods, this object is now painted in blue or black and is usually inscribed with the name of Osiris followed by the name of the deceased. Clearly, in this context, the amulet is used as a symbol of the osirification of the deceased and it can be seen as an important iconographic feature among those referring to Osiris.[47]

As an Osirian symbol of justification, the amulet is also used by the deceased in a variety of vignettes depicting the hereafter. Playing the *senet* game[48] and being refreshed by the powers of life bestowed by the tree goddess are only two of the many pleasant situations that can be available in the afterlife to the rightful ones. Going forth by day, travelling on the solar bark[49] to the paradisiacal fields of Iaru[50] and giving praise to the divinities of the beyond are among the many situations in which the deceased is frequently depicted with the heart amulet.[51] By means of the representation of the amulet, all these situations of the hereafter were connected to the osirification of the deceased, the true cause of the happiness experienced in the beyond.

Nevertheless, the ultimate privilege bestowed by the amulet was to be able to participate in the great mysteries of the Duat, such as the regeneration of the solar disk or the triumph of the solar bark over Apopis.[52]

Generally speaking, this kind of iconographical use of the heart amulet is intended to identify the deceased as a justified one, someone who had successfully overcome the trial of the beyond and from that point on could be welcomed into the presence of the gods and go forth by day. In this way, the amulet was viewed as an Osirian symbol, a sign of purity and virtue that allowed the deceased to participate in the mysteries of the beyond. Most probably it is precisely as a symbol of the victory of Osiris over death (Seth) that the heart amulet is used in a rather unusual and later context: in some mummy sandals we can observe the enemies of Egypt adorned with the heart amulet.[53] Positioned in this pictorial context, the heart amulet, as a symbol of the justification of the deceased, displayed the victory of Osiris over the Sethian powers of death in a similar way that in earlier depictions the hearts of the enemies were depicted wripped off out of their bodies as a symbol of the annihilation of Seth.

The depiction of the heart amulet on ostraca

Contrasting with the above-mentioned pictorial contexts, a few contemporary *ostraca*, most of them from Deir el-Medina, present a very different picture of the use of the heart amulet. Instead of the highly elaborated meaning that the amulet seems to have in the tombs of the elite, surprisingly enough, here we see the amulet being worn by humble shepherds,[54] or even, something that is very rare among contemporary sources, by girls. An *ostracon* preserved in Berlin depicts the amulet being used by a naked girl who is riding a horse.[55] This is an exceptional depiction since the advent of horseback riding in Egypt seems to be a later phenomenon and certainly restricted to a military context and therefore to an adult and male use. If the use of the amulet by a girl, by itself, is strangely enough, the entire picture depicted in this *ostracon* is a compilation of bizarre features.

Another strange situation is contained on an *ostracon* preserved in the Louvre Museum. Once again we see what seems to be the heart amulet being used by a naked girl.[56] She addresses a tender gesture to a monkey while he plays a double flute, which clearly invests the object with a satirical character, a common feature among contemporary *ostraca*.

DAVIS, *The Funeral Papyrus of Iouiya*, 1908, Pl. I.

[45] See H. FRANKFORT, *The Cenotaph of Seti I*, II, 1933, Plate LXXIII

[46] See lid of the exterior coffin of Pinedjem II (JE 26197, Cairo Egyptian Museum), but also the coffin of Padiamun (CG 6233, Cairo Egyptian Museum), the coffin and mummy cover of Pakharu (CG 6122/6121, Cairo Egyptian Museum, now in National Museum of Alexandria), the coffin of Tjenetethatnetjeru (CG 6191, Cairo Egyptian Museum) and other coffins (CG 6153, Cairo Egyptian Museum).

[47] See Fig. 93. These coffins, dated from the reign of Pinedjem II, usually have a great *usekh* necklace, in the centre of which is depicted the heart amulet. See typology of these coffins in A. NIWINSKI, *21st Dynasty Coffins from Thebes*, 1988, pp. 67-96.

[48] In the tomb of Nebenmaet (TT 219), from 19th Dynasty, the deceased is depicted playing the *senet* game with his wife, Meretseguer. See C. MAYSTRE, *Tombes de Deir el-Médineh: La tombe de Nebenmât (n° 219)*, Cairo, 1936, pl. V.

[49] See Fig. 85: in the tomb of Irinefer (TT 290) the deceased wears the amulet in front of the *benu* bird while travelling in the solar bark.

[50] In the tomb of Amenemopet (TT 41) the deceased is depicted with the heart amulet in several situations of the Afterlife: while he visits the Fields of Iaru, among the navigation of the solar bark and in the combat with Apopis. See J. ASSMANN, *Das Grab des Amenemope (TT41)*, 1991, tl. 40.

[51] In the tomb of Khakhebenet (TT 2), the deceased, adorned with the amulet, prays in front of Thoth. See also Fig. 86.

[52] Depictions like these show that the heart amulet was seen as a symbol of the Osirification of the deceased. As such, it allowed the deceased to participate in the mysteries where the sun would triumph over the powers of darkness and death. As a result of these ideas, in the 21st Dynasty, pictorial compositions with the heart amulet became highly elaborate, turning into the way to express complex theological notions. To this iconographic trend see A. NIWINSKI, "The solar-Osirian unity as principle of the theology of the 'State of Amun' in Thebes in the 21st Dynasty", *JEOL* 30 (1987-1988), 91.

[53] See Fig. 90.

[54] See N 1562 (Louvre Museum) – Fig. 91.

[55] See *ostracon* n° 728 (Berlin Egyptian Museum) – Fig. 92.

[56] See E 25309 (Louvre Museum).

When compared to the formal contexts found in tomb decoration, depictions such these seem to reveal, clearly with satirical purposes, a completely contrary picture: instead of being used by male high officials in religious scenes of the hereafter, the heart amulet is used by humble men or, even more strangely, by naked girls performing phantastical activities. Due to the extremely reverential religious meaning that the object appears to be invested with during the Ramessid Period, it seems at least plausible that a satirical view of the judgement of the dead could be illustrated by means of the images depicted on these *ostraca*.

4. The heart of divine birth

From the beginning of the 18th Dynasty, the heart amulet was used to distinguish royal princes. The oldest record of such use can be found on the Donation Stela, where it is worn by the young prince while his father leads him into the presence of Amun-Ra.[57]The amulet is also present in a group statue of royal princes found at Zagazig that shows a nurse with four princes adorned with the amulet.[58] The significance of the use of the amulet in this context is not clear. As we have seen, in the early 18th Dynasty the amulet did not seem to carry the strong funerary significance that it attained in later times. It seems likely that, at the beginning of the 18th Dynasty, the amulet was used by the royal family as a symbol of purity. That would explain the later use of the amulet as a royal decoration: it symbolized the rise in status of the officer to the inner and intimate circle of the "family" of the Pharaoh.

In a certain perspective, all of the previously discussed contexts in which the amulet is used can also be connected to the idea of purity: while it was used as a royal decoration, it was also a symbol of the purification required to be in the presence of the Pharaoh. The same idea of purity is also underlined in the amulet of justification, since it was the symbol of purity measured in the weighing of the heart.

Perhaps reflecting this original *locus* of beliefs related to the heart amulet, from the Late Period on, the object became a typical iconographical element of the divine children. Horpakhered is frequently depicted with the amulet when he takes control over savage beasts.[59] In this context, the amulet stands as a symbol of the purity which triumphs over corruption and poison. It was perhaps this apotropaic power that explains the wide range of situations in which divine children wear this amulet in temple decoration. Very frequently, the divine children seem to be identified with the Pharaoh, being depicted with royal attributes such as the sceptres *heka* and *nekhakha*, or the crown *pshent* and the *nemes* headdress.[60] In other cases, these gods are depicted above the lotus[61] or the *sema-taui* motif, which on the other hand, may allude to another attribute of the divine child: he assures the re-creation of the world and a return to the mythical time of the creation. The wide use of the amulet by these gods may, in fact, be related to the intention to provide a cosmic renewal. Although used as a religious and political statement in the context of temple decoration, these same images could also be used in the funerary context as symbols of regeneration. In the vignettes of the weighing of the heart of the Greco-Roman Period, the deceased is often depicted as a newborn solar child: although still connected to the weighing of the heart, the amulet comes to be invested with a wider obstetric meaning, being regarded as a sign of rebirth and of a new life. This subtle change in meaning is also accompanied by a change in the depiction of the heart, which assumes the typical features of the cornice heart amulet,[62] and which we will discuss later in this book.

It is perhaps as a symbol of regeneration that the amulet appears above mummiform gods produced in this period, where it is depicted on the centre of the *usekh* necklace and not above its layers, as it was the usual procedure in earlier depictions. Such is the case of some corn mummies.[63] In addition, the amulet is no longer used on coffins and sarcophagi as a royal or even an Osirian decoration but purely as a symbol of rebirth and regeneration.[64] Depictions of the heart amulet found amongst the later vignettes of the cardiac chapters of the *Book of the Dead* carry this same meaning.[65] In other words, during the first millennium BCE, the heart amulet seemed to be valued as a symbol of new life and rebirth, being a tangible sign of the power of light and purity of a new and divine childhood. As a symbol of the purity of the divine children, the amulet was then invested with prophylactic power against evil and demons.

[57] See I. HARARI, "Nature de la Stéle de Donation de Fonction du roi Ahmôsis a la reine Ahmès-Nefertari", *ASAE* 56 (1956), Pl. II – Fig. 94.

[58] See JE 98831 (Cairo Egyptian Museum), in C. SHEIKHOSLESLAMI, *The Egyptian Museum at the Millenium: a Special Exhibition in honor of the VIIIth International Congress of Egyptologists*, 2000, pl. 22.

[59] See Fig. 98 - CG 9402 (Cairo Egyptian Museum), in É. CHASSINAT, *Textes et dessins magiques*, Cairo, 1903, pl. II. See also Fig. 96 - (N 4434, Berlin Egyptian Museum).

[60] See decoration of the temple of Dendera: F. DAUMAS, *Les Mammisis de Dendara*, 1959. Many statuettes of the god depict him with these symbols. See Fig.104 – (SR 46380, Cairo Egyptian Museum). See also CG 38182/CG 38176 (Cairo Egyptian Museum).

[61] See Fig. 103. To the depictions of the god over the *sema-taui* motif see A. VARILLE, "La grande porte du temple d'Apet à Karnak", *ASAE* 53 (1956), pl. II and also J. HALLOF, H. VAN DEN BERG and others, *Le Temple de Dendara: La Porte d'Ísis*, 1999, pl. 34-35.

[62] See R. SOUSA, "The heart amulet in Ancient Egypt: A typological study", in *Proceedings of the Ninth International Congress of Egyptologists*, I, 2007, pp. 713-721. In fact, most of the amulets produced in Late Period have the shape of the cornice heart amulet. Besides the obvious funerary use, the heart amulet seems to have been highly regarded to be used by the living. However, this later use of the heart amulet by the living ones seems to be connected more to its power to keep evil apart and to grant good health than as a sign of high rank, as previously happened. In order to be used in earthly life, amulets became smaller and, in many circumstances, much more cheaper, as it can be inferred through the quality both of the raw materials used and of the craftsmanship.

[63] See E 12183 (Louvre Museum).

[64] See Fig. 108 - sarcophagus of Setueret (23/1/21/9, Cairo Egyptian Museum) or the coffin of Duasahotep (21/11/16/11, Cairo Egyptian Museum).

[65] See R. SOUSA, "The cardiac vignettes of the Book of the Dead (Late Period)", *BAEDE* 17 (2007), 39-53.

5. General implications of the meaning of the heart amulet

These distinct contexts of the representation of the heart amulet demonstrate that the prominent meaning of the heart amulet must be focused on its mental and psychological sense, which is, in fact, is the usual understanding of the word *ib*, "heart" in hieroglyphic writing.[66] We must also stress that the heart amulet is nothing more than a three-dimensional rendering of this same hieroglyph. Thus, the hieroglyphic reading of the object as the word *ib* is mandatory in the bi-dimensional pictorial context. As such, although the physical image of the bull's heart (hieroglyph F 34) is used, the metaphorical use of the term *ib* as the seat of the mind is undoubtedly primary. Therefore, the heart amulet must be seen as a depiction of the mind of the individual but most assuredly not of his ordinary mind. The use of gold, especially in the earliest examples, must lead us to consider this "heart of gold" as an immortal and solarised mind that was formed thanks to the practice of *maet* and thus symbolized wisdom.

We also should stress that although red is the colour traditionally associated with the heart amulet, the fact is that we can equally identify yellow and black/dark blue as typical colours of this object, especially when it is depicted in the pictorial context of the heart of wisdom (yellow) and of the heart of justification (dark).

Following these ideas, we can admit the following development of the meaning of the heart amulet: first, it seems to have been invested with a strong "political" status: it could be earned in earthly life, as the result of a successful career in the service of the Pharaoh. However, by the end of the 18th Dynasty, the heart amulet was mainly associated with the hereafter where it was expected to be given by Osiris as a moral distinction. In fact, as a symbol of wisdom and purity, the heart amulet was central to the weighing of the heart, when it was given to the deceased as a symbol of the triumph of purity and wisdom over death and corruption. Finally, from the Late Period on, a time that was witness to the mass-production of heart amulets[67], this object seems to incarnate the power of the child divinities and, as such, it seems to have been disinvested from its distinctive function that had been so highly regarded in earlier periods. The widespread use of the amulet, even by the lower levels of the Egyptian population, seems to be explained by the increase in its apotropaic power which was based on the power of purity to control darkness and evil and to grant good health both in earthly life and in the beyond.[68]

However distinct they might be, these various semantic contexts of the use of the heart amulet should not lead us to lose sight of the fact that they all share some common features. In all of them the heart is depicted as the seat of the mind and illustrates the responsibility of each man to keep the *maetic* order in motion. In fact, the innermost meaning of the heart amulet lies in its ability to symbolize the pure heart as an embodiment of the *maetic* order. As such, "illumination", wisdom, purity and renewal are all aspects of the heart filled by *maet*.

[66] That does not exclude that sometimes the amulet could be used, quite parsimoniously, to depict the physical organ.

[67] These objects indeed started to be produced massively employing glass and mould casts. Roughly finished, certain heart amulets found in late burials attest a much wider use of apotropaic objects by the Egyptian population. See W. PETRIE, *Dendereh*, Egypt Exploration Fund, 1900, pl. XXVI

[68] That explains the prodigality of the use of the amulet in late mummies: far from the centrality and uniqueness of the amulets used in former periods, heart amulets used to the protection of the mummies are numerous and may be placed in any part of the body.

CHAPTER TWO

THE TYPOLOGY OF THE HEART AMULETS

Heart amulets are among the most common funerary apotropaic objects in ancient Egyptian burials. In her work on Egyptian amulets, Claudia Müller-Winkler accurately describes a wide variety of shapes, sizes, materials and symbols found on heart amulets and concludes that it is not possible to identify a single amulet considered as 'typical'.[1] According to her, the wide variety of formal features and symbolic depictions found on these objects do not allow a general reading of the symbolism of the heart amulet beyond the generally accepted idea that it embodies the power of life.[2] Nevertheless, as we have seen in the first chapter, analysis of iconographic sources alerts us to a broader meaning of the object: connotations related to wisdom and virtue being prevalent.

Thus, to better understand the significance of heart amulets, we must proceed to a more detailed analysis of these objects. The first step in this analysis should be to differentiate categories of objects. Previously, Flinders Petrie attempted such categorization but the typology thus created was based more on symbolic categories rather than on formal criteria with the predictable result that the same amulet could be placed in several different categories, an outcome that does not provide much assistance when the intent is to define a single class of objects.

We realized that the establishment of formal criteria that could assist in the identification of different types of objects was a critical step. Our analysis of the formal features of the heart amulet and their variations has demonstrated that neither the shape of the body of the amulet nor the shape of the side projections were useful in creating categories. The variations detected among these features do not seem consistently related to a change in the general shape of the object. On the contrary, variations in the shape of the top and of the border of the object seemed to have a significant effect on the general shape of the object, affecting its size, decoration, the choice of materials and many other features.

Based solely on these formal criteria (shape of the top and shape of the border) we then proceeded to the characterise of the various types of heart amulets. In this chapter we will focus on a discussion of the types of amulets that we were able to identify by the shape of their upper border of the amulet.[3] We have proposed the following categories:

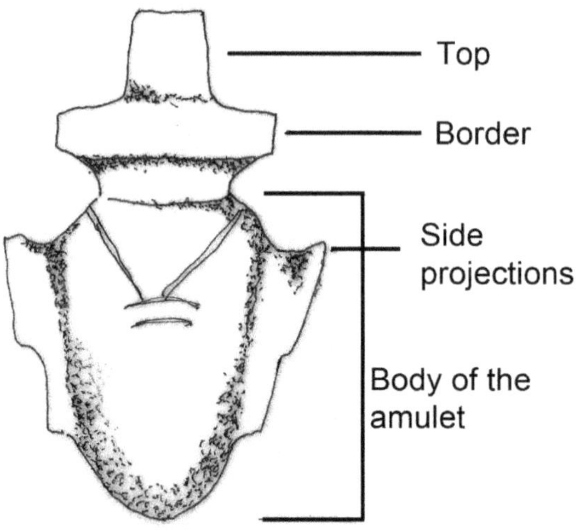

Morphology of heart amulet

amulets with a rounded border (vase heart amulets), amulets with a square border (cornice heart amulets) and amulets without a border (pendulum heart amulets). Surprisingly enough, we have found that within each category, internal variations both in formal features, such as the shape of the body or the shape of the side projections, and symbolic depictions were indeed much more limited in scope, which may allow us to conclude that in antiquity they could actually be seen as distinct types of heart amulets.[4]

1. The pendulum heart amulets

The objects that we group as 'pendulum amulets' do not have an upper border. For this reason, the eyelet for suspension is carved directly onto the top of the body of the amulet. Curiously enough, this group of amulets also displays an exceptionally elongated body that clearly gives to these artefacts the shape of a pendulum. Side projections are rarely found among these artefacts.[5] Another uncommon feature is the great variation in size of these objects: they can be as small as one centimetre[6] but

[1] See C. MÜLLER-WINKLER, *Die Ägyptischen Objekt-Amulette*, 1987, p. 214. In any case the author could not find a feature considered as 'typical': nor the materials, nor the colours, nor the shape of the side projections, not even the nature of its symbols provided clues in order to establish a typical meaning of the object.

[2] *Idem*, p. 212.

[3] This classification is unavailable to the heart amulets headed by a human or animal head or by a solar disk. Each one of these types of amulets needs to be understood as a category on its own, as we will see in the Third Chapter.

[4] Our classification of the heart amulets was first published in R. SOUSA, 'The heart amulet in Ancient Egypt: A typological study', in Goyon, J.-C., Cardin, C., *Proceedings of the Ninth International Congress of Egyptologists*, 2007, Vol. I, p. 713-721.

[5] Such projections can be detected on a few pendulum heart amulets: see SR 10813 (Cairo Egyptian Museum): in Z. GONEIM, *Excavations at Saqqara*, p. 26. See also Fig. 2 - SR 9205/CG 12127 (Cairo Egyptian Museum): in G. REISNER, *Amulets*, I, 1907, pp. 121-122. Also SR 9213/ CG 12128 (Cairo Egyptian Museum): in *ibidem*, p. 122.

[6] See UC 38420 (Petrie Museum). Also CG 53221 (Cairo Egyptian Museum): E. VERNIER, *Bijoux et Orfévreries*, 1927, pl. XCV. Also E 16221 (Louvre Museum).

they can frequently reach six[7] or even nine centimetres in size,[8] remarkable large for this type of object.

Datation

The small amount of information available in museological records, makes it very difficult to obtain a clear idea about the dating of these objects. Taking into consideration the scarcity of such data, it appears that the use of the pendulum heart amulet came to be favoured during the Ramessid Period,[9] particularly in the funerary context, but that it only became more common in burials of the 21st Dynasty.[10] This particular kind of heart amulets disappears after this period.

Materials

Materials used to produce these amulets may differ significantly: unidentified green stones,[11] schist[12] and glass[13] stand out as the most frequently used, but materials such as cornelian[14] and gold[15] were also used.

Decoration

Some of the largest objects are richly decorated. The most magnificent objects are superbly carved with depictions of the solar scarab. On the reverse of most of them a version of chapter 30 B of the *Book of the Dead* was inscribed.[16] Less commonly, other solar symbols such as the *benu* bird can also be found,[17] as well as other funerary symbols, such as the *ba* bird.[18] More complex representations, such as as the splendid object presenting a winged scarab holding the heart *ib* and the *akhet* hieroglyph in its legs,[19] are seldom found.

Use

In addition to the funerary use that seems to be the most important function of the pendulum heart amulets described above, an alternative and surprising use was made of these artefacts: certain measurement instruments used the pendulum heart amulet with pragmatic and (perhaps) with symbolic intent. Instruments with the heart amulet acting as a pendulum were used to level architectonic structures. Two types of levels are known to us. The triangular-shaped one was used on horizontal surfaces and it was made of two pieces of wood connected in a straight angle.[20] A small crossbar, with a mark in the middle connected the two boards, forming a sort of hypotenuse. Hanging from the straight angle of this triangle, the plumb line consisted of a pendulum, which was very similar to the heart amulets described above. A different type of level was created to check vertical surfaces. In this case, the plumb line was hung from the end of a board with two wooden saliencies and when the pendulum heart amulet inclined to one sides, it would indicate construction defects.[21]

The pendulum heart amulet was also used in certain sun dials. They were made of a wooden board which needed to be exactly parallel to the ground. It was the plumb line, again in the shape of a pendulum, that allowed the instrument to be correctly oriented so as to determine the time by means of the shadow projected onto the scale. In some cases, the plumb line would extend from a baboon statuette.[22]

However interesting these uses of the heart amulet as a measurement instrument may be, its most striking use is as a needle on scales. Documented in funerary vignettes that depict the weighing of the heart, this use is also corroborated by representations showing these scales in scenes of the daily life.[23] In the Theban tomb of Ipuki (TT 181), for example, we see one of these scales being used to weigh precious materials such as gold. Although intended for a very clear practical purpose, this scale exhibits exactly the same shape as on the scales depicted in contemporary vignettes of the weighing of the heart: the top of the scale is in the shaped of the head of the goddess Maet and the pendulum is actually very similar to those that are depicted in funerary scales. In the *Book of the Dead* of Neferuebenef,[24] for instance, we find a scale with similar features. Note that, in both images, the pendulum is depicted in red, a colour traditionally associated with the heart amulet.

It can be argued that the pendulum used in these scales can in fact be identified as a heart amulet. The evidence that this identification is correct can be found in the vignettes of the weighing of the heart. While, until the 21st dynasty, the needle of the scale is shaped like a pendulum heart amulet, from the Late Period on it is clearly shaped like

[7] See Fig. 2 - SR 9205/CG 12127 (Cairo Egyptian Museum): in G. REISNER, *Amulets*, I, 1907, pp. 121-122. Also AF 2578 (Louvre Museum).

[8] See Fig. 6 - SR 10813/JE 41826 (Cairo Egyptian Museum).

[9] See JE 92635 and also SR 10813, both from Cairo Egyptian Museum. Archaeological reports on Z. GONEIM, *Excavations at Saqqara*, p. 26 and G. STEINDORFF, *Aniba*, 1937, II.

[10] See SR 9217/CG 12131 (Cairo Egyptian Museum): in G. REISNER, *Amulets*, I, 1907, p. 123. Also SR 9262/CG 12129: in *ibidem*, p. 123. See also Fig. 2 - SR 9205/CG 12127: in *ibidem*, p. 121 & pl. IX. All of these objects were discovered among the wrappings of the priests of Amun found in the collective tomb of Bab el-Gasus. The tomb of Pinedjem II also delivered a pendulum-heart amulet: CG 53220 (Cairo Egyptian Museum)

[11] See again Fig. 2 - CG 12127 (Cairo Egyptian Museum). See also SR 9213/CG 12128 (Cairo Egyptian Museum): in G. REISNER, *Amulets*, I, 1907, p. 122.

[12] See AF 2578 (Louvre Museum), SR 10813 (Cairo Egyptian Museum).

[13] See JE 92635 (Cairo Egyptian Museum): in Z. GONEIM, *Excavations at Saqqara*, 1957, p. 26. Also UC 52194 (Petrie Museum) – Fig. 1.

[14] See UC 38420 (Petrie Museum).

[15] See collection of amulets from the mummy of Sheshonk I, in Cairo Egyptian Museum.

[16] See Fig. 2 - CG 12127 - and CG 12128 (Cairo Egyptian Museum): in G. REISNER, *Amulets*, I, p. 121-122. See also AF 2578 (Louvre Museum).

[17] See JE 92635 (Cairo Egyptian Museum).

[18] See Fig. 6 - SR 10813/JE 41826 (Cairo Egyptian Museum).

[19] See Fig. 5 - G. LEGRAIN, *Collection Hoffmann*, 1894, p. 13. A short version of chapter 30 B is inscribed on the reverse of this object.

[20] See JE 27258 (Cairo Egyptian Museum), from the tomb of Senedjem, 19th Dynasty.

[21] See CG 2005 (Cairo Egyptian Museum), 19th Dynasty.

[22] See sun dial from the Louvre Museum (without number) dated from the reign of Amen-hotep III.

[23] See Fig. 3 - depiction of a scale used to measure the weight of gold, in tomb of Ipuki (TT 181). The scale is depicted with a pendulum and, as the funerary scale used in the weighing of the heart,

[24] See Fig. 3 - N 3092 (Louvre Museum), vignette of chapter 125 of the *Book of the Dead.* See S. RATIÉ, *Le Papyrus de Neferoubenef*, 1968, p. 41.

a typical heart amulet, with the side projections clearly visible. Curiously enough, archaeology shows that scales from the Late Period did in fact use a typical *ib*-shaped heart amulet instead of the pendulum heart amulet used in earlier periods.[25] The use of the typical heart shaped amulet in these later depictions can only be attributed to the decline in the use of the pendulum heart amulet. This decline in use can be corroborated by its absence in later archaeological contexts.

Symbolism

The change in the shape of the scale needle suggests that the development of the iconography of the weighing of the heart, which occurred during the 18th dynasty, pointed to a moral reading of the scales' components. As in the funerary scale used in the court of Osiris, measurements that used ordinary scales were actually made via the interposition of the heart that, by its movement along the crossbar of the scale, would give the desired result. In this earthly context, the amulet could be used as a reminder of the value of truth and honesty since those qualities would be measured in the weighing of the heart. Therefore the scribe should avoid making false measurements since, once in the court of Osiris, he would be confronted with his own heart testifying against him, showing his bad deeds to the divine assembly. In this way, the pendulum heart amulet could have been used in two different yet related ways. In instruments of earthly life it could remind the scribe of the possibility that any false or dishonest operation would be revealed in the weighing of the heart. On the other hand, when used in the funerary context, the pendulum heart amulet was clearly served to insure a positive outcome in the weighing of the heart through the identification of the heart of the deceased with the *maetic* needle of the divine scale.

Pendulum heart amulets used in construction levels could also have been invested with a similar wisdom reading. Since the heart was the seat of wisdom, not only could the pendulum heart amulet be adapted for practical use but it would also constitute a permanent challenge to the user – reminding him that, when measuring the foundations of a new building, he should align himself with the cosmic order, so that his work and achievements would be built upon truth, wisdom and harmony. This spiritual reading of practical instruments could be rooted in the need to insure that buildings created by man would express the divine order of the universe.[26] In other words, the pendulum heart amulet can be regarded as a symbol of the heart that is aligned with the cosmic order. As such it was probably seen as a physical representation of the equilibrium required to express the *maetic* harmony in human actions and constructions.

Viewed in this light, the pendulum heart amulet poses some interesting questions related to the creation of meaning around magical artefacts such as amulets. We know that the pendulum was already in use as a measurement instrument in the Old Kingdom. However, the heart amulet does not seem to have been in use during this period.[27] In fact, it seems that the association between the heart amulet and the pendulum was only established toward the end of the 18th dynasty, when the development of the iconography of the vignette of the weighing of the heart occurred. Therefore it seems quite plausible that the identification between the heart amulet and the pendulum was developed as another iconographical expression of the set of religious beliefs related to the weighing of the heart. As such, the pendulum heart amulet certainly served the magical purpose of promoting the identification of the heart of the deceased with the needle of the divine scale, that is to say, with the very symbol of truth and *maet*. By means of that identification a positive outcome for the weighing of the heart would be virtually assured.

2. The vase heart amulets

The main morphological feature of the vase heart amulet is the round border carved immediately below the top of the amulet, usually provided with a suspension ring. We have chosen to describe these objects as 'vase heart amulets' because of the rounded shape of the border which gives them a form typical of a vase. Curiously enough, certain of these amulets were hollowed out, giving them the shape of an actual vase.[28] At times, the resemblance between the vase heart amulet and the vase amulet is so pronounced that it is only the existence of side projections,[29] a typical feature of heart amulets, that can help us to distinguish them.

[25] Although equal in shape to the amulets manufactured to apotropaic use, these objects were made of bronze, thus being bigger and much heavier. See bronze heart amulet E 18224 (Louvre Museum) or CG 1930 (Cairo Egyptian Museum): in A. WEIGALL,*Weights and balances*, 1908, pl. IX . Also object nº inv 13493 (Museu da Farmácia de Lisboa): in L. ARAÚJO, P. BASSO, *A Farmácia no Mundo Pré-Clássico e nas Culturas Tradicionais*, 2008, p. 118-119.

[26] The fact is that similar and even more complex spiritual readings of apparently mundane elements are well known in ancient Egypt. Just to quote an example, we can refer to the columns known as the Memphite *djed*-pillar, an architectural element that was seen as an embodiment of Shu, sustainer of the universe. See J. VAN DIJK, 'The symbolism of the Memphite Djed-pillar', *OMRO* 66 (1986), pp. 7-17

[27] Amulets in the shape of parts of the human body or organs are characteristic of burials of the late Old Kingdom and First Intermediate Period. See C. ANDREWS, *Amulets of Ancient Egypt*, 1998, p. 69

[28] See Fig. 11 - SR 9203/CG 12914 (Cairo Egyptian Museum): in G. REISNER, *Amulets* I, 1907, pl. IX. See also Fig. 9 - SR 9199/JE 28490/ CG 12053 (Cairo Egyptian Museum): in *ibidem*, p. 106. Müller-Winkler pointed out to the existence of heart amulets fully carved as vases. See C. MÜLLER-WINKLER, *Die Ägyptischen Objekt-Amulette*, 1987, p. 225. We don't include in our study the collored glass objects typical of the 18th Dynasty for its identification as heart amulets is doubtful, although not impossible. Iconographic sources also did not provided any support to help to identify these objects as heart amulets.

[29] Among vase heart amulets, side projections usually have the shape of a button or a cardiac vein. Amulets with button side projections exist since the Middle Kingdom times. Amulets with side projections shaped as a cardiac veins became prevalent only from the New Kingdom on. Elongated and pointed side projections are typically found on amulets from the Late Period. This later configuration of side projections thus can be very useful to the dating of the objects. As to the earlier types of side projections they can also appear in later periods.

Datation

The earliest recorded vase heart amulets (dated from the 5th and 6th Dynasties) must be approached with some care: their direct connection with the heart is not clear.[30] Rather, it seems that these amulets must be considered as vase amulets in *stricto sensu*, being simply depictions of the offering vase *nw*.[31] It is only when side projections, evocative of cardiac veins, are added to the vase amulet that we can accurately use the term 'heart amulet'.[32] In fact available archaeological information does not allow us to date the 'invention' of the heart amulet any earlier than the beginning of the 11th Dynasty when, for the first time, we can see a clear association between the side projections and the offering vase. The first object known to us that can be properly termed a heart amulet is the golden amulet inscribed with the cartouche of Nebhetepre Mentuhotep II.[33] Clearly the object does not bear any resemblance to the hieroglyph F 34 (from Gardiner's list). On the contrary, it is fully conceived as a vase, including the shape of its side projections in the form of small pierced buttons. However strange they might seem anatomically speaking, these small buttons, as well as the inscription of the royal cartouche, will remain typical features of heart amulets. Notwithstanding this early occurrence, in archaeological sources heart amulets only begin to appear in numbers from the New Kingdom on, a phenomenon that is also documented in iconographic sources.[34]

Due to the close resemblance between the vase amulet *stricto sensu* and the early vase heart amulet, side projections can be helpful in distinguishing them. Side projections can also help us with the task of dating, although with a very limited degree of accuracy. Typically, in earlier vase heart amulets, side projections are shape like buttons and not like the veins we see in the hieroglyph *ib* (F 34). Full resemblance to this hieroglyph only became more evident during the 18th Dynasty, particularly after the Amarna Period. From that point on, side projections traditionally assumed the shape of the cardiac veins. Another change in the shape of side projections occurred during the Late Period: they came to be extremely elongated, with sharp edges, and in some instances bearing a greater resemblance to a pair of ears.[35]

In later burials, the vase heart amulet was a very common object and, most often, a very modest one. Nonetheless, this later use leads to misconception about its role in earlier times, when, on the contrary, it seems to have assumed a very exclusive character. The first attested heart amulets known to us reveal demonstrate a particularly strong connection to the Theban royal elite. The heart amulet has been found within the wrappings of the few un-plundered royal mummies discovered thus far. Queen Ah-hotep's mummy, for instance, wore it on a bracelet.[36] The mummy of the king Ahmose, found at Dra Abu el-Naga, revealed a superb heart amulet crafted in lapis lazuli and suspended from a gold chain.[37] Tutankhamun's mummy also wore a pair of pectorals that displayed such heart amulets.[38] In the Third Intermediate Period, heart amulets were still a precious item in royal burials as is demonstrated by the mummy of the king Psusennes, in Tanis, where an important collection of large heart amulets was found.[39]

From the reign of Hatshepsut on we observe the use of the heart amulet by those outside of the royal family, but this use remains the prerogative of a very exclusive elite. The 'demotisation' of the heart amulet only becomes evident after the Amarna Period and would only attain its 'golden age' during the Late Period. This 'demotisation' generated a much broader use of heart amulets among a larger cross-section of the Egyptian population, as well as a significant deterioration in their quality.[40] It is not uncommon to see unpierced amulets in later burials; this clearly shows that they were made strictly to be used within the wrappings of the mummy.[41]

---

[30] See Fig. 7 - A. MINAULT-GOUT, *Balat II: Le mastaba d'Ima-Pepi*, 1992, 90; M. VALLOGGIA, *Balat I: Le mastaba de Medou-nefer*, 1986, fig. 13; G. BRUNTON, *Mostagedda and the Tasian culture*, 1937, pl. LVIII. The identification of these objects as heart amulets is also contested in C. MÜLLER-WINKLER, *Die Ägyptischen Objekt-Amulette*, 1987, p. 225.

[31] These vases were shaped to suggest the vase *nw* which, indeed correspond to a trend detected among late Old Kingdom amulets to depict ritual objects on amulets. See C. ANDREWS, 'Amulets', in D. Redford, *Oxford Encyclopedia of Ancient Egypt*, 2001, Vol. I, p. 79. Note that this vase amulet can also be regarded as a three dimensional rendering of the hieroglyph *nw* and, as such, it has strong connotations with the ritual meaning of the water. See, for instance, that this hieroglyph was used to write the word *nwn* and also the name of Nut, both with a strong affinity with water. See A. GARDINER, *Egyptian Grammar*, 1994, p. 530-531.

[32] In fact it is actually a possibility that the vase heart amulets may have derived from the vase amulets dated from the late Old Kingdom. Although very similar with later versions of the vase type heart amulet, these older versions of the object do not seem to have been understood as a heart amulet at all. See M. VALLOGGIA, 'Rapport préliminaire sur la troisiéme campagne de fouilles du mastaba V à Balat (Oasis de Dakhleh)', *BIFAO* 80 (1980), p. 97-128;

[33] See Fig. 8 - N 551 (Louvre Museum).

[34] The first occurrences of the heart amulet on iconographic sources are well documented on royal children since the beginning of the 18th Dynasty. See chapter I.

[35] Despite the importance of the side projection among earlier heart amulets, we agree with Müller-Winkler that, especially on later objects, they are not an important feature to identify a heart amulet since in fact they can be totally absent. See C. MÜLLER-WINKLER, *Die Ägyptischen Objekt-Amulette*, 1987, p. 225.

[36] See JE 28606/CG 52091 (Cairo Egyptian Museum): in E. VERNIER, *Bijoux et Orfévreries*, pl. X. The Donation Stela, from the temple of Karnak, also show the association between the Theban royal princes with the heart amulet. To this document see I. HARARI, 'Nature de la Stéle de Donation de Fonction du roi Ahmôsis a la reine Ahmès-Nefertari', *ASAE* 56 (1956), pl. II.

[37] See heart amulet from king Ahmose's burial, SR 9386 (Cairo Egyptian Museum).

[38] The lunar winged scarab pectoral and the falcon pectoral, from the group object nº 256. See N. REEVES, *The Complete Tutankhamun*, 1990, p. 113 (these objects are identified in the illustration by letters *uuu* and *qqq*). Another golden heart amulet decorated with the *benu* bird, CG 62067 (Cairo Egyptian Museum) – Fig. 13, was found in a chest.

[39] See P. MONTET, *Les constructions et le tombeau de Psousenès à Tanis*, 1951, pl. CXIX

[40] These objects indeed started to be produced massively employing glass and mould casts. Roughly finished, certain heart amulets found in late burials attest a much wider use of apotropaic objects by the Egyptian population. See F. PETRIE, *Dendereh*, 1900, pl. XXVI

[41] See UC 38441 (Petrie Museum), UC 38442 (Petrie Museum), CG 5226 (Cairo Egyptian Museum in M. REISNER, *Amulets*, I, p. 2), CG 5240 (Cairo Egyptian Museum in *ibidem*, p. 4), CG 5257 (Cairo Egyptian Museum in *ibidem*, p. 7), just to quote a few examples.

Materials

The range of materials used in the production of these amulets is extremely wide. In the Late Period the use of stone is always prevalent (nearly 80% of those amulets are made of stone) and more than 30 different kinds of stone can be identified. Red stones such as cornelian and red jasper are particularly abundant. In earlier periods, however, the use of gold in the production of vase heart amulets is not uncommon.[42] Surprisingly, the use of materials such as faience or glass did not play an important part in the considerable growth witnessed in the production of vase heart amulets during the Late Period.[43]

Decoration

Royal cartouches and titulatures are very common, especially on earlier amulets.[44] Funerary inscriptions, such as chapter 30 of the *Book of the Dead*, also played an important role in the decoration of larger amulets, especially during the Ramessid Period and among the 21st Dynasty Theban clergy. Nevertheless short inscriptions are the rule, mainly limited to the name of the deceased, which that can be understood if we take into account the belief that the heart was the seat of identity and memory.

Iconographic details are also frequently depicted on the bodies of vase heart amulets. Especially after the 18th Dynasty, the iconographic motifs used on these amulets became increasingly complex and sophisticated. Solar symbols are often found, especially on the large funerary versions of the vase heart amulet. Scarabs are also present, depicted either quite elaborately[45] or more simply, using representations or in simpler depictions consisting of just three incised lines depicting the elytra of the insect.[46] Nevertheless, the Heliopolitain *benu* bird is the symbol most often connected with the heart amulet.[47] The prevalence of these solar symbols in the decoration of the heart amulet definitely echoes their meaning in the *Book of the Dead*, since the scarab and the *benu* bird evoke chapters 30 B and 29 B respectively, and play an important role in securing the rebirth and regeneration of the deceased.[48] Although infrequent, the full depiction of Osiris also occurs.[49]

During the Late Period, the typical geometrical patterns of the hieroglyph *ib*, such as the crescent and the mound, took precedence in the decoration of the vase heart amulets. These patterns, of course, derived from the anatomical representations of the cardiac organ. Nevertheless, at least in certain instances, the auricle and the ventricle seem to acquire a more transcendent meaning and become allusions to cosmic elements. In some cases the auricle is explicitly identified with the hieroglyphic symbol for the moon, the *Ah* sign.[50] The ventricle could also be used to suggest the primordial mound.[51]

Use

Unlike the heart scarab (which had an exclusively funerary use), most of vase heart amulets (especially the smaller versions), seem to have been made to be used during earthly life. It is possible that the objects decorated with a royal cartouche may have been offered by the king to his subjects as an official decoration, particularly the golden ones. This offering could be understood as a tangible way of concretising the bureaucratic ideal of being in the king's heart, which is often mentioned in autobiographical texts. Nevertheless, objects such as these could also be included among the funerary equipment of the deceased and carried into the afterlife.

Other vase heart amulets were carefully hollowed out in order to be properly seen as ritual vases.[52] Made of faience or of stone, they were probably intended to receive unguents and could have been used as votive objects before being included with the funerary equipment of the deceased.

Symbolism

Curiously enough, archaeology has provided evidence of the use of ritual vases in the shape of the heart, some of them of monumental size. In a private context, we know of a set of eleven identical vases from the 19th Dynasty (from Abydos) dedicated by a priest of the cult of Osiris to this deity. These heart-shaped vases are decorated with incised depictions of the priest praying to Osiris.[53] Other heart-shaped vases seem to have been used as a mortar. [54] Some

[42] See AF 9101 (Louvre Museum), UC 38422 (Petrie Museum), UC 58020 (Petrie Museum), CG 5259 (Cairo Egyptian Museum). Royal amulets are also known, such as the golden heart amulet from the tomb of Tutankhamun, CG 62067 (Cairo Egyptian Museum) – Fig. 13.

[43] Cornice heart amulets, on the contrary, were very often crafted on rough materials such as clay or glass. Vase heart amulets keep to be carved in stone. A good sample of later heart amulets can be found in C. MÜLLER-WINKLER, *Die Ägyptischen Objekt-Amulette*, 1987, tf. XV-XXI.

[44] Early on there already were royal cartouches that were used as the main decoration motif on such objects. See Fig. 8 – golden amulet with the cartouche of Nebhepetre Mentuhotep II, N 551 (Louvre Museum).

[45] See CG 12054 (Cairo Egyptian Museum): in M. REISNER, *Amulets*, I, pl. VII. See also Fig. 60 - CG 12056 (Cairo Egyptian Museum): in *ibidem*.

[46] See Fig. 12 - CG 5233 (Cairo Egyptian Museum): in M. REISNER, *Amulets*, I, p. 3). Also CG 5234 (Cairo Egyptian Museum): in *ibidem*, p. 3. See also AF 2589 (Louvre Museum).

[47] Depictions of the *benu* bird can be seen among vase heart amulets since the late 18th Dynasty. We can find it in the object EA 50742 (British Museum) and in the superb amulet from the tomb of Tutankhamun, CG 62067 (Cairo Egyptian Museum) – Fig. 13. More often it is found among vase heart amulets of the 21st Dynasty: N 4619 (Louvre Museum), CG 5235 (Cairo Egyptian Museum): in M. REISNER, *Amulets*, I, p. 3. Also in object nº 22.2.24/54831 (Metropolitan Museum of Art).

[48] The scarab and the *benu* bird are particularly abundant among the heart amulets found among the 21st Dynasty's funerals of the priests of Amun.

[49] See Fig. 14 - JE 34409/SR 9219 (Cairo Egyptian Museum).

[50] See Fig. 10 - E 14708 (Louvre Museum), inscribed with the name of Ahmose.

[51] See the amulet AEO 9644 (Louvre Museum) where the sign of the ventricle is used as the primordial mound as suggests the *benu* bird that rests upon it.

[52] See Fig. 11 - SR 9203/CG 12914 (Cairo Egyptian Museum): in G. REISNER, *Amulets*, I, pl. IX). Also SR 9258/CG12067/JE 27170 (Cairo Egyptian Museum): in *ibidem*, p. 108.

[53] See E 21801 (Musée Champollion). The objects are described in M. DEWATCHER, *Musée Champollion: La collection égyptienne*, 1986, p. 25.

[54] See Nº Inv. 8881 (Museu da Farmácia de Lisboa): in L. ARAÚJO, P. BASSO, *A Farmácia no Mundo Pré-Clássico e nas Culturas*

are inscribed with short dedicatory inscriptions. Some stone vases, in the same shape but of much larger size, may have been used in the context of the temple ritual. Of monumental size, some of these vases are inscribed with royal cartouches while others, from later periods, are inscribed with dedication inscriptions of private individuals.[55] Their large size and rough carving seem to indicate that these objects were positioned within the sacred precinct of the temple, most probably in its outer areas.

Other heart-shaped vases, although also inscribed with the royal titulature, were clearly crafted as very exquisite objects. This is the case with the alabaster heart-shaped vases inscribed with the cartouches of Queen Hatshepsut.[56] Another superb heart shaped vase belongs to a later period, and it was inscribed with the cartouches of King Apries (26th Dynasty).[57]

As to the purpose of these vases, it seems plausible that most of them, especially the rough monumental vases, were used as containers. We know that, when they were discovered, the eleven vases of Abydos did not show any trace of being used to store substances.[58] Nevertheless it is possible although difficult to identify, that the finest objects, such as the vase of Apries, may have served a different use.

A clue to understanding the ritual purpose of such heart-shaped vases may be provided through iconography. In the context of the divine cult, temple decoration presents interesting depictions of ritual vases shaped as hearts.[59] Such objects seem to have been used as containers for water and other liquids used in the divine cult. Therefore, it remains a possibility that the hollow vase heart amulets could be regarded as miniatures of those ritual artefacts used in the divine cult. As with other miniature amulets,[60] they could have been used as tributes to the god and, as such, they could have been hung in some part of the temple as testimonies of devotion. This use supposes that, at least in certain contexts, the vase heart amulet could have allowed a spiritual reading concerning the inner cult performed in the heart, a typical feature of the "personal piety" cultural trend.[61] Hollow heart amulets in particular may have been used in this context as an illustration of the ideal of "being in god's water" so well known from liturgical hymns and wisdom literature. 'Being plunged into the water of the god' hints at the reanimation of the individual by the action of the divinity. Even the late Petosiris wisdom tells us that the waters of life guide the heart towards the god's way and by doing so this text establishes a relationship between the purification of the heart and virtue.

Also in religious texts, 'to put god in the heart' is extremely important in the context of a personal relationship with god:

> Blessed is he who puts you in his heart! Woe to him who attacks you! For your display of might is so powerful, your plans so effective, your grace so swift.[62]

Being formulated as a vase, the heart probably illustrated the role of the human mind in the context of the personal relationship with god. As the ritual vase was filled with life-giving water, so also should the mind be filled with new life. In other words, one should be filled by god's presence in order to be strengthened by the power of life.

Thus, it is possible that a subtle shift in the religious meaning of the vase heart amulet occurred: the wisdom reading of the object as a symbol of a *maetic* mind could have gradually evolved to become an image of the inner presence of god.

3. The cornice heart amulets

The objects that we group within the classification of 'cornice heart amulets' have a square border. Interestingly enough, this feature is carved in such a way that it is remarkably similar to the cornice that usually adorns the edge of a sanctuary or a temple gateway. In this particular class of objects the top of the cornice, always flattened, is carved with an eyelet for suspension. This cornice gives the heart amulet a significant visual impact, especially when it is attached to the body of the amulet by means of a very elongated 'neck'[63] Usually, cornice amulets are quite small in size, the average being no larger than 2,5 cm[64], but many are even smaller.[65] Taking this into account, an object measuring 3,5 cm is obviously of significant size[66] and an object larger than this appears only infrenquently.[67]

Another distinctive feature of cornice heart amulets is the shape of their side projections. Instead of being shaped like a button or the cardiac veins (as they appear in the *ib* hieroglyph) the side projections typically found in cornice amulets are elongated and pointed, bearing a resemblance

Tradicionais, 2008, p. 102. Substances used in pharmacopoeia as well as other diverse preparations could be mitigated and transformed using these vases.

[55] See JE 86848 (Cairo Egyptian Museum).

[56] See JE 57203 (Cairo Egyptian Museum).

[57] See Fig. 16 - CG 829 (Cairo Egyptian Museum).

[58] See M. DEWATCHER, *Musée Champollion: La collection égyptienne*, 1986, p. 25.

[59] See, for instance, the depiction of the heart-shaped offering vases in the funerary temple of Seti I, north-western chapel of the hypostyle hall, west wall.

[60] See O. PERDU, 'Des pendentifs en guise d'ex-voto', *Rd'E* 54 (2003), p. 155-166.

[61] See J. ASSMANN, ‚Zur Geschichte des Herzens im alten Ägypten', in *Die Erfindung des inneren Menschen: Studien zur reliogiösen Anthropologie*, 1993, pp. 81-113

[62] Block statue of Ramose, in J. ASSMANN, *The Search for God in Ancient Egypt*, 2001, p. 232

[63] See Fig. 18 - UC 38428 (Petrie Museum)

[64] See CG 13216 (Cairo Egyptian Museum): in G. REISNER, *Amulets* II, 1958, p. 90.

[65] See AEO 23346 (Louvre Museum) with 1,9 cm or SR 9245/CG 5227 (Cairo Egyptian Museum) with 1,8 cm. To this last object see *idem*, *Amulets* I, 1907, p. 2.

[66] See Fig. 17 - AF 11531 (Louvre Museum), with 3,13 cm. Also CG 12062 (Cairo Egyptian Museum) with 3,3 cm: in *idem*, p. 108. The largest object that we are aware of (nearly 9,0 cm) can be found in W. PETRIE, *Historical Studies*, 1911, pl. XIX. It is now exhibited in Cairo Egyptian Museum.

[67] See 10.130.1806 (Metropolitan Museum of Art).

to a pair of ears. Unlike the other side projections, these may extend completely along the amulet's body. Usually they are decorated with an incised pattern of parallel lines, similar to that which is frequently found on Hathoric bovine ears.

Datation

Although cornice heart amulets are very common objects in ancient Egyptian collections, only a few of them can be dated with any accuracy. Of those that we have studied, not one can be dated earlier than the 21st Dynasty. In fact known examples of this particular class of heart amulets were found within the wrappings of Psusennes I[68] and Amenemope.[69] After this, during the Late Period, a 'demotisation' of cornice heart amulets seems to occur, evidenced by the huge numbers found in later burials.

Materials

Materials used to the produce these amulets may vary. A vast array of different stones can be identified from the commonplace cornelian[70] to, most frequently, darker stones such as lapis lazuli[71] steatite[72], obsidian[73], schist[74], green jasper[75], and many others. The use of lapis lazuli and darker stones is surprisingly widespread in this particular type of heart amulets which could indicate that blue and darker colours had a distinct connection to this particular category of heart amulets, as opposed to the traditional use for these objects. Notwithstanding the prevalence of the use of stone, other raw materials such as faience and glass were also heavily used in the production of these amulets. The very rough quality of many such objects made of glass suggest the use of mass production techniques[76] such as using moulds to facilitate the production of large quantities of objects. These materials and techniques certainly played an important role in the considerable growth witnessed in amulet production and in the 'demotisation' of their use by a wider population.

Nevertheless we can also identify finely carved objects made of stone, especially lapis lazuli[77] and darker stones[78] such as amazonite,[79] serpentine,[80] greywacke[81] and schist[82]. Some fine examples of objects made of glass exist as well.[83]

Decoration

Cornice amulets are very simply decorated, if they are decorated at all. Unlike earlier types of heart amulets, such as pendulum heart amulets or vase heart amulets, there is a clearly evident simplification in cornice heart amulets; instead of complex decorations such as the scarab or the *benu* bird, we find simple geometrical patterns in the shape of stars. These particular patterns do not seem to bear any resemblance to anatomical features in the shape of the crescent and the mound that are so typical in depictions of the *ib* hieroglyph (F 34).[84] Usually the geometrical patterns are V-[85] or X-shaped[86] and are sometimes combined with a depiction of the mound.[87] More complex depictions are rare. An exceptional object was found in the wrappings of Psusennes I depicting the solar triad of Re, Atum and Khepri.[88] As far as we are aware only one other cornice amulet was carved with depictions of gods and these were also solar gods: Atum and Re.[89] Both amulets were carved in lapis lazuli. Another interesting and very rare depiction shows the image of an ibis, the sacred bird to Thoth.[90]

Use

The small size of cornice heart amulets may well indicate that, although found in a funerary context, these amulets could certainly be used by the living, which is definitely not the case with the heart amulets most commonly used in mummies from earlier periods.[91] Nonetheless, in some objects, the eyelet for suspension is not even pierced. In these situations, such objects were made only to be placed within mummy bandages.

---

[68] See JE 85804 (Cairo Egyptian Museum). A good sample of this kind of amulets was found in the mummy of the king. See P. MONTET, *Les constructions et le tombeau de Psousennès I à Tanis*, 1951, pl. CXIX.

[69] See JE 86044 (Cairo Egyptian Museum). See *ibidem*.

[70] See UC 38417 (Petrie Museum) and Nr. 195 (Roemer and Pelizaeus Museum). Also CG 53191 (Cairo Egyptian Museum): in E. VERNIER, *Bijoux et orfèvreries*, 1927, pl. LXXXV.

[71] AF 8828 (Louvre Museum), AF 8822 and AEO 23438 (Louvre Museum). Also SR 9267/CG 12068 (Cairo Egyptian Museum): in G. REISNER, *Amulets* II, 1958, p. 108. See also N. 321 (Liebieghaus): B. SCHLICK-NOLTE, V. HULSHOFF, *Aegyptische Bildwerke*, Band I, p. 324.

[72] See 247 (Musée de Picardie): in O. PERDU, N. MAHEÓ, E. RICKAL, *La collection égyptienne du Musée de Picardie*, 1994, n° 247.

[73] See n° 192172 (Michael Carlos Museum): See P. LACOVARA, B. TROPE, *The Realm of Osiris: Mummies, Coffins and Ancient Egyptian Funerary Arts in the Michael C. Carlos Museum*, 2001, p. 60.

[74] See AEO 10284 (Louvre Museum)

[75] See SR 9266/CG 5253 (Cairo Egyptian Museum): in G. REISNER, *Amulets* I, 1907, p. 6.

[76] Some of these objects show not only that they were made by the use of mould but also that they were very quickly finished while the glass was still soft. See CG 13297 (Cairo Egyptian Museum): in *idem*, *Amulets*, II, 1958, pl. XV.

[77] See AEO 23438 (Louvre Museum). See also SR 9267/CG 12068 (Cairo Egyptian Museum): in *idem*, *Amulets* I, 1907, p. 108. See also SR 9280/CG 5247 (Cairo Egyptian Museum): in *ibidem*, p. 5.

[78] See unidentified brown stone in E 18237 (Louvre Museum), Fig. 19.

[79] See CG 53212 (Cairo Egyptian Museum): in E. VERNIER, *Bijoux et orfèvreries*, Tomes I-II, 1927, pl. XCI.

[80] See AEO 31504 (Louvre Museum).

[81] Se AF 9903 (Louvre Museum).

[82] See AF 8826 (Louvre Museum).

[83] See Fig. 17 - AF 11531 (Louvre Museum). Also SR 9245/CG 5227 (Cairo Egyptian Museum): in G. REISNER, *Amulets* I, 1907, p. 2.

[84] See SR 9264/CG 5250 (Cairo Egyptian Museum): *ibidem*, p. 6.

[85] See CG 13302 (Cairo Egyptian Museum): in *idem*, *Amulets* II, 1958, pl. XXIX

[86] See UC 22527 and Fig. 18 - UC 38428 (all from Petrie Museum). Also BM 8128 (British Museum): in J. COONEY, *Catalogue of Egyptian antiquities in the British Museum*, IV: *Glass*, 1970, p. 16.

[87] See AF 11553 (Louvre Museum). Müller-Winkler also pointed out that these patterns cannot be identified with the anatomical features typical of the hieroglyph F 34 (from the Gardiner's list). See C. MÜLLER-WINKLER, *Die Ägyptischen Objekt-Amulette*, 1987, p. 214.

[88] See JE 85804 (Cairo Egyptian Museum): in P. MONTET, *Les constructions et le tombeau de Psousennès à Tanis*, 1951, pl. CXIX.

[89] See Fig. 22 - AEO 28353 (Louvre Museum).

[90] See Fig. 23 - UC 38447 (Petrie Museum).

[91] Such is the case of the human and animal-headed heart amulets. Pendulum-heart amulets also seem to be used only in the funerary context.

As opposed to earlier funerary uses of this amulet, beginning with the Late Period heart amulet came to be used in great numbers within the same mummy; it is not uncommon to find three, four or even more heart amulets within the same mummy, most often distributed over the entire body and not particularly related to the position of the heart, as was the rule in earlier periods, especially during the Ramessid Period.[92] This may be related to a subtle change in the magical purpose of the object.

Symbolism

The cornice heart amulets and iconography

Curiously enough, the spread of the cornice heart amulet that we find in the archaeological records seems to be related to the contemporary use of the heart amulet as an iconographic attribute of the divine children. In fact, from the Late Period on, the heart amulet is shown as an attribute of Horpakhered and Ihy and, as such, it is often depicted in the context of temple decoration. It is sometimes difficult to identify the type of heart amulet depicted on the chests of the divine children but, when the quality of the sculptural work is good enough, the clear features of the cornice heart amulet are quite evident: an elongated neck linking the cornice to the body of the amulet which may even be decorated with the typical geometrical pattern in the shape of an X.[93] Elongated side projections may also be visible. Divine children are depicted with the heart amulet in late statuary as well. In some finely-carved statues we can easily recognize the features of the cornice heart amulet.[94] The object is also found in the chest of the divine child depicted in the context of the vignettes of the weighing of the heart produced from the Late Period on. As a result of this pictorial information, in our interpretation of the cornice heart amulet we must consider the use of the amulet as an iconographic attribute of divine children.

However, before we proceed, we need to understand the significance of the cornice that makes these amulets singular. First, we must bear in mind that this particular element is a common feature of depictions of divinities such as Bes and Hathor.[95] In fact, statues of Bes wear a similar cornice on their heads. Interestingly enough, on some Bes amulets, the eyelet for suspension is carved on top of the cornice, just as it appears in cornice heart amulets. The cornice also appears in Hathoric objects, such as amulets and *systra*, just above the head of the goddess, where it usually supports a model of a temple.[96]

It is also interesting to note that both gods are in fact symbolically related, especially in the temple structures known as *mammisi*, where the tops of the Hathoric columns are usually carved with the depiction of the god Bes or with scenes related to the divine birth. Such motifs could thus be seen as symbolic of the Duat and the sky, where the regeneration and rebirth of the divine children took place.[97] This symbolic meaning suggests that the cornice could have been incorporated into the heart amulet in order to provide for the regeneration of the user's heart. Ergo, when used by the living, the amulet could be considered as an apotropaic object with healing and regenerative powers.[98] On the other hand, when used by the dead, in mummy wrappings, the object could insure regeneration and rebirth. The prodigal use of this amulet in later mummies may also reflect an intention to provide the deceased with purification and healing.

This meaning seems to be supported by the X- or V-shaped incisions found on the amulet itself. Although their meaning is quite obscure, they bear an intriguing similarity to the symbols that the Hemsut goddesses wear above their heads in scenes of the divine birth of the Pharaoh.[99] If this is the case, these marks, when carved on the heart amulet, may have been used as further symbols of protection for the divine birth.

The meaning of the cornice heart amulets

Cornice amulets did not become common until the Late Period. However, from that point on they became the most prevalent form of heart amulet.[100] Astonishingly, the mass production of cornice heart amulets began at precisely the same time that the iconography of the divine children seemed to expand. This broad use of the heart amulet in the iconography of these gods may, in fact, be related to the intent to initiate a cosmic renewal in the world. Since the divine children are, in the context of temple decoration, the embodiment of the divine nature of the Pharaoh, such cosmic renewal can be regarded as a political statement, especially during a period when a return to Egypt's origins was highly valued. Divine children could also be used in iconography as symbols of resurrection or rebirth. In vignettes of the weighing of the heart from the Greco-Roman period, the deceased is often depicted as a newborn solar child; in this context, although still connected to the weighing of the heart, the heart amulet seems to be invested with a broader obstetric meaning.[101] In fact, there is a strong possibility that the heart amulet

[92] Among contemporary anthropoid coffins, this little version of the heart amulet is also a common attribute, sometimes in several occurrences. We know of a very interesting wooden anthropoid coffin from the Late Period with the depiction of a collar with three heart amulets. It is conserved in the Medelhavsmuseet (Stockholm), but unfortunately without number to identify it.
[93] See Fig. 20.
[94] See the bronze statue SR 46380 (Cairo Egyptian Museum).
[95] See Fig. 24.
[96] See F. FRIEDMAN, *Gifts of the Nile: Ancient Egyptian Faience*, 1998, p. 102.

[97] To the meaning of the cornice on hathoric amulets see Y. EL SHAZLY, 'Pendant in the form of a hathoric head' in E. Hornung & B. Bryan, *The Quest for Immortality: Treasures of Ancient Egypt*, 2002, p. 116.
[98] This use could be stimulated through the depiction of the heart amulet on the iconography of Horpakhered among the magical *cippi*, so much popular from the Late Period on.
[99] See Fig. 21.
[100] During Late Period cornice amulets replaced older features of heart amulets such as the pendulum heart amulets used on scales. See R. SOUSA, 'Symbolism and Meaning of Pendulum Heart Amulets', *GM* 221 (2009), p. 69-79.
[101] To the meaning of the heart amulet in later vignettes of the *Book of the Dead* see R. SOUSA, 'The cardiac vignettes of the Book of the Dead (Late Period)', *BAEDE* 17 (2008), p. 39-53

came to be considered as a divine attribute of the infant gods and, as such, was used to insure rebirth and a new life. In other words, during the first millennium, the heart amulet, especially the cornice version, came to be valued as a symbol of new life and rebirth, being a tangible sign of the power of light and purity of the divine children.

Being quite small, such amulets appear to have been used in earthly life as well as in the beyond, which, therefore, significantly extended their magical scope. Their increasing popularity is evidenced by the existence of crudely produced artefacts, most likely intended to be less costly and thus more available for use by commoners. On the other hand, very finely crafted artefacts show that the amulet was also highly regarded by the elite of that time.

Considering the elements collected thus far, we can assume that the magical scope of cornice heart amulets seems to be largely connected to the symbolism of the divine children. In fact, it seems likely that the cornice heart amulet was used specifically as an attribute of the divine children and, as such, it can be understood as a symbol of magical protection *per se*. On later *cippi* of Horpakhered, the god wears the heart amulet while he is defeating the beasts that embody the evil forces of Seth.[102] Therefore, it is possible that the amulet was used as an embodiment of the apotropaic power of the infant gods, and thus was used by the living as a healing and apotropaic symbol. On the other hand, when used in the funerary context, the amulet could serve to protect the rebirth that resulted from the weighing of the heart, a rebirth understood as provided by a cosmic mother goddess, such as Isis or Hathor.

Finally, the cornice heart amulets exemplify a subtle change in the representation of the heart. The image of the heart as a temple seems to have been added to the rendering of the heart as a vase. When personal piety absorbed the reflection about *maet*, the cornice came to be preferred over the vase as the symbol of the heart, which certainly reflected the idea that the heart was the inner temple where the supreme god resided.

[102] See CG 9402 (Cairo Egyptian Museum): in É. CHASSINAT, *Textes et dessins magiques*, 1903, Pl. II..

CHAPTER THREE

COMPOSITE FORMS OF THE HEART AMULET

Human head	Animal head	Flower	Solar disk
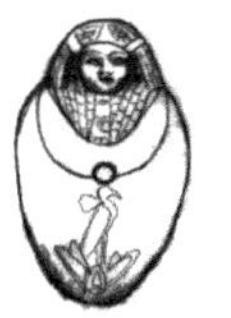	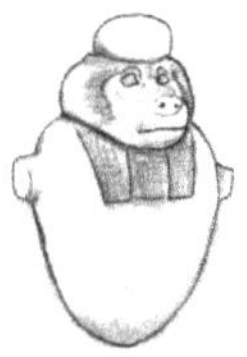	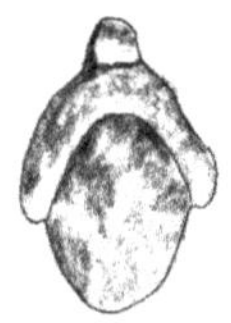	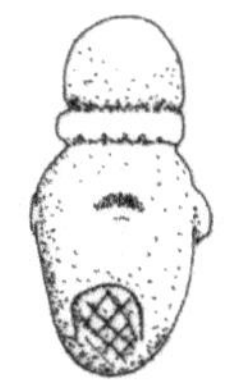

Classification of the heart amulets according to the dominant feature of the top

In the previous chapter we studied amulets with a standardized top, consisting of only a suspension ring. In this chapter we will focus on the study of composite forms of the heart amulet. Ordinarily a human or animal head would be added to the body of the amulet, but in some cases the addition would be in the form of a solar disk or some other unusual feature.[1] Unlike the amulets previously discussed, amulets with any of these features are very rare, particularly those having animal heads.

1. The human-headed heart amulets

Human-headed heart amulets are usually the largest of heart amulets, as much as five to seven cm in height. Unlike the standard versions, human-headed amulets do not possess any side projections[2].

Datation

The human-headed heart amulet seems to have assumed great importance as a funerary artefact during the Ramessid Period. This type of object was used less often after that period. Interestingly, a similar class of objects reappeared in the Greco-Roman Period.

Materials

Ramessid human-headed heart amulets were carved out of a great variety of raw materials: faience,[3] glass[4], alabaster[5], quartz[6] and steatite[7] were among the most commonly used.

Decoration

A tripartite wig, an attribute commonly associated with the depiction of the deceased as an Osirian divinity, usually frames the head. The wig is sometimes carefully incised with vertical lines intended to suggest hair. In some stone amulets the wig is formed using an incrustation of some darker stone,[8] while the hair of some faience or glass amulets may be coloured with a black or dark blue pigment.[9] Additional decoration is rarely found anywhere other than the head in the earliest forms of this amulet.[10] However, the decoration of these amulets appears to become increasingly heavy. The most common decoration of this particular category of amulets seems to consist of the two hands of the deceased, suggesting a mummiform attitude.[11] The *usekh* collar also came to play an important part in their decoration.[12] More rarely, the *ba* bird,[13] the winged scarab[14] and the *benu* bird[15] are among the symbols depicted on the body of these objects. A *naos*, sometimes flanked by the gods Re and Osiris, may be depicted as well.[16]

Inscriptions take the form of the Osirian name of the deceased,[17] and short versions of chapter 30 B of the

[1] The heart amulet found in the mummy of prince Khaemwaset, for instance, provided a strange object. Sculpted in red jasper, the amulet presents tree protuberances at its top, resembling to veins. See Fig. 62 - AF 2333 (Louvre Museum). Without paralel and because this depiction do not consists on a composite addition of other features than the heart itself, we didn't create an additional category.

[2] We have found only one object with a suspension ring, SR 9221/CG 5237 (Cairo Egyptian Museum): in G. REISNER, *Amulets* I, 1907, p. 4.

[3] See JE 34448 (Cairo Egyptian Museum)

[4] See object nº 26807 (British Museum): in C. ANDREWS, *Amulets of Ancient Egypt*, 1998, fig. 61

[5] UC 69861 (Petrie Museum).

[6] See CG 12052 (Cairo Egyptian Museum).

[7] UC 52606 (Petrie Museum).

[8] See AF 12141 (Louvre Museum) or Fig. 25 - DP136533 (Metropolitan Museum of Art).

[9] See again SR 9221/CG 5237 (Cairo Egyptian Museum). Also SR 9196/JE 34412 (Cairo Egyptian Museum).

[10] See, for instance, Fig. 25 - DP136533 (Metropolitan Museum of Art), N 4622 (Louvre Museum) or UC 69861 (Petrie Museum).

[11] See BM 15598 (British Museum) or SR 9215/JE 34448 (Cairo Egyptian Museum).

[12] See SR 9204/CG 5238 (Cairo Egyptian Museum): in G. REISNER, *Amulets* I, 1907, p. 4. Also SR 10824 (Cairo Egyptian Museum): in G. STEINDORFF, *Aniba*, II, 1937, tf. 50. Also EA 29440 (British Museum).

[13] See object nº 26807 (British Museum): in C. ANDREWS, *Amulets of Ancient Egypt*, 1998, fig. 61.

[14] See again SR 10824 (Cairo Egyptian Museum). Also UC 52612 (Petrie Museum).

[15] See Fig. 27 - B326 (Rijksmuseum van Oudheden): in *Leben und Tod im Alten Ägypten*, 1999, p. 92. The *benu* bird is depicted in this amulet over a lotus flower and topped by a solar disk. See again object EA 29440 (British Museum).

[16] See Fig. 26 - UC 52605, UC 13212 (Petrie Museum).

[17] See Fig. 27 - B326 (Rijksmuseum van Oudheden).

Book of the Dead may also occur on the reverse of some objects.[18]

Use

The heads of some amulets are pierced in order to provide for a suspension device, but many other objects have no piercing, which clearly indicates an exclusive funerary use. In addition to their use within the wrappings of the mummy, these amulets could also be inserted into large funerary pectorals. For example, a human-headed heart amulet functions as the centerpiece for the superb pectoral of the lady Kiemneferui found at Saqqara. The entire pectoral is shaped like a *naos* inside of which is found a heart amulet above a solar barque where the gods Re and Osiris are also visible.[19] While in some pectorals the human-headed heart amulet seems to be identified with the sun disk,[20] in other objects it seems to be more decidedly associated with Osiris.[21]

Greco-Roman objects with flattened bases seem to have been used in a different fashion. In fact, while they might seem similar to the Ramessid objects, these later amulets served a votive purpose indicated by the inclusion of a base at their bottom end.[22]

Symbolism

Both the formal and iconographic features of Ramessid human-headed amulets definitely suggest a funerary purpose. Their size, weight and suspension method simply do not allow for their use by the living. Also, their iconographic attributes clearly show the deceased as an Osirian entity: a divine wig, hands carved in a manner suggestive of the features of contemporary anthropomorphic coffins, and the addition of traditional funerary symbols such as the *ba* bird or the winged scarab. These elements and the writing of the Osirian name of the deceased confer both an Osirian and a funerary significance on these objects.

In order to clarify the meaning of these artefacts we must bear in mind the meaning of heart amulets in general. It is often suggested that the heart amulet is an apotropaic object intended to present a physical substitute for the heart organ. This is not our interpretation of the available data concerning its use in iconographical contexts. In fact, as we have seen in previous chapters, during the Ramessid Period the main symbolism of the heart amulet is concerned with the weighing of the heart and the justification of the deceased. The funerary vignettes that illustrate this event frequently show the deceased receiving the heart amulet as recompense for the positive outcome of the judgement. During the Ramessid Period and even in the 21st Dynasty, the object seems to have been used as a symbol of the deceased's virtue and wisdom or, in other words, as a symbol of his pure and *maetic* heart (in a spiritual and not a physical sense). This general meaning of the object makes it clear that human-headed heart amulets were intended to depict the deceased's justified heart, i.e., the divine heart fully identified with Osiris.

The increasing complexity of the solar-Osirian theology of the Ramessid Period is also reflected in the decoration of these amulets. Some of them depict a *naos* flanked by the gods Re and Osiris[23], which demonstrates that the pure heart of the deceased was seen as a temple where the mythic union of Re and Osiris took place. Symbols such as the *benu* bird[24] and the solar scarab[25] also show that the deceased was supposed to experience a solar rebirth. This idea is also suggested in some of the pectorals where the amulet was framed: the amulet is found in the centre of a *naos*, where the union of Re and Osiris leads to a solar rebirth of the deceased.[26]

A very different meaning seems to be associated with the human-headed heart amulets crafted in later times, especially during the Greco-Roman Period. The formal features of these objects, made with a plain base, show that they were conceived as miniature forms of a divine statue. It would seem that these amulets were no longer seen merely as an image of the justified heart of the deceased but as an image of the sacred heart of Osiris, i.e., the sacred vase of Athribis. In fact, the decoration of the body of the amulet follows the iconography of Osiris Canopus. The central element of the decoration is a *naos,* which is sometimes associated with a winged scarab and two child divinities. The head is also often adorned by a tall crown, a common attribute in the iconography of Osiris Canopus.[27] Therefore, these amulets should be understood as a demonstration of a personal relationship with a god and not as a funerary symbol.

2. The animal-headed heart amulets

Animal-headed amulets are extremely rare. They are amazing examples of the fine miniaturist work done by Egyptian craftsmen. Unfortunately, we have only identified three objects that fall into this category.

[18] See G. STEINDORFF, *Aniba*, II, 1937, tf. 50

[19] See Fig. 28 - JE 92638 (Cairo Egyptian Museum): in Z. GONEIM, *Horus Sekhem-khet, the unfinished step pyramid at Saqqara*, 1957, pl. LXVIII. This object was found in the Ramessid coffin of the lady Kiemneferui, which was found at the precinct of Sekhememkhet, in Sakara.

[20] See J. TAYLOR, *Death and the afterlife in Ancient Egypt*, 2001, p. 204. Here, the amulet rises from the solar bark, and it is greeted by Isis and Nephtys.

[21] See B. VOGEL, *Meisterwerke Altagypsicher Keramik: 5000 jahre kunst und kunstlandwerk aus Ton und Fayence*, 1978, nº 318

[22] According to Julia Falkovitch the presence of a base in an amulet indicates that the object could be used as a divine statue See J. FALKOVITCH, 'L'usage des amulettes égyptiennes', *BSEG* 16 (1992), pp. 20-26

[23] See Fig. 26 - UC 52605, UC 13212 (Petrie Museum).

[24] See Fig. 27 - nº Inv. B326 (Rijksmuseum van Oudheden). See also EA 29440 (British Museum)

[25] See again SR 10824 (Cairo Egyptian Museum). Also UC 52612 (Petrie Museum).

[26] See again Fig. 28 - JE 92638 (Cairo Egyptian Museum). Also J. TAYLOR, *Death and the afterlife in Ancient Egypt*, 2001, p. 204.

[27] See UC 52618, UC 52616 (Petrie Museum). See also Fig. 29.

The one from the Cairo Egyptian Museum was found within the wrappings of Amenemope, in the tomb of Psusennes I.[28] The amulet measures only 3,5 cm in height and is carved out of chalcedony. The upper portion of the amulet is a baboon head framed by a tripartite wig and a collar and topped by a suspension ring. The body of the amulet has two side projections and is inscribed with a short version of the titulature of the Pharaoh Amenemope.

The object from the Louvre Museum, which appears to date from the Ramessid Period, is carved out of schist and measures 4 cm in height.[29] The lower end of the object is shaped like the lid of a vase topped by a canine head. The body has two side projections.

The object from the British Museum is moulded from clay as an avian head[30] that clearly resembles that of a falcon framed by a tripartite wig. The body of the amulet has two side projections.

Symbolism

The few examples of animal-headed heart amulets known to us do not permit us to make definite assumptions about their symbolism. However, it is possible to formulate certain hypotheses based on the available information.

The way in which these objects were carved precludes the possibility that their cardiac configuration was accidental. In fact, the side projections that they all possess clearly identify these artefacts as heart amulets. Their animal features serve as divine attributes. As a result, two alternative readings of these objects can be proposed. In the first place, we can consider the heads of the baboon, the dog and the falcon as examples of the typical iconography of Thoth, Anubis and Horus. However, the gods most commonly associated with such attributes are the four sons of Horus. Instead, it seems more plausible that the features of the baboon, the jackal and the falcon may in fact be intended to depict Hapi, Duamutef and Khebehsenuef, respectively. This reading of animal-headed amulets admits the possibility that some of the human-headed amulets previously discussed may in fact represent Imsety. This is possibly the case with the simplest unadorned human-headed heart amulets. Like their animal counterparts, the human-headed amulets that could depict Imsety would not have any decoration besides the name of the deceased.[31]

Admitting the possibility that some heart amulets were associated with the imagery of the four sons of Horus requires us, therefore, to pay some attention to the significance of such symbolism. As protectors of the viscera, the four sons of Horus were magically related to the heart *ib* of the deceased which, according to the interpretation of Thierry Bardinet, was a symbol of the inner part of the body cavity and not of the cardiac muscle.[32] This is one possible explanation for the depiction of the four sons of Horus, not merely as miniatures of the canopic jars, but specifically as heart amulets. However reasonable this explanation may be, one other possibility may explain the association of the four sons of Horus with the heart amulet. In the iconographical compositions of the Ramessid Period we can see a clear connection between these four gods and the weighing of the heart. In the funerary papyrus of Amenemuia (Berlin Egyptian Museum, nº P 3127), for example, these deities are depicted in close association with the heart amulet, which forms the central element of the composition.[33] The reason for the four gods to appear to be so closely connected to the heart amulet may be found in the depiction of the amulet itself that is inscribed with chapter 30 B of the *Book of the Dead*. Additionally, the four sons of Horus are a regular iconographic element of vignettes of the weighing of the heart, where they are usually depicted beside the throne of Osiris. When we examine the iconography of the papyrus of Amenemuia, these gods seem to play the role of guardian deities who protect the justified deceased during his journey through the Duat.

Curiously, the text of chapter 27 of the *Book of the Dead* also mentions that the deceased stands before an assembly of gods and tries to persuade them not to speak against him in the court of Osiris:

> Paroles dites par N.: 'O vous qui enlevez les coeurs (...) salut à vous maîtres de l'éternité, organizateurs de la perennité! Ne m'ôtez pas ce coeur qui est le mien, ne critiquez pas ce viscére de mon coeur![34]

In certain vignettes the deceased stands before a single deity. In this case, it is possible that this god may figure as his personal god or as the 'great god', as mentioned in the text. Nevertheless, three is usually the number of gods depicted which, in fact, may be read as the plural form of the word 'god'.[35] This was the simplest way of depicting the deceased before an assembly of gods. However, there can be four deities and, in that case, they usually represent the four sons of Horus,[36] which provides us with another argument concerning the depiction of these gods in heart amulets. Their role is clearly expressed in the text:

> Paroles dites par N.: 'O vous qui enlevez les coeurs, vous qui dérobez les viscères du coeur, vous qui faites se manifester le coeur de l'homme dans ce qu'il a fait, alors qu'il ne se reconnaît pas par suite de ce que vous avez fait(...)'.[37]

[28] See Fig. 30 - JE 86045 (Cairo Egyptian Museum): in P. MONTET, *Les constructions et le tombeau de Psousennèes à Tanis,* 1951, pl. CXXXVI.
[29] See Fig. 31 - E 11682 (Louvre Museum).
[30] See Fig. 32 - the object nº 35412 (British Museum)
[31] This could be the situation of the amulet DP136533 of the Metropolitan Museum of Art (Fig. 25) or the object N 4622 from the Louvre.

[32] See T. BARDINET, *Les papyrus médicaux de l'Égypte pharaonique,* Paris, 1995
[33] See Fig. 48 (nº P 3127, Berlin Egyptian Museum).
[34] Chapter 27 of the *Book of the Dead,* in P. BARGUET, *Le Livre des Morts,* 1967, p. 72.
[35] See Fig. 34.
[36] See M. MOSHER, 'Theban and Memphite *Book of the Dead* Traditions in the Late Period', *JARCE* 29 (1992), p. 145, note 19.
See Fig. 33.
[37] Chapter 27 of the *Book of the Dead,* in P. BARGUET, *Le Livre des Morts,* 1967, p. 72.

The gods watch over the heart of the deceased and transform it according to his personal deeds. This sentence has interesting implications since it can only be understood in the light of beliefs about the weighing of the heart. Without being aware of it, a man could see his heart transformed as a result of his own deeds, exposing him to attack by the gods who punish sinners and steal their hearts.

Thus, the animal-headed heart amulets emphasize the connection between the heart amulet and the imagery of the weighing of the heart. This typically corresponds to the religious direction of the Ramessid Period, during which a complex iconographical set of symbols and beliefs concerning the afterlife was elaborated. This iconographical exploration of the judgement of the dead seems to be a funerary development of the cultural trend so typical of personal piety. The significance of animal-headed heart amulets seems to be primarily related to the protection provided by these stellar gods to the deceased on his secret journey through the Duat: a protection made possible only through the purity of his heart. The fact that so few of these items have come down to us most probably also indicates that such objects were probably known only to a very exclusive elite (we should recall here the royal origins of the baboon-headed amulet) and, therefore, the symbolism that underlies these amulets may be seen as the actual reason for the scarcity of these artefacts: perhaps their religious meaning was too particular to be known to a larger portion of the population.

3. The flower heart amulet

A unique category of heart amulet consists of objects in which the top is configured strangely: it folds down over the body, which assumes the shape of a seed, bearing a striking resemblance to a hazel nut. As with other categories of rare heart amulets it is very difficult to date such objects accurately, although iconographic sources indicate that they were used in a funerary context mainly from the Late Period on.

Some of these objects are made of wood and covered with gold leaf.[38] Others are made of glass.[39] They usually have no decoration or texts which would make it easier to identify them as heart amulets, since their shape does not particularly resemble that of the typical heart amulet. Also, side projections, another typical feature of heart amulets, are rarely found in this category of object.

The only evidence that can help us to understand that these are indeed heart amulets is found in the vignettes of chapter 28 of later copies of the *Book of the Dead*. Some of these vignettes depict the deceased kneeling before a god who holds a divine staff with a heart in front of him.[40] A peculiar appendage consisting of two lobules is usually depicted above the heart, bringing to mind the shape of the hieroglyph *sema*, the lungs united with the cardiac organ.

It is interesting to note that both this type of object and this type of vignette seem to have been produced during the Late Period. The use of gold leaf on the objects suggests a solar symbolism.[41]

Symbolism

The significance of this strange representation of the heart must necessarily be connected to the presence of the god depicted in the same vignette. In Egyptian iconography, the depiction of a deity and a standard usually means that the god is concealed within the sacred object. If this reading is correct, the figure shows the god that lives inside the totem of the heart. Unlike other vignettes of the *Book of the Dead* here the deceased does not hold the heart in his hand: both his arms are raised in adoration. This is certainly the depiction of the adoration of the inner god that lives in the 'temple' of the heart. The magical concern of the vignette seems less focused on the 'possession of the heart', as in contemporary vignettes in chapters 26 and 27, and instead seems to have a wider spiritual scope, since it pays greater attention to the heart as the seat of the inner god.

Although well-documented in Egyptian literature, this god of the heart is rarely depicted, especially in contexts other than the *Book of the Dead*. The *mammisi* of the temple of Isis at Philae houses the only known depiction of such a 'god of the heart'. He is depicted as an anthropomorphic god who holds a vase with a heart on top of his head. The god is shown in the context of the presentation of Horpakhered to an assembly of gods. This personication of the heart seems to provide protection for the young Horpakhered at the moment of his birth, undoubtedly as an embodiment of the divine conscience and wisdom.

The text of chapter 28, although very obscure, gives us some clues for understanding the magical function of the vignette. In the text, the deceased identifies himself with the primordial flower in order to be protected against the enemies of light and cosmic order:

> O lion, je suis la fleur-*ouneb*! Mon abomination est la salle d'abattage. Que ce viscère de mon coeur ne me soit pas enlevé par les combattants dans l'Héliopolis![42]

The word *uneb* simply means 'flower'[43] and it was an allusion to the mythic primordial lotus of the Hermopolitan

[38] See AEO 30798, Fig. 35 - AEO 30053, Fig. 36 - AF 11524 (Louvre Museum).

[39] See 10.130.2538 (Metropolitan Museum of Art) and also AF 10447 (Louvre Museum).

[40] See Fig. 37, 38 and 39.

[41] Solar symbolism is also detected suggested in the depiction of the 'flower' heart in the vignettes of chapter 28 of the later copies of the *Book of the Dead*, through the use of red ink in the coloration of the heart. We must point out that among later copies of the *Book of the Dead*, the use of colour is very rare, even among the depiction of the heart. When it happens, it must have a special significance. See M. MOSHER, 'Theban and Memphite *Book of the Dead* Traditions in the Late Period', *JARCE* 29 (1992), p. 172.

[42] Chapter 28 of the *Book of the Dead*, in P. BARGUET, *Le Livre des Morts*, 1967, p. 73.

[43] See R. FAULKNER, *A Concise Dictionary of Middle Egyptian*, 1999, p. 61.

cosmogony. Therefore, the *uneb* flower symbolizes the power of light and the allusion to it seems to be connected to a particular kind of threat: certain Heliopolitan 'demons' could remove the hearts of those who were impure. By means of this identification with the *uneb* flower the deceased probably aimed to insure the pristine purity of his heart, which could keep him safe from attacks by the guardians of the hereafter.

For undetermined reasons, it is possible that this particular type of anatomical representation of the heart and the lungs eventually gained an iconographic value as a symbol of the identification between the heart and the *uneb* flower.[44] It is most probably this meaning that gave shape to the 'flower' heart amulet.

4. The solar heart amulets

Solar amulets are rare artefacts as well. Side projections, intended as a depiction of the cardiac veins, are a common feature in these amulets. As to the body of the amulet, it is usually decorated very simply, the most common anatomical features being the shape of the crescent and the mound. Although such decoration does occur, most known heart amulets have no decoration whatsoever on their body.

Datation

Most of the objects known to us date from the Late Period, although, due to the small amount of data available in museum records, dating can be quite a difficult, if not impossible, task.

Materials

Faience is the most common raw material used to mould these objects. Crystal rock, which was not commonly used to carve standard heart amulets, is found with surprising frequency in solar amulets.[45] Amulets like these, carved in crystal rock, make a strong visual impact thanks to the light effects produced by the material. Gold and, more rarely, cornelian were also used to manufacture these objects.[46]

Decoration

The top of these artefacts is usually square in shape, suggesting the motif of a cornice.[47] The sun disk, or at times the body of the amulet, may be pierced to allow the object to be suspended.[48] The sun disk is usually shaped as a full circle. However, some objects may actually be more nearly semicircular in shape, thus suggestive of the form of the sun at sunrise.[49] A highly interesting variation on this theme is the depiction of the head of a scarab on top of the amulet, in place of the solar disk.[50] Since the scarab is the symbol of the rising sun, we are once again presented with the same symbolism: the rising of the sun in the heart of a man. Note that the similarity between the head of the scarab and the hieroglyph *kha*, "rise up" or "emerge", makes this symbolism even stronger.

Another intriguing object, probably dating from the Late Period, may be related to this category of amulets. It consists of a vase heart amulet with the strange and somewhat uncommon depiction of two arms instead of the usual side projections. The arms hold a bowl in a typical offering gesture. The top of the amulet is broken but the remaining traces suggest that it was surmounted by a solar disk.[51]

Symbolism

The solar heart amulet is a common attribute of the avian form of the god Horus. In fact, especially among bronze statuettes of the Late Period, the solar heart amulet was frequently depicted on the chest of Horus, who also sometimes wears a royal crown, such as the *pa-sechemty*, and a *usekh* collar.[52] Interestingly, the earliest known depiction of the solar heart amulet dates from the reign of Hatshepsut and can actually be seen in the funerary temple of this queen in Deir-el-Bahari, in the context of the Punt expedition relief.[53] Afterwards, during the 21st Dynasty, similar depictions where used mainly as funerary symbols. The pectoral depicted on the mummy cover of Padiamun is especially interesting due to its complex symbolism.[54] The centre of the composition consists of a heart topped by a solar disk and flanked by two cobras, thus resembling the royal pectoral of Hatshepsut/Thutmosis III. The difference between these objects is that the later figures display a superb, large winged scarab with a ram's head. We cannot ignore the ritual and symbolic distinction between these objects: while the pectoral of Hatshepsut is used in the context of the divine cult, a royal prerogative, the

[44] See P. BARGUET, *Le Livre des Morts*, 1967, p. 73, note I. Its determinative shows that the flower is a lotus. See the hieroglyphic version of the text in the coffin of the lady Gautsechenu, in Ny Carlsberg Glyptotek, in Copenhagen (AEIN 1522). M. JORGENSEN, *Catalogue Egypt II (1550-1080 B.C.)*, 1998, p. 204. The solar significance of this flower is also suggested by the fact that among some versions of this chapter, the deceased identifies himself with Re, as an equivalent form of the lotus. See P. BARGUET, *Le Livre des Morts*, 1967, p. 73, note I. Chapter 71 also speaks about that flower and establishes a parallel with the plant *nebheh*: 'Je suis la fleur-*ouneb* de Naref, la plante-*nebheh* de la butte cachée'. See *idem*, p. 110, note 4. The plant *nebheh* symbolizes the sacred mound that stood over the tomb of Osíris, in Busiris. Also here the primordial meaning of the flower seems to be prevalent.

[45] See SR 9214 (Cairo Egyptian Museum), AEO 10164 (Louvre Museum) and also amulet no. 142877 (Warsaw National Museum).

[46] See C. MÜLLER-WINKLER, *Die Ägyptischen Objekt-Amulette*, 1987, p. 216-217.

[47] See SR 9261/JE 37120 (Cairo Egyptian Museum). Also SR 9263/CG 5249 (Cairo Egyptian Museum): in G. REISNER, *Amulets* I, p. 6. Also SR 9269/CG 5248 (Cairo Egyptian Museum): in *ibidem*, p. 8.

[48] See SR 9261/JE 37120 and SR 9269 (Cairo Egyptian Museum).

[49] See UC 22526 (Petrie Museum).

[50] See heart amulet with the head of a scarab, Fig. 43 - 37.492E (Brooklyn Museum).

[51] See Fig. 42 - N. Inv. 50.353 (Museum of Fine Arts, Budapest): in I. NAGY, *Guide to the Egyptian Collection, Museum of Fine Arts of Budapest*, 1999, p. 64.

[52] See avian statue of Horus, Fig. 44 - Cairo Egyptian Museum, JE 30335.

[53] See Fig. 45.

[54] See E. HORNUNG, B. BRYAN, *The Quest for Immortality: Treasures of Ancient Egypt*, 2002, p. 158. See Fig. 49.

pectorals used by the clergy of Amun have a clear funerary significance. Therefore, we need to clarify the meaning of the object in each context.

The funerary meaning of the solar heart amulet

If we are to gain a clear picture of the funerary symbolism of the solar heart amulet we cannot ignore those iconographic motifs where the solar heart is depicted not as an amulet but as a symbol. In fact, the solar heart is often used in the iconography of 21st Dynasty anthropoid coffins. We will now comment briefly on some of these compositions.[55]

On the coffin 24793 (British Museum), the solar heart is repeatedly depicted on the central vertical axis of the coffin. In the lower registers, the solar heart stands between two enthroned gods. Above the head of each god, a *shendjit* shrine is depicted, an image frequently used as a symbol of the Osirian underworld. Interestingly, the coffin of the lady Direpu, in the Cairo Egyptian Museum,[56] is composed in a similar fashion: although the enthroned gods may be absent, the solar heart is still flanked by two *shendjit* sanctuaries.

One frequently sees another type of composition. The solar heart is shown above the *nub,* or "gold", sign. Once again, this is the case with coffin 24793 (British Museum), where two solar hearts appear above a *nub* and a *heb* sign.[57] This composition clearly alludes to the iconographical depiction of the "Horus of gold", where the god Horus stands above the *nub* sign to symbolize the triumph of Horus over Set. This triumph is, in fact, the reason for the justification of Osiris and the cause of his resurrection.[58] Therefore, due to the funerary context of the composition, the black heart can only be seen as a symbol of the resurrection of Osiris.

This interpretation can indeed be corroborated by other iconographic details. In contemporary coffins, we find depictions of the heart amulet, always black, inscribed with the Osirian name of the deceased. The association between depictions of the *shendjit* and the solar heart also emphasizes the Osirian significance of this object.

Furthermore, because of the presence of the solar disk, the symbolism of the object is enriched by an obvious solar significance. In fact, the solar heart can be seen as an iconographic rendering of the mythic union of Re and Osiris. As one of the most important theological issues of the period, the cosmic union of Re and Osiris was the subject of many iconographic compositions.[59] Therefore, particularly in this funerary context, the solar heart can be regarded as another symbol of the solar-Osirian union that was supposed to occur in the Duat.

In fact, we can also find the same symbolic articulation between the heart amulet and the solar disk in contemporary funerary papyri. In the funerary papyrus of Nesipautitaui, which we will study in detail in the Chapter Five, we find a depiction of both a large heart amulet and a solar disk[60] However, instead of being shown together, these symbols are placed at opposite ends of the scroll. The heart amulet is depicted at the beginning of the document and is inscribed with chapter 30 B, functioning as a symbol of the justification of the deceased. On the other hand, the solar disk is depicted at the end of the scroll and stands as a symbol of the rebirth of the deceased.[61] It is between these two symbols with more or less the same rounded shape that the path of transformation in the beyond is depicted.[62]

These elements lead us to the assumption that the juxtaposition of the sun disk and the heart amulet was regarded as a symbol of the solar-chthonian union of Re and Osiris[63] and, as such, as a symbol of the two possible ways by means of which the deceased could achieve immortality in the afterlife: he could be justified and therefore could live as an Osiris in the *djet* dimension of time, as an Uennefer, or he could be reborn, identifying himself with the solar god and thus being integrated into the renewing cycles of time, *neheh.*[64] Seen in this light, the solar heart amulets depicted on the chest of the anthropoid coffin of Theban clergy could express this complex set of beliefs and thus could have played a decisive role in the afterlife since they could help the deceased to be united with both the chthonian realm of Osiris and the solar rebirth of Re. The late and funerary origin of most of the solar heart amulets known to us suggests that this latter reading is highly probably.

The "royal" meaning of the solar heart amulet

As we have already seen, outside of its funerary context, the solar heart amulet seems to be a divine attribute of the god Horus and, as such, can be considered as a royal attribute. As with many other amulets, this particular category of object should be read in relation to the hieroglyphic value of its symbols: *ib* and *Re*. "Solar heart" is thus a possible interpretation of this composition that could be seen both as a royal attribute and as a symbol of the illuminated heart of the Pharaoh which enabled him to perform *maet*

[55] In all the quoted depictions the heart is always coloured in black with anatomical features coloured in red.

[56] See Fig. 47 - JE 29669/CG 6028 (Cairo Egyptian Museum).

[57] Around the central composition we see the signs *ankh*, *djed* and the *tjet.*

[58] See J. ASSMANN, *Mort et au-delà dans l'Égypte ancienne*, 2003, p. 114. The resurrection of Osiris is expressed in this composition by the hieroglyphic signs of *ankh*, *djed* and the *tjet.*

[59] See A. NIWINSKI, "The solar-osirian unity as principle of the theology of the "State of Amun" in Thebes in the XXI dynasty", *JEOL* 30 (1987-1988), pp. 87-106

[60] See A. PIANKOFF e N. RAMBOVA, *Mythological Papyri*, 1955, pl. 77.

[61] For the study of these religious papyri of the 21st Dynasty, see A. NIWINSKI, *Studies on Illustrated Theban Funerary Papyri of the 11th and 10th centuries B.C.*, 1989, pp. 38-42.

[62] Interestingly enough, some heart amulets also display an iconographic relation between the heart and the solar disk. The heart amulet of Khaemwaset (Fig. 5), in the Collection Hoffmann, depicts a scarab holding on its legs the heart and the rising sun, thus expressing the solar rebirth from the Duat where the heart stands. See Fig. 5 - G. LEGRAIN, *Collection Hoffmann Catalogue des antiquités égyptiennes*, 1894, p. 13.

[63] These depictions follow the iconographic trend of the period that was significantly enriched by motifs that celebrated the duality between the symbols of Osiris and Re. See A. NIWINSKI, "The solar-osirian unity as principle of the theology of the "State of Amun" in Thebes in the 21st Dynasty", *JEOL* 30 (1987-1988), 87-106.

[64] For the importance of the notions related to the union of Re and Osiris on the funerary beliefs system of the afterlife, see J. ASSMANN, *Mort et au-delà dans l'Égypte ancienne*, 2003, pp. 282-292.

as the earthly manifestation of the god Horus. The use of the amulet in the context of the dedication of offerings performed by the king to the god Amun, at Deir el-Bahari, clearly provides this object with a royal significance. This splendid piece of jewellery is used by Hatshepsut/ Thutmosis III in a ritual context that aimed to prove her/ his ability to perform the divine cult. Depicted in this context, the solar heart amulet could help to demonstrate the successful action of the king in performing the divine cult, thus connecting the divine realm and the earthly world literally through his heart. Topped by a solar disk, the amulet might have been a symbol of the identification of the king's heart with the sun, and could therefore express the illumination of his heart/mind (i.e., his ability to perform *maet* following the model of the sun god, which also achieved the same goal on the cosmic level). At least during the 18th Dynasty, the solar heart amulet seems to have been a tangible sign of the divine status of the Pharaoh and of his identification with Horus. It is most probably with this meaning that the solar heart amulet is used in avian depictions of Horus. As the divine model of the Pharaoh, the iconography of Horus showcased *par excellence* his *maetic* control over all of creation by means of his solar heart. It is also possible that the use of solar amulet on the 21st Dynasty coffins of the Theban priests of Amun can be seen as an appropriation of an object that, in the past, had been given clear royal status. However marked a political reading may have been given to this object, in burials of the 21st Dynasty priests of Amun, it was used mainly as a funerary symbol of resurrection, a significance that it most probably maintained until the Late Period. At this time, the votive use of these amulets is not precluded; they might actually have been used in the context of a personal relationship to god.

CHAPTER FOUR

THE RITUAL USES OF THE HEART AMULET

In this chapter we shall study the use of the heart amulet in the context of temple and funerary rituals. Beginning with the use of the heart amulet in the leonine locks of temple gates, we will also study the depiction of the heart amulet in the context of the weighing of the heart and in the context of the journey through the underworld. Although originating in different ritual contexts, these uses of the heart amulet share the belief that, as a symbol of knowledge and virtue, this object was pivotal in insuring the progress of the deceased into the sacred territories of the temple or the Duat.

1. The heart amulet in leonine locks

The leonine locks of the monumental gates that once stood in temple gateways are among the most surprising artefacts from ancient Egypt figures. These large objects, measuring approximately 40 cm in length, depicted superbly modeled reclining lions formed out of massive pieces of bronze.[1] They were usually imbedded in the wall, so that they might be slid out to prevent the door in the gate from being opened. Several models dating from the Late Period or the Greco-Roman Period are equipped with a chain holding a heart amulet. Pulling the heart amulet would cause the lion to slide from its niche, thus blocking the door.[2] As part of the temple structure, this device undoubtedly performed a magical or ritual function. In order to gain an understanding of this function, and of the locks' symbolic purpose, we must develop an iconographic reading of these objects.

The architectural context: the sacred gates

In the first place, we must consider the architectural context of the leonine locks. Since they were imbedded in the walls of the monumental gate, their purpose must be directly related to the functioning of its doors. Monumental gates played an ambivalent symbolic role: if, on one hand, they granted access to the inner sacred space, they were, on the other hand, a protective barrier that insured the holiness and purity of the divine address. Thus, the tension between sacred and profane spaces was concretized in these architectonical structures.[3] Not surprisingly, these structures bring to mind the gates of the netherworld guarded by monstrous entities that were intended to bar those who were not eligible for admission as followers of Osiris. Indeed, both the sacred gates of the temple and the gates of the netherworld shared a comparable symbolism: the Duat was seen as a temple but the temple was also seen as a progression into the territories of the Duat.

From a symbolic point of view, monumental gates marked the access to the ritual path that led into the presence of the god, which was architectonically represented by means of a *maetic* ramp leading to an upper floor. In fact, the ramp that facilitated the "ascent" of the visitor was inspired by the hieroglyphic sign *maé*. In this way, the inner path to the temple and contact with the god was placed under the sign of justice and truth. This also means that admission to the temple's inner chambers depended on ritual purity, sacred knowledge and even on the moral character of the priest. Closely regulated, the contact with the divine that was insured by the priests demanded a consistent 'professional' preparation.[4] We also know that the sacredness of the divine presence required the protective veil of mystery and isolation. The most secret areas of the temple were reserved solely for those who possessed sacred knowledge, those who would carry out the divine ritual and would watch over the image of the god.[5] As he moved forward in this process, the Egyptian priest would certainly be challenged to demonstrate his preparation for performance of the divine cult.[6]

As special structures that established frontiers between different temple areas, temple gates provided an ideal setting in which to enhance the ritual progression through the inner chambers of the temple. If access to restricted areas of the temple required an examination to ascertain the candidate's merits as well as his purity, it is not surprising that this passage would be concretized in the immediate vicinity of the monumental gates.[7]

---

[1] See the leonine lock in Cairo Egyptian Museum (CG 37765) found in Kom el-Kalaah, in Mit Rahina. See also Fig. 50 from Berlin Egyptian Museum (N 15424).

[2] Several of these objects are described in A. VARILLE, 'La grande porte d'Apet À Karnak', *ASAE* 53 (1956), pp. 79-118. In the Egyptian Museum of Berlin, a rigorous reconstitution, shown on picture 1, was made by Ludwig Borchardt. The lion slides out of the wall from a hole in the shape of a pylon and there is a heart chained to the lion

[3] See A. LOPRIENO, *La Pensée et l'Écriture: Pour une analyse sémiotique de la culture Égyptienne*, 2001 p. 14.

[4] *Idem*, p. 23.

[5] See J. ASSMANN, *The Search for God in Ancient Egypt*, 2001 p. 32.

[6] While passing through the doors, which had been closed untill then, the priest could be in the presence of the god, who would grant him knowledge of his mysteries. This phenomenology of the revelation of the divine presence is also found among funerary imaginary. Because the Beyond was faced as a temple, funerary literature was inspired to create texts connected to the passage of the Gates of the Beyond. This passage was surrounded by a great danger, as the Gates of the Beyond were guarded by threatening demons that would kill whom wasn't worthy of this passage. In love poems, but with a more mundane appearance still connected to religious concepts, the door of the house of the beloved one is praised like a divinity, like a way of conquering her complicity for a romantic date. See *Chester Beatty I*, III, 7, in SOUSA, *Doces Versos*, 2001, p. 101.

[7] Even the raw material used in these gates, wood from the tree *ache*, had a specific symbolism referring to the protection of the sun and its ability to keep any harmful influence away. See V. LORET, 'Quelques notes sur l'arbre *âch*', *ASAE* 16 (1916), pp. 33-51

The meaning of the lion

The lion was one of the protective symbols most commonly associated with the border of the cosmos: the mythic lions of the horizon, the lion of Yesterday and the lion of Tomorrow were supposed to protect the sun on its way to the underworld. Similarly, the alleys of sphinxes that preceded the pylons protected the border between cosmos (the temple) and chaos (the outside world) and were meant to protect the entrance of the temple. These iconographic details aside, the reclining lion shape is undoubtedly the central element of the lock's symbolism.

The following inscription, from the gate of the temple of Opet at Karnak, reinforces the magical role of the lock by its association with a leonine goddess:

> *Je suis l'épouse de Celui qui apparait en Or, la femme du Ka nefer. Je suis le verrou de la grande porte de la demeure du seigneur. Je suis quiconque s'approche de lui. Je suis la grande* uraeus, *maitresse terrifiante, qui repousse le demuni, qui refoule l'opposant. J'attaque au couteau l'Ennemi vil. Je (...) ses compagnons. Je mange leurs coeurs. Je dévore leurs foies en ce nom de Sekhmet-Mehit. J'avale leur sang et je ne laisse pas monter dans ce temple d'éternité.*[8]

According to this inscription, the entrance to the temple was guarded by the terrifying leonine goddess Sekhmet. The leonine lock that was imbedded in the gate was most assuredly connected to the guardian role traditionally associated with that goddess, as well as with lions in general.[9]

The meaning of the (pendulum) heart amulet

Although the original meaning of the heart amulet may have been quite broad in its symbolic connotations, the leonine locks employ this object in close connection to imagery of justification, so typical of the Ramessid Period.[10] In fact, the heart amulet used in the locks brings to mind the meaning of this object in the vignettes of the weighing of the heart, where it functions as a symbol of the positive outcome achieved by the deceased.

Interestingly, we can ascertain that the chain on the leonine lock from which the heart amulet is suspended recalls the device used in the scales depicted in vignettes of the weighing of the heart. In fact, a similar heart amulet appears frequently in the scales depicted in the court of Osiris. Another interesting detail is that the heart amulet in these depictions is attached to the scale by a chain in a fashion akin to its attachment to the leonine lock. A corresponding use of the heart amulet as the needle of scales also occurs in objects intended for use in daily life. Here, the heart amulet used in the scales was also suspended from a chain and was usually made of bronze.[11] Just as in the funerary scale of Thoth, the measurement was made through the interposition of the heart, since its movement along the crossbar of the scale would yield the result. This use of the heart amulet in the scales of daily life appears to have had a didactic purpose since, in all probability, it reminded those who manipulated the scales that a false measurement would be inscribed in the heart of the measurer and that this heart would eventually be weighed on the scale of Thoth, where it would be denounced as heavy and corrupted. Thus, the heart amulet of the leonine locks can be seen as a monumental, large-scale version of the small heart-shaped bronze needles used in contemporary scales.

This type of use of the heart amulet in daily life may be linked to the power of the concept of the judgment of the dead: the purpose for the use of the heart amulet in the scales of daily life was undoubtedly as a reminder to its user of the necessity of being guided by the ethical principles of *maet* and of putting them into practice. Similarly, the heart amulet used in the monumental locks may have some affinity with the heart amulet used on the scales of the weighing of the heart. It is also possible that a similar ritual was performed in divine temples in order to 'evaluate' the candidate. The recitation of a version of the negative confession used for admission to the priesthood may have been a part of this ritual, as occurred with the funerary weighing of the heart in the Duat. In fact, according to Jan Assmann, it is actually possible to identify textual evidence of the use of a negative confession in the context of priestly initiation to the cultic service:

> Je ne mangerai rien de ce qui est interdit aux prêtres
> Je ne couperai pas avec un couteau (...)
> Et ne chargerai pas un autre de faire ce qui est interdit.
> Je n'ai coupé la tête d'aucun être vivant,
> Je n'ai tué aucun homme,
> Je n'ai eu aucun commerce avec des hommes impurs,
> Je n'ai couché avec aucun garçon,
> Je n'ai pas couché avec la femme d'un autre, (...)
> Je ne mangerai ni ne boirai ce qui est interdit ou est signalé dans les livres.
> Rien ne prendra plus à mes doigts
> Je ne peserai pas de grain sur l'aire de battage.
> Je ne prendrai aucune balance en main.
> Je n'arpenterai aucune terre.
> Je ne foulerai aucun lieu impur.
> Je n'effleurerai aucune laine de mouton.

---

[8] Adapted from the French version proposed by A. VARILLE, 'La grande porte du Temple d'Apet à Karnak', *ASAE* 53 (1956), pp. 90-91

[9] Based on this animal's symbolic reputation amongst Egyptian priests, Horapollo wrote: 'Voulant écrire celui qui veille, ou bien le gardien, ils dessinent une tête de lion, parce que le lion ferme les yeux quand il veille et les tient ouverts quand il dort, ce qui est le signe qu'il fait bonne garde ; c'est pourquoi ils mettent des lions aux serrures des temples pour symboliser des gardiens', *Hierogyphica* (I, 19), in *idem.*, p. 86. In this way, Horapollo established a direct connection between the lion shaped locks and the protective vigilance ensured by the mythical animal.

[10] See R. SOUSA, 'The heart amulet in Ancient Egypt: A typological study', in Goyon, J.-C., Cardin, C., *Proceedings of the Ninth International Congress of Egyptologists*, 2007, Vol. I, pp. 713-721. See also R. SOUSA, 'The cardiac vignettes of the Book of the Dead (Late Period)', *BAEDE* 17(2008), pp. 39-53.

[11] See heart amulets used in scales: Cairo Egyptian Museum (CG 1930), Fig. 4 - Louvre Museum (E 18224), or Museu da Farmácia de Lisboa (53): L. ARAÚJO, P. BASSO, *A Farmácia no Mundo Pré-Clássico e nas Culturas Tradicionais*, 2008, p. 119.

> Je ne toucherai à aucun couteau jusqu'au jour de ma mort[12]

Resemblance to chapter 125 of the *Book of the Dead* may be not accidental: the admittance of the priest to the higher levels of the temple hierarchy may have been dependent on ethical values, since it was intended to occur in the court of Osiris, where the deceased could also participate in the cultic service of the temple of the Duat. Thus, there is a strong possibility that admittance to temple service was, in fact, inspired by the funerary ritual of the judgement of the dead.[13] In sum, admittance to the temple's cult was depended on following a way of life that was inspired by the *maetic* ideal of truth and justice. The 'measuring of the heart' was certainly the best means of evaluation, which may explain the heart amulet being attached to the lock, as this would otherwise be considered a peculiar addition to a lock. In this light, the heart amulet of the monumental locks may have been used to symbolize a ritual 'weighing of the heart' that, since it took place in the court of Osiris, would separate the individual from his faults. Such a procedure was required to fulfill the individual's cultic obligations in the temple. As in the Duat's temple, this 'weighing of the heart' allowed the 'god to be seen'.

2. The heart amulet in the weighing of the heart

The depiction of the weighing of the heart is one of the most important vignettes of the *Book of the Dead*. Although the first known instances of the depiction of the weighing of the heart occur no earlier than the 18th Dynasty, the earliest literary allusions to this measurement process date to the 11th Dynasty.[14] The autobiographical text of Antef, from the 11th Dynasty states:

> Offrande que donne le roi ...pour l'*imakhu* Antef juste de voix. Que le glorifient (sakh) les Grands de Busiris et (?) les Courtisans du Seigneur d'Abydos; que Ceux-qui-sont-dans-l'abondance lui tendent leur main dans la nécropole (...) que le défunt arrive au tribunal du dieu, à l'endroit où sont les dieux. Que son *ka* soit avec lui, que ses offrandes soient devant lui. Que sa voix soit (reconnue) juste dans l'évaluation de l'excès (*hesebet au*).[15]

The expression 'measurement of the excess', *em hesebet áu* (*m ḥsb.t ꜥꜣw*), was used in mathematical texts as a reference to the result of a measurement operation.[16] The measurement operation referred to in these texts cannot be anything other than the weighing of the heart. From the beginning, the scale seems to have been the symbol of the court of the dead, to such an extent that the deceased compared himself to it:

> Je fus un homme doux pour l'irrité et indulgent pour l'ignorant, afin d'écarter la dispute, je fus un homme calme, exempt de précipitation, en apprenant les résultats et en envisageant les consequences. (...) je fus un homme équitable comme la balance, exact et juste comme Thot. [17]

The measurement of the heart by means of the scale is, primarily, a statement of the fairness and objectivity of divine justice. The heart, i.e., the individual conscience of the deceased, is measured against *maet*. Personal virtues such as 'kindness', *neferu* (*nfrw*), 'character', *bia* (*biꜣ*), or patience, *uah ib* (*wꜣḥ-ib*), were qualities that were believed to lighten the heart.[18] Behaviour could also transform the heart of a man during his lifetime. Several inscriptions are quite clear about the utility of such good behaviour upon entry into the afterlife:

> S'il peut être vrai qu'on désire qu'un bon comportement soit utile à celui qui en fait preuve, (alors) c'est à la suite d'Horus et du divin Isi, le vivant, que je serais.[19]

> S'il est vrai qu'on devient un glorifiè à cause d'un comportement excellent, mon *ba* accomplira des transformations en phênix.[20]

According to these texts, good behaviour was a decisive factor in the afterlife: it empowered the *ba* of the deceased and most certainly lightened his heart when it was placed on the scale, thus identifying it with the feather of Maet and predicting a positive outcome in the weighing of the heart. Conversely, sin weighed the heart down and corrupted it.

The growing importance of beliefs related to the judgement of the dead led to the iconographical depiction of the process of the weighing of the heart, largely from the 18th Dynasty on. In early versions of the *Book of the Dead* the depiction of the weighing of the heart seems to have been referred for use with chapter 30, although by the Ramessid Period it had come to be more frequently associated with chapter 125.

Early vignettes of the weighing of the heart are quite simple, their main feature being their static character. The depiction is clearly focused on the measurement operation:

[12] J. ASSMANN, *Mort et au-delà dans l'Égypte ancienne*, 2003, p. 135. In fact this text remarkably resembles chapter 125 of the *Book of the Dead*. However there is a subtle difference: while the negative declarations of the *Book of the Dead* are always formulated in the past tense (since the deceased's actions among the living were supposed to have been performed in the past) they are formulated both in the past and in the future tense in this text (as they enforce a commitment to the future life of the priest). To Assmann this text was clearly recited by the priests in their admission to cultic service in the temple. This conclusion was strengthened by the discovery of a hieratic version of this later text by Joachim Quack, see *ibidem*.

[13] So it is possible that the negative confession that was formulated in the initiation of the priest to the temple's cult followed the model of the 'weighing of the heart'. *Ibidem*.

[14] See A. MORET, 'La doctrine de Maât', *RdÉ* 4 (1940), p. 5.

[15] M. J. CLÈRE, 'Un passage de la stèle du général Antef (Glyptothèque Ny Carlsberg, Copenhagen)', *BIFAO* 30 (1931), p. 426

[16] *Ibidem*, p. 429.

[17] É. DRIOTON, 'Le jugement des âmes dans l'ancienne Égypte', *RdC* (1949), p. 11.

[18] H. SMITH, 'Maet and Isfet', *BACE* 5 (1994), pp. 70-80

[19] Stela of Userhat, 13th Dynasty: in P. VERNUS, 'La formule du bon comportement', *RdE* 39 (1988), p. 148.

[20] See *idem*, p. 154.

the deceased is positioned near the scale,[21] at times even set on one of its plates.[22] Thoth may be found nearby, in the form of an ibis-headed human figure or a baboon, in close association with the scale. The top of the scale may be decorated with a baboon, a canine head or the head of Maet. Osiris, usually seated on a throne, presides over the weighing of the heart. Less often, two silhouettes of Maet may also preside over the operation.[23] Interestingly, the deceased is depicted grasping one of his shoulders with the other hand, a gesture of submission typically associated with earthly courts of justice. Sobriety is the rule for the rest of the vignette: sometimes only columns of text fill the spaces between the figures. The static character of these early scenes reflects their magical purpose, which is focused on the positive outcome of the measurement process. As early as the reign of Amenhotep III, the vignette of the weighing of the heart came to be used in the context of tomb decoration, particularly in the Theban necropolis,[24] but it only became common in this context in the Ramessid Period.[25]

The heart amulet in the Ramessid vignettes

By the end of the 18th Dynasty a growing need to fill the vignette of the weighing of the heart with new iconographic details led to further development in the arrangement of the scene, particularly in tomb decoration.[26] It is in this context that we encounter to the depiction of the heart amulet as an Osirian decoration. Curiously, this innovation seems closely connected to the global transformation that affected the composition of contemporary vignettes of the weighing of the heart. As opposed to a simple juxtaposition of elements of equal importance and size, a clear distinction was made between the main register, where the measurement of the heart takes place in front of the enthroned Osiris, and the secondary registers, where an assembly of gods is depicted in a much smaller size. In addition to this enhancement of the formal arrangement of the scene, a new sense of forward motion gives these vignettes a dynamism that had been absent. Anubis introduces the deceased to the court. Near the scale are the fearsome Ammut and Horus, who manipulates the needle of the scale. Thoth communicates the verdict to Osiris. Osiris, enthroned in a pavilion, is usually flanked by Isis and Nephtys. Sometimes the four sons of Horus are depicted on a lotus blossom positioned near the throne. The Imiut is also frequently depicted in close association with the Osirian pavilion. An assembly of enthroned gods, usually depicting the Heliopolitan Ennead, is placed in the secondary register.[27]

The dynamic sense of these depictions is often strengthened by the repeated depiction of the deceased, portrayed at different stages in this process. The 'classic' vignettes of the weighing of the heart clearly belong to this category of documents, as is the case with a scene depicted in the *Book of the Dead* of Hunefer.[28] Here the deceased appears three times.[29] First he adores the Heliopolitan Ennead in the secondary register. Then Anubis leads him by the hand towards the place where the weighing of his heart will occur. It is again Anubis who performs the measurement, while the presence of Ammut seems to add a certain 'tension' to this critical moment. In some cases, a number of new elements may be included surrounding the scale: the *ba* bird, the human-headed brick of Meskhenet, Shai (the personification of destiny) and the goddess Renenutet.[30] Obviously, the operation is supervised by the imposing figure of Thoth. Once this measurement is taken, the deceased is led by Horsaiset into the presence of Osiris.[31] Before Osiris the deceased assumes a humble and fearful demeanor in order to show reverence towards the god. Vignettes of the weighing of the heart no longer depict the measurement process alone, but also the full justification of the deceased.

Usually, in order for it to be seen as a symbol of this justification process, the heart amulet is put to work by the deceased after the weighing of the heart.[32] The vignette of the weighing of the heart now appears to be more focused on the personal approach of the deceased to the god Osiris. At this point, it seems that the depiction of the measurement on the scale is merely a step in this process and no longer the central feature of the composition. In other words, this new arrangement of the scene appears to demonstrate the same integration of *maetic* morality within the context of

[21] See *Book of the Dead* N 3073 (Louvre Museum).
[22] See *Book of the Dead* of Maherpa, reign of Thutmosis IV, CG 24095 (Cairo Egyptian Museum).
[23] See *Book of the Dead* N 3073 (Louvre Museum).
[24] See tomb of Menna (TT 69), reigns of Thutmosis IV and Amen-hotep III.
[25] Nevertheless, we can see that this kind of depiction was recovered periodically in later periods, probably with the intent to provide an 'older' look to the scene. See *Book of the Dead* of Nedjmet, 21st Dynasty, E 6258 (Louvre Museum). See also *Book of the Dead* of Nedjmet, 21st Dynasty, EA 10541 (British Museum). By the late 18th Dynasty an interesting process began to occur: further elements were progressively juxtaposed to the nuclear scheme of the depiction composed by the scale, the deceased, the god that assures the measurement process and the god that presides over the judgement, without any apparent degree of differentiation between the main register and the secondary ones. The lake of fire, Apopis, Anubis and Horus make their first appearances in this context creating sometimes a second, but not secondary, register since the size of both registers is equal. Although not achieving a full integration, the additions of these elements, which will have an important place in the vignettes of the weighing of the heart from the Ramessid Period, attest the need for a further elaboration of the iconographical features of the depiction. See *Book of the Dead* of Nebked, reign of Amen-hotep III, N 3968 (Louvre Museum), the *Book of the Dead* of Neferuebenef, reign of Tutankhamun (?), N 3092 (Louvre Museum), *Book of the Dead* JE 95652 (Cairo Egyptian Museum) and *Book of the Dead* AEO 23825 (Louvre Museum).
[26] To our knowledge the earliest depiction of this kind of vignettes can be found in the decoration of the tomb of Horemheb (TT 78), reign of Amen-hotep III. See U. BOURIANT, 'Tombeau de Harmhabi', *MMAF* 5 (1891), Pl. V
[27] See tomb of Nefersekheru and Pabasa (TT 296), tomb of Neferenpet (TT 178).
[28] N 9901 (British Museum).
[29] In certain vignettes the deceased may even be depicted four times: see tomb of Khonsu (TT 31).
[30] See *Book of the Dead* of Ani, 19th Dynasty, N 10407 (British Museum).
[31] See tomb of Userhat (TT 51), tomb of Rai (TT 255), tomb of Nakhtamun (TT 341), tomb of Amenemopet (TT 41). The same scheme can be found in further contemporary necropolis, such as in Aniba (tomb of Penniut).
[32] See tomb of Rai (TT 255).

personal piety that we find in the contemporary literary wisdom texts of the period.[33]

In this light, the weighing of the heart can be seen as a purification procedure that allows the god to be revealed to the deceased, the most desirable outcome of this process. It is interesting to note that, when depicted in this context, the heart amulet serves as a sign of the pure heart of the deceased that allows him to come into the presence of the god.

The heart amulet in the vignettes of the 21st Dynasty

This meaning seems to retain all of its importance in the complex iconography of the 21st Dynasty.[34] Instead of a qualitative change, we witness a quantitative development. As the classic type, the typical vignettes of the 21st Dynasty possess a dynamic and even 'narrative' structure through which the justification process of the deceased is described and illustrated. The deceased may be depicted one,[35] two[36] or even three[37] times during this process. Unlike earlier vignettes, the deceased may appear in a multitude of new attitudes. The gesture of raising *maetic* feathers in his arms is used to illustrate his joy as the result of a positive outcome in the weighing of the heart. A new gesture exhibited by the deceased consists of the offering of his mouth, eyes and heart to the scale. These two gestures seem to be closely related, since the offering of the heart to the scale is followed by the depiction (in a gesture of joy) of the heart amulet in the chest of the deceased as a sign of his justification.[38] In these vignettes, this joyful gesture is indeed the attitude most closely connected to the possession of the heart amulet, which seems to corroborate the idea that such an object was presented to the deceased as a decoration.

The role of the deceased's escorts into the court of Osiris, assigned to female deities such as the Mistress of the West,[39] Isis[40] and Maet,[41] is another distinctive feature of these vignettes. More often, a multitude of animal-headed gods and goddesses may also perform this role, making these vignettes appear strangely 'crowded'.[42]

However, the depictions surrounding the *maetic* scale are some of the most important iconographical innovations of these vignettes.[43] In fact, a multitude of new depictions appear beneath the arms of the scale: the cobra and the vulture that embody the mother goddesses of the Upper and Lower Egypt, Meskhenet's brick in the shape of the hieroglyph *pet*, 'sky', and a seated god with royal sceptres.[44] Sometimes Meskhenet's brick is replaced by a chest adorned with the head of Maet and followed by the word 'Duat'.[45] The sign Wedjat is also commonly used.[46] This multiplicity of signs suggests that, by this point, the divine scale was very clearly connected to the symbolism of redemption, regeneration and the cosmic rebirth of the deceased.[47] Indeed, the seated god depicted with royal sceptres can be seen as the new manifestation of the deceased as a newborn god since we find the name of the deceased associated with this figure.[48] Later, in vignettes of the Late Period, this recumbent god will be depicted as a solar child seated on a *heka* sceptre, sometimes wearing the heart amulet. Curiously, the deceased of these later vignettes no longer uses the amulet. This iconographic shift seems to reflect a subtle change in the meaning of the heart amulet: the former Osirian decoration it has become a symbol of the rebirth of the deceased as a solar child.

3. The heart amulet and the journey through the Duat: the iconographical reading of the papyrus of Nesipautitaui (SR 1025)

From the late Ramessid Period on, especially during the 21st Dynasty, new types of funerary papyri were produced. Instead of the traditional composition of the *Book of the Dead* which combined a great deal of text with carefully designed vignettes, the new books of the hereafter emphasised the magical power of the images, paying little attention to the texts themselves. These books became elaborate iconographic compendia, sometimes

[33] See J. ASSMANN, *The Mind of Egypt*, 2002, pp. 229-231.

[34] In the funerary papyrus of Nesitanebetacheru (BM 10554, British Museum), two scenes are depicted, both of them following the old pattern from the Ramessid Period. The same can be said about the vignette of the weighing of the heart of the funerary papyri of Horemakhbit (see A. NIWINSKI, *Studies on Illustrated Theban Funerary Papyri*, 1989, p. 86) and of Maatkaré. Also the vignette of the *Book of the Dead* of Pinedjem I (SR 11488, Cairo Egyptian Museum) follows the archaic pattern typical of the first half of the 18th Dynasty. Among the decoration of funerary artefacts it is also possible to see the archaic vignettes (see funerary chest of Tjauen-hui, N 4124, Louvre Museum) or classic vignettes (see coffin of Sesekhneferu, 1908 E 118, Ny Carlsberg Glypotek).

[35] See coffin of Padiamun (CG 62233/6235, Cairo Egyptian Museum) or the coffin of Pakharu, CG 6122/6121 (now in National Museum of Alexandria).

[36] See inner coffin of Nesikhonsu (SR 10325/CG 61030, Cairo Egyptian Museum).

[37] See coffin of Amenempermut (CG 6153, Cairo Egyptian Museum).

[38] See funerary papyrus of Nesipakachuti (E 17401, Louvre Museum), the funerary papyrus of Nesitanebet-taui (SR 40017, Cairo Egyptian Museum), the coffin of Senu (JE 29651, Cairo Egyptian Museum), the inner coffin of Tanethereret (E 13034, Louvre Museum) or even the inner coffin of Paser (N 2570, Louvre Museum).

[39] See coffin of Padiamun (CG 62233/6235, Cairo Egyptian Museum).

[40] See *Book of the Dead* of Nani (0.3.31, Metropolitan Museum of Art).

[41] See coffin of Tauheret, CG 61032 (Cairo Egyptian Museum), coffin of Pakharu, CG 6122/6121 (now in National Museum of Alexandria).

[42] See Fig. 46 - coffin of Unet, AF 9593 (Louvre Museum).

[43] An innovation is the depiction of its strings with the shape of *djed* and *tjet* signs. See *Book of the Dead* of Nani (0.3.31, Metropolitan Museum of Art). See also the funerary papyrus of Tawedjatré (Cairo Egyptian Museum) in A. PIANKOFF, N. RAMBOVA, *Mythological Papyri*, 1955, pp. 133-142.

[44] See coffin of Djedmaetiuesankh (Cairo Egyptian Museum), in A. NIWINSKI, *The Second Find of Deir el-Bahari*, vol. I, 1°, 1999, p. 29.

[45] See coffin of Padiamun, CG 62233/6235 (Cairo Egyptian Museum).

[46] See outer coffin of Pakharu, CG 6122/6121 (now in National Museum of Alexandria).

[47] The new 'obstetric' symbolism of the divine scale is perhaps the reason why we find among the vignettes of the period a number of them in which the scale is the dominant feature. In one of these scenes the depiction of the scale is followed by the primordial couple, Nut and Geb, and the creative manifestations of Amun, which gives the depiction of the divine scale a meaning that is closely related to the purification and recreation. See funerary papyrus of Djedkhonsuiuefankh and funerary papyrus of Tawedjatré, in *idem*, p. 133-142.In these vignettes the depiction of the judge is omitted and the divine scale is sometimes integrated in complex iconographical compositions. See funerary papyrus SR 10232 (Cairo Egyptian Musem).

[48] See funerary papyrus of Djedkhonsuiuefankh, in A. PIANKOFF, N. RAMBOVA, *Mythological Papyri*, 1955, pl. 19.

labelled under the designation of 'mythological papyri'. In this rubric we will focus on the study and interpretation of the papyrus of Nesipautitaui (Cairo Egyptian Museum, SR 1025), which presents an interesting iconographic programme in that which is concerned with the magical purpose of the heart amulet in the journey of the deceased in the hereafter.[49] The symbols depicted in this document seem to be used to represent a specific selection of chapters of the *Book of the Dead*. Thus the document is an excellent example of the ultimate development of the *pars pro toto* rule in 21st Dynasty funerary papyri[50]. In fact, whole chapters seem to be represented by a single vignette: we can easily identify chapters 145/146 (figures of the guardians), 149/150 (the depictions of the mounds), 148 (the four paddles) and 186 (the divine cow)[51] among others. In addition to these symbolic allusions to those texts, chapter 30 B of the *Book of the Dead* is also written on the heart amulet depicted in the papyrus.

Although this symbolic repertoire is clearly inspired by the *Book of the Dead*, such compositions carried a different title, the *Book of the Amduat*. This title is of interest since it provides a clue to the book's primary focus: a depiction of the journey of the deceased in the Duat. In fact, we believe that the idea of a dynamic process and of a path is clearly expressed in the horizontal arrangement of the symbols, starting on the right border of the papyrus, with the introduction of the deceased to the serpent-god, and ending on the opposite side with the depiction of the rising sun.

The vignettes that represent particular points on the deceased's path through the Duat stand between these two moments. First, in order to enter the underworld, the deceased must prove the purity of his heart. The heart amulet and related images (the *benu* and the scarab) symbolize the weighing of the heart and the possibility of regeneration. The large heart amulet depicted in the papyrus of Nesipautitaui is therefore a sign of the positive outcome of the weighing of the heart and its large-scale depiction is probably due to its important role of assuring the deceased a good journey through the Duat in order to be regenerated. This path serves as a kind of initiation of the deceased into the mysteries of the underworld. The guardians of the gates and mounds of the beyond are elements of the mystical topography of the Duat, which is understood as a temple where the regeneration of the sun takes place in the secret chambers of Osiris.

[49] Curiously enough, its iconographic programme presents a particularly careful sequence of symbols and images that follows what seems to be a very well established pattern which is also found in other contemporary documents such as the following papyri: papyrus of Padikhonsu (British Museum, 10004), 21st Dynasty, papyrus of Isetemakhbit (Cairo Egyptian Museum, JE 95657), 21st Dynasty, papyrus of Tabaketenkhonsu (Louvre Museum, N 3287), 21st Dynasty, papyrus of Mashitsekebet (Turin Egyptian Museum, 1769), 21st Dynasty, papyrus of Amememwya (Berlin Egyptian Museum, Inv. Nr. P 3127), Ramessid Period.

[50] See A. NIWINSKI, *Studies on the Illustrated Theban Funerary Papyri*, 1989, p. 38. See also, *idem*, 'Iconography of the 21st dynasty', in Uehlinger (dir), *Images as Media: Sources for the cultural history of the Near East and the Eastern Mediterranean (Ist millennium BCE)*, 2000, p. 27.

[51] See *Idem*, p. 193

The demons of the underworld are depicted in the fourth scene of this book, most probably with the same magical purpose that we have noted in the leonine locks. In exactly the same way that the locks of a temple protected the inner sanctuary from intruders and led the priest into the presence of the gods, the gates of the netherworld blocked the way to those who did not possess the secret knowledge: only those who were endowed with the magical power of this knowledge were allowed to be led into the most sacred region of the Duat where their regeneration took place. In a manner most likely comparable to the earthly initiation in the temple, in the hereafter the deceased had to prove his knowledge of the sacred mysteries so that he could pass through the doors of the beyond, a situation described in chapters 145 and 146 of the *Book of the Dead*. In some of the vignettes in these chapters,[52] the deceased is depicted with the heart in his hands, showing it to the guardians of the gates, in the precise attitude in which it is depicted at the beginning of the papyrus of Nesipautitaui. The act of presenting the deceased's pure heart to the guardians served to open the gates and allowed him to be separated from his own sins.[53] Thanks to his purity and knowledge, the deceased would then be able to enter the secret domain of Osiris, symbolized by the sacred mounds, where his regeneration would take place. In this way, mystery and purity were intimately connected to regeneration.

Passing through the gates could be interpreted as a process of entering the womb of the cow goddess that bestowed the powers of life upon the deceased. Each gate was, in fact, an embodiment of the womb of the cosmic mother. In this way, the deceased entered the fourteen mounds or crypts where mysterious gods were buried. Thus, the depiction of the *iats* corresponds to chapters 149-150[54]. In each one of these *iats*, the deceased was able to regenerate a specific spectrum of vital powers.

The depictions of the wild dog and the mummiform god with a lamp's head, symbols of the East and South, allude to the burial chamber of the deceased, also evoked in chapters 151-160 of the *Book of the Dead*. Therefore the funerary chamber of the deceased was also seen as one more secret hill of the beyond, where his powers could be regenerated.[55] In the final portion of the scroll we find the

[52] See Fig. 52 - *Book of the Dead* of Userhatmose (SR 10249, Cairo Egyptian Museum), vignette of chapter 145-146.

[53] The role of those entities was to guarantee a moral dissociation of the deceased towards death. The weighing of the heart, the Ammut monster and the keepers of the gates were steps in the path of the deceased, which granted him the removal of all his sins. Once he passed through those gates, the deceased would be safe and protected. See J. ASSMANN, *Mort et au-delà dans l'Égypte ancienne*, 2003, p. 196.

[54] The image of death as a path is also present in the *senet* game. In front of the adversary, the deceased must follow a path through thirty squares, in order to reach the opposite side of the table. If he gets there, he obtains the renewal. See *Idem*, p. 290.

[55] Especially in the royal tombs, the funerary chamber is a highly symbolic place which is identified with a crypt of Osiris. Some of the architectural layout of the funerary chamber originated with the desire to identify it with an Osirian crypt. The L shaped plan of the Tuthmosid tombs built in the Valley of the Kings has been understood as a way to give to the royal tomb the configuration of the Osirian crypt. See N. REEVES & R. WILKINSON, *The Complete Valley of the Kings*, 1996, p. 25

four heavenly paddles, a visual allusion to chapter 148 of the *Book of the Dead*, where the deceased was supposed to meet the seven sacred cows and their divine bull.[56] Finally, the depiction of Hathor as a sacred cow is an allusion to chapter 186 of the *Book of the Dead.* Its function is to give birth to the deceased as a solar manifestation of the rising sun. The mythic cycles of Re and Osiris were, at this stage, perfectly united.[57] The beginning and the end were bound together, just as life and death were perfectly joined. The path in the Osirian underworld led to a rebirth into the light. This concept is expressed at the very end of the scroll through the depiction of the sun disk between the words Re and Duat.

4. The heart amulet and ritual: some clues from iconography

Now that we have examined several contexts of the use of the heart amulet, it is time to turn our attention to its ritual purpose. For the above-mentioned reasons, we must consider the leonine locks and the depictions of the heart amulet in the hereafter as evidence of rituals that were performed in order to 'examine' the virtue and knowledge of the priest (in the temple context) or of the deceased (in the funerary context). The common ground in both contexts is the notion of a symbolic 'weighing of the heart' through which the priest or the deceased was to unlock the sacred doors of the Duat.

The heart amulet in the temple ritual

In this context, the magical operation of the lock must be interpreted in the knowledge that the heart amulet was the piece that ruled this mechanism. It was in fact the heart amulet that operated the mechanism– it would cause the leonine guardian either to come out of its carved stone *naos* to block the way, or to remain hidden there instead, granting access to the interior of the temple to the newly invested priest. This was a didactic message: the key to the admission of the priest to the secret areas of the temple was his own heart. The lion would "devour" all those who were not ready but it would grant safe passage to all those who possessed the knowledge and purity required to continue their meeting with the deity in their hearts.

Iconographic evidence of the connection between the leonine locks and the revelation of the divine mysteries can be found in an interesting depiction in Adrian's Gate at Philae's temple of Isis.[58] There, the operation of the gate follows a specific sequence. The Pharaoh presents himself in front of the gate holding a chest, a symbol of mystery and transformation. Then, as is his usual practice in the funerary scenes of the weighing of the heart, Thoth makes an enigmatic register and reports it to Isis, who handles the leonine lock. The shape of this lock is identical to those mentioned earlier: a heart amulet is suspended from the chain attached to a carved lion. Placing one hand on the chain, the goddess puts the lion depicted in the gate's rabbet in motion. Next, there are three more gates that lead the Pharaoh inside and into a chamber carved in the bedrock. We find important cosmologic symbols inside the crypt, under the watchful eye of Isis. Submerged in the waters of the flood from which lotus flowers spring, the crocodile that signifies Sobek carries Osiris' mummy on his back. Above the swamp flowers, a solar disk emerges from the horizon, carrying within it the image of the enthroned Osiris and the child Horus over a lotus flower. Finally, the sun, the moon and the stars, appear in the upper register. There can be no doubt that this complex representation illustrates the revelation of the mysteries of creation and resurrection. This revelation was undoubtedly made in the sanctuary, under the protection and vigilance of the goddess Isis. By pulling the leonine lock, it was Isis who, in a fashion similar to that of the goddess Sekhmet-Mehit in the temple of Opet, allowed the king to proceed into the temple, granting him a vision of the cosmic mysteries.[59] This revelation, however, depended on the mysterious register made by Thoth, which bears a strange resemblance to his gesture in the vignettes of the weighing of the heart.

This important depiction clearly shows how close the imagery associated with the temple 'initiation' was to the funerary imagery of the 'initiation' of the deceased in the Duat. As was supposed to happen in the afterlife, the leonine lock of the temple gateway seems to be closely connected to a ritual in which the moral worth and sacred knowledge of the priest were measured in order to introduce him to the mysteries of the deity. Hence, it was only natural that a symbol of the priest's purity and moral virtue, such as the heart amulet, became an important iconographic feature of these objects. On the other hand, the lion serves as a symbol of the divine guardian who stood in front of the gate's entrance. As in the gates of the beyond, the priest would display his heart before the divine guardian in order to gain admittance to the inner chambers of the temple, the secret domain of the Duat. Vignettes with the deceased showing his heart before the funerary guardians can, in fact, be seen as the funerary counterpart of such a ritual.

The most interesting result of this iconographical achievement is that it extended beyond the production of the funerary heart amulets and began to influence the production both of objects used in daily life (such as the scales used for everyday weighing) and objects used in temple architecture. Placed on the scales, the pendulum heart amulet was used as a reminder to the scribe that he

[56] The four paddles of the sky are symbols of the limits of the world, the frontiers through which the sun must run its course. As they link the underworld to the world of the living, they are also frontiers between life and death. For chapter 148 See P. BARGUET, *Le Livre des Morts*, pp. 207-208.

[57] Viewed from this perspective the entire book displays an iconographic composition that plays with the solar and Osirian symbols, as many other funerary compositions.

[58] See Fig. 51.

[59] Both goddesses (Isis in Philae and Sekhmet-Mehit in Opet) might also be seen as divine personifications of the temple sacred gates: they are able to protect from contamination both the primordial world encrypted in the innermost regions of the temple and the outside world. By pulling the leonine lock, Isis should be seen as the goddess that lead the king through that passage, revealing to him the mysteries of the Duat.

should prepare the outcome of the weighing of his heart in the afterlife by making accurate measurements in this life. On the other hand, when used in the leonine locks, the pendulum heart amulet reminded the neophyte that his path to the revelation of the mysteries of the temple was perhaps only a precursor to the path that he would be faced with in the hereafter.

Combining symbol and function, these pendulum heart amulets demonstrate a clear 'contamination' of the realm of the living by the funerary belief system, thus showing how much influence the idea of the judgment of the dead had and how life and death in ancient Egypt were lastingly united by this belief set.

The heart amulet and the funerary ritual

The large heart amulet depicted in the papyrus of Nesipautitaui seems to be intended to protect the deceased against all the dangers that he might encounter along the path of the Duat. Here, the heart amulet seems to be the key element that guaranteed the success of the deceased's journey in the Osirian underworld, leading to a rebirth through his identification with the rising sun depicted at the end of the scroll.[60] Curiously, the composition of the images seems to be symmetrical: the heart amulet at the beginning of the book has the rising sun as a counterpart at the end of the book. It is between these two symbols, which have more or less the same rounded shape, that the path of transformation in the beyond is depicted. Over and above this 'geometrical' symmetry of the heart amulet and the sun disk, we can also understand these symbols as different manifestations of the deceased. The large heart amulet explicitly refers to the Osirian identity of the deceased: the Osirian name is written on the surface of this amulet. On the other hand, the rising sun showcases the solar manifestation of the deceased as a result of the regeneration performed in the womb of Hathor, the mother goddess. The great stability and almost rigid replication of this iconographic programme in several documents points to its deeply revered religious significance. In fact, the ultimate message of the papyrus seems highly relevant: through a pure heart, the deceased could be justified as an Osiris, and through (sacred) knowledge, he could also be reborn as fully identified with the rising sun. Then, as a result of to its purity and knowledge, the two principles of the universe, Re and Osiris, could be united in the deceased's heart.

Another point must also be emphasized. According to Andrzej Niwinski, the major part of the iconographic programme of Theban coffins of the 21st Dynasty can be understood in light of the funerary ritual. Sharing many of the features found in contemporary coffins, the iconographic programme of the papyrus of Nesipautitaui may, in fact, allude to a particular set of rituals in which the consecration and offering of a large heart amulet would be the main focus. This could explain the large size of the depiction of this object as well as some of the symbols associated with it. Perhaps it is not by chance that, in the papyrus of Nesipautitaui, the *benu* bird and the scarab were depicted next to the heart amulet, since their images were quite often engraved on the surface of large heart amulets, frequently with an inscription with chapter 30 B of the *Book of the Dead* on the reverse.[61] Thus, these depictions found in front of the heart amulet in the papyrus of Nesipautitaui may very well evoke the symbols that were supposed to be represented on the reverse of the object, following the inscription. Therefore, it seems highly plausible that this entire composition could be used to recall the consecration ceremony of the heart amulet, which embodied the purity and knowledge of the deceased required in the court of Osiris in order to be admitted to the underworld and to undergo a solar rebirth.

Curiously, depictions of a large amulet surrounded by solar symbols, such as the one that we find in the papyrus of Nesipautitaui are also a common feature in 21st Dynasty Theban coffins, where the amulet is surrounded by identical solar symbols.[62] Depicted in this context, these representations of the heart amulet most probably lend support to the idea that there may have been specific funerary rituals involving the presentation of this amulet to the mummy, which, in fact, seemed to be the aim of chapter 26 of the *Book of the Dead.*[63] In this context, the heart amulet was given to the deceased not so much as a substitute for the cardiac organ, but as an Osirian decoration that could testify to his purity and knowledge. As such, due to the iconographical programme that surrounds it, both in the coffins of the Theban priesthood and in the papyrus of Nesipautitaui, we can venture to state that it was this Osirian heart that could lead the deceased through the Duat in order to be reborn as a solar manifestation. This dual articulation of the heart as a solar and an Osirian entity is also found in 21st Dynasty coffin decoration. In the external coffin of Pinedjem II, for instance, we find a ravishing depiction of a heart, a winged scarab and a solar disk.[64] Similar depictions are also found in the coffins of Nesikhonsu[65] and Padiamun,[66] among others. We can assume that the scarab (as well as the solar disk) and the heart amulet (or simply the heart) were used in this context in order to define the heart as a solar-Osirian entity.

[60] With regard to the study of the religious papyri of the 21st Dynasty see A. NIWINSKI, *Studies on Illustrated Theban Funerary Papyri of the 11th and 10th centuries B.C.*, 1989, pp. 38-42.

[61] Depictions of the *benu* bird: See CG 5235 and CG 5231 (in G. REISNER, *Amulets*, I, p. 4). Depictions of the scarab: See Fig. 60 - CG 12056 (*idem*, I, pl. VII)

[62] See coffin of Tjenetethatnetjeru, Cairo Egyptian Museum (CG 6191), in A. NIWINSKI, *The Second Find*, 1999, fig. 113. The depiction of sacred objects is a common iconographical feature among 21st Dynasty coffins. See *idem*, 'Iconography of the 21st dynasty', in Uehlinger (dir), *Images as Media: Sources for the cultural history of the Near East and the Eastern Mediterranean (Ist millennium BCE)*, 2000, p. 27.

[63] See R. SOUSA, 'The cardiac vignettes of the Book of the Dead (Late Period)', *in BAEDE* 17 (2007), p. 43

[64] See Fig. 66 (CG 61029C, Cairo Egyptian Museum) and Fig. 67 (JE 29668, Cairo Egyptian Museum)

[65] Cairo Egyptian Museum (SR 10325, JE 26199, CG 61030) in *ibidem*, pl. XLV

[66] See Fig. 49 - Cairo Egyptian Museum (CG 6235). Drawing after E. HORNUNG, B. BRYAN, *The Quest for immortality*, 2002, p. 158.

Analysis of these documents suggests that the heart amulet was believed to be a pivotal piece, intended to guarantee both contact with the divine (in the temple ritual) and regeneration (in the Duat). Such beliefs demonstrate a strong religious reflection related to the dualistic nature of the heart.

CHAPTER FIVE

THE CARDIAC AMULETS AND DUALISM

As noted in the previous chapter, large funerary versions of the heart amulet were produced, especially from the Ramessid Period on. We find iconographic evidence of the use of this particular type of heart amulet in pictorial decoration of tombs. In Sennefer's tomb (TT 96), for instance, the depiction of a dark heart amulet, due to the context in which it is found (a funerary procession), has a clear funerary purpose. But the most important of these depictions are found in the decoration of the yellow anthropoid coffins of the 21st Dynasty . Dark, usually black or dark blue, depictions of these funerary heart amulets are usually positioned over the chest of the deceased, suspended from a large chain. In some cases it is even possible to distinguish the Osirian name of the deceased inscribed on the surface of the amulet. Solar symbols, such as the *benu* bird and the scarab, are usually displayed around it. These symbols are not randomly depicted in this context since they are very often used in the decoration of funerary heart amulets.[1] Thus it is possible the depiction of the *benu* bird and the scarab next to the heart amulet in the papyrus of Nesipautitaui, a pattern found in contemporary coffins, did not occur by chance. There is a distinct possibility that the symbols displayed around the amulet allude to typical features used in its decoration. In fact, there are examples of heart amulets decorated with the depiction of a scarab.[2] Amulets such as these may also be inscribed with chapter 30 B of the *Book of the Dead* and seem to have flourished from the late Ramessid Period on, particularly among the Theban 21st Dynasty priesthood of Amun.[3]

Although to a much lesser extent, the addition of features typical at the heart amulets to heart scarabs is further evidence of the symbolic association between amulets related to the heart. It became customary to carve the base of the heart scarab in the shape of a heart amulet, particularly from the Ramessid Period on.[4] We even find this feature in human-headed scarabs.[5] Chapter 30 B is usually inscribed on this heart-amulet-shaped base.

Objects like these seem to add, as decoration, a depiction or inscription that is a reminder of the magical function of a related amulet is often added to these objects as a decoration.[6] This is a process frequently used in the production of Egyptian amulets and was intended as a means of enriching their magical powers. While this process of magical 'addition' did not change the shape of the heart scarabs significantly (this addition simply consisted of the insertion of the heart-shaped base), the same can not be said for the heart amulets, which became darker and larger in order to be inscribed with chapter 30 B of the *Book of the Dead* and decorated with symbols, such as the scarab. Thus, the reshaping of cardiac objects through the process of addition reflects a search for further magical 'empowerment' of the objects through additive or substitutive arrangements.[7]

This process reached its peak on a particular type of amulet that commingled the features of the heart amulet and the heart scarab in so perfect a way that it can be very difficult to classify them either as heart amulets or as heart scarabs. At first glance amulets such as these may not seem very different from the common heart scarab. The scarab is usually perfectly sculpted in a very organic style. However, unlike ordinary heart scarabs, these objects have an elongated base, much larger than the scarab itself. The base is carved in the shape of a large heart amulet. The heart amulet is usually the largest element of the composition. Amulets such as these are rare and they only seem to have been produced for a short period of time. One such object dates from the reign of Amenhotep III and was found in the 18th Dynasty tomb of Yuya (KV 46), the father of queen Tiye.[8] A similar object, inscribed with the name of Iui, also dates from the New Kingdom.[9] Both objects are made of green stone: the amulet of Yuya is carved in feldspath, while that of Iui is made of serpentine. The size

---

[1] See coffin of Tjenetethatnetjeru, Cairo Egyptian Museum (CG 6191), in A. NIWINSKI, *The Second Find of Deir el-Bahri (Coffins)*, 1999, fig. 113. The depiction of sacred objects is a common iconographical feature among 21st Dynasty coffins. See *idem*, 'Iconography of the 21st dynasty', in Uehlinger (dir), *Images as Media: Sources for the cultural history of the Near East and the Eastern Mediterranean (Ist millennium BCE)*, 2000, p. 27.

[2] See SR 9201/CG 12054, Cairo Egyptian Museum, in G. REISNER, *Amulets* I, 1907, pl. VII. See also SR 9213 (CG 12128), Fig. 2 - SR 9205 (CG 12127), both from the Cairo Egyptian Museum, and AF 2578 (Louvre Museum).

[3] See Fig. 60 - CG 12056 (Cairo Egyptian Museum). See also SR 9213 (CG 12128), Fig. 2 - SR 9205 (CG 12127), both from the Cairo Egyptian Museum. From an unknown provenance see also AF 2578 (Louvre Museum).

[4] Michel Malaise pointed out the fact that some heart scarabs were sculpted in order to resemble to the heart amulet: 'il existe des scarabées de coeur dont le plat a été aménagé pour revêtir un aspect cordiforme évident.' (in *Les Scarabées de coeur dans l'Égypte ancienne*, 1978, p. 41.) The base of the amulet, being a flat surface, is normally carved with the shape of the heart amulet, including two little side projections. See AF 6981 (Louvre Museum).

[5] See object n° 1595 (Sammlung Ägyptischer Kunst, Munich). In N. SEIPEL, *Ägypten: Götter, gräber und die Kunst*, 1989, p. 228. See also G. STEINDORFF, *Aniba*, 1937, Tl. 50.

[6] C. MÜLLER-WINKLER, *Die Ägyptischen Objekt-Amulette*, 1987, p. 217.

[7] We use here the conceptual frame of Claudia Müller-Winkler. A additive process consists of an addition of some features from a class of objects to another, without changing significantly the shape and the general features of the object. A substitutive process consists of a massive appropriation of the features of one particular class of objects, changing significantly the general shape (and probably the symbolism) of the object. See *ibidem*.

[8] See Fig. 59 - SR 95301/CG 51165, Cairo Egyptian Museum. In J. QUIBELL, *The Tomb of Yuaa and Thuiu*, 1908, PL. XLIX

[9] See BM 7925, British Museum, in C. ANDREWS, *Amulets of Ancient Egypt*, 1998, p. 57

of the objects is also very similar: 11,4 cm for Yuia's amulet and 9,8 cm for Iui's. Both objects were heavily inscribed with hieroglyphs: chapter 30 B of the *Book of the Dead* was inscribed on the flattened surface of the heart amulet, while solar hymns, namely prayers for sailing across the heavens and seeing the gods, were inscribed over the elytra of the scarab. Only the amulet of Iui has additional inscriptions: the signs *tjet*, *djed* and *ankh* were carved on the surface of the heart amulet. Although very rare, these objects testify to an important phenomenon of symbolic convergence between the heart scarab and the heart amulet. In her work on Egyptian amulets, Claudia Müller-Winkler refers to these objects as the result of a substitutive process where a massive appropriation of the features of the heart scarab by the heart amulet came about.[10]

If such additive and substitutive processes took place in the two categories of cardiac amulets, then different magical powers must have been attributed to each of them. Taking this into account, it becomes necessary to understand the specific magical purpose of each of them.

1. The distinction between the heart amulet and the heart scarab in iconography

By the simple fact that both the heart scarab and the heart amulet have a clear connection to the magical protection of the heart, we can easily understand that a strong symbolic affinity could be established between these two categories of objects. Despite this common ground, the two objects could not be more different. Although selecting a particular heart amulet as a 'canonical' object can be a difficult, if not impossible, task, the same does not apply to its depiction in Egyptian art. So, in order to establish a preliminary basis for discussion about the distinctions between heart-related amulets, we will focus our attention on their depiction in tomb decoration.

The pictorial decoration of Sennefer's tomb (TT 96) provides us, once again, with interesting clues for purposes of our discussion. The large funerary heart amulet painted on the antechamber walls aside,[11] we are dealing with a small yellow object in all other occurrences of the object. The depiction, side by side, of the heart scarab and the heart amulet, on the west wall of the northwest pillar of the funerary chamber is of particular interest to us.[12] Here we see Sennefer adorned with the double heart amulet while he receives two necklaces with amulets from Merit, one of which is adorned with a large heart scarab. Here, the typical 'canonical' features of both amulets are clearly present: the yellow heart amulet is a small object, while the heart scarab is a large object made of green stone and framed by a golden chain. Not surprisingly, this pattern follows the 'prescription' for the production of cardiac amulets that is found in chapters of the *Book of the Dead*. Chapter 29 B states that the heart amulet should be crafted of *sehert* stone (i.e., cornelian),[13] while chapter 30 B states that the heart scarab should be crafted of *nemehef* stone (green jasper or green basalt).[14] In the scene depicted in the above-mentioned pillar of Sennefer's tomb, the funerary purpose of the heart scarab seems obvious: Merit gives it to Sennefer in order to provide reanimation of his vital powers. Note that the scarab is offered along with other typical funerary amulets such as the snake-headed amulet, the *djed* pillar and the *tjet* sign. On the other hand, we know that the double-heart amulet was worn by Sennefer during his lifetime, since the same object was depicted in a group statue found at Karnak.[15] In this statue he is also portrayed wearing the typical "gold of honour" necklace, which suggests the use of the double-heart amulet as a royal decoration. This interpretation is also supported by the fact that, in his tomb, this amulet is inscribed with the cartouches of Amenhotep II. In fact, rather than an object made with a strictly funerary purpose, the heart amulet seems to have been used in earthly life as a distinctive sign of high rank and royal favour due to the virtue and wisdom of this powerful governor of Thebes, as we have seen in the first chapter. It is interesting to note that this symbol of social status and wisdom also seems to be invested with funerary significance as it is repeatedly depicted in scenes in the funerary chamber.

A similar distinction between the heart amulet and the heart scarab can be seen in other pictorial contexts. In the tomb of Ramose (TT 55) the two amulets also seem to be dedicated to different purposes. The heart amulet is depicted next to the entrance of the tomb in the ritual context of lustral purification and seems to be related to the 'going forth by day'. On the other hand, a scarab shaped amulet is depicted next to the corridor that descends to the burial chamber, which places it in the context of the entrance to the underworld. In other words, the reading of both amulets seems to be related to the two paths of the hereafter.[16]

In the first chapter, we have seen that some of the king's highest officials used the heart amulet as a sign of status and wisdom as well, at least in the Theban area. From the

[10] C. MÜLLER-WINKLER, *Die Ägyptischen Objekt-Amulette*, 1987, p. 217. This phenomenon of magical convergence originated other interesting pieces where the distinction betwen the heart amulet and the heart scarab is virtually impossible and where the 'classical' features either from one category of objects and the other are surprisingly absent. See as an example, the human-headed 'heart scarab' which in fact is hard to distinguish from a human-headed heart amulet, since it does not present any trace of a typical scarab. See Fig. 61 - object nr inv.1951,5 (Kestner Museum): in G. STEINDORFF, *Aniba*. II, Nr 19-20 Tfl 49, S. 88. In the same way, the contemporary ramesside 'heart amulet' of prince Khaemwaset present a rather strange configuration exceptionally reminding the anatomical features of the cardiac organ, presenting the depiction of three large protuberances at the top, loosely reminding cardiac veins. For the rest its features are totally exceptional to a heart amulet, except the use of red jasper. See Fig. 62 - AF 2333 (Louvre Museum).

[11] See Fig. 56.

[12] See Fig. 55.

[13] C. ANDREWS, *Amulets of Ancient Egypt*, 1998, p. 72. Red and yellow are complementary colours, magically speaking, since both have solar connotations.

[14] See L. ARAÚJO, *Antiguidades Egípcias*, 1993, p. 273. Also J. HARRIS, *Lexicographical Studies*, 1961, pp. 114-115.

[15] Cairo Egyptian Museum, JE 36574, see E. HORNUNG, *The Quest for Immortality*, 2002, pp. 95-96

[16] See N. DAVIES, *The Tomb of the Vizier Ramose*, 1941, Pl. and XV-XXVIII

Ramessid Period on, one can see substantial changes in the iconographical context of the depiction of this amulet since it becomes associated mainly with vignettes of the weighing of the heart,[17] where the deceased appears to receive it as the sign of a positive outcome obtained in the court of Osiris. The fact that the deceased raises *maetic* feathers in his hands in a gesture of joy[18] makes it very clear that, when used in this pictorial context, the heart amulet was seen as a reward given by the court of Osiris to the deceased.[19]

As for the heart scarab, its depictions usually focus on the object itself. It can be represented in the context of a frieze of objects, particularly among other funerary amulets,[20] but most of its depictions are largely restricted to the vignettes of chapter 30 B of the *Book of the Dead*, whose magical purpose consists mainly in the reanimation of the heart.[21] At this point we must also consider that the cardiac chapters (26-30) of the *Book of the Dead* constitute a sequence of texts concerned with the reanimation of the vital powers of the deceased. Further funerary scenes related to the heart scarab usually show the object being offered to the mummy, a gesture that typically stands for the restoration of the heart to the deceased. Surprisingly, the depiction of the heart scarab does not play any significant role in vignettes of the weighing of the heart, in contrast to the heart amulet. This clear asymmetry in the depiction of both amulets suggests the following reading of the magical purpose of these objects: if the heart scarab seems to be closely connected to the reanimation of the vital powers of the mummy, the heart amulet appears to be a symbol of the justification of the deceased.

2. The magical purpose of the heart scarab in the *Book of the Dead*

We know that the location of the heart scarab within the mummy seems to be closely connected to the location of the cardiac organ. While the object was usually located on the exterior of the mummy and placed on a large collar over the chest of the deceased during the 18th Dynasty,[22] during the Ramessid Period it came to be placed in direct contact with the corpse.[23] This practice persisted until the 21st Dynasty and subsequent periods, when the amulet was actually placed inside the thoracic cavity.[24] Because of the usual location of the heart scarabs, it is only natural to conclude that one of its most important magical purposes may well have been to protect the cardiac organ or indeed to substitute for it, in case it was corrupted. In fact, the importance of the heart scarab precludes its religious meaning from being reduced to a single dimension. Just as we are unable to identify a precise rule governing the placement of the amulet in the mummy, neither can we say that its meaning remained the same over time. As with many other religious topics in ancient Egypt, it appears that this object may have served a variety of magical purposes. Although chapter 30 B of the *Book of the Dead* could provide protection against negative testimony in the weighing of the heart, the magical role of this object as a potential substitute for the heart and, above all, as a symbol of rebirth seems much more important.[25] Ultimately, our understanding of this amulet as a symbol should focus on its most evident feature, the god Khepri, the scarab itself, 'The one who transforms' or 'The one who manifests'.[26] This provides the heart scarab with its symbolism of self-engendered life and resurrection.[27] As an image of the sun god, the scarab embodied the transformation or reanimation of the heart and its identification with the god Khepri. Thus, the main function of the heart scarab was to provide identification between the cardiac organ and the rising sun in order to assure the awakening of the deceased to a new life.

In addition to this primary purpose, it seems plausible that the heart scarab performed further functions connected to the stages of the journey of the deceased in the netherworld. In fact, the heart scarab is also supposed to be connected with several other chapters of the *Book of the Dead*. Along with chapter 30 B, the rubrics following chapters 64 and 148 also state that those texts should be read during the offering of the heart scarab to the mummy. It is of interest that these particular texts do not seem to have been selected randomly. In fact, each of these chapters might represent a whole thematic cycle within the journey of the deceased

[17] The scene of the weighing of the heart is a common theme depicted among the tombs of Theban necropolis. This is the case of the tombs of Amenemuia (TT 178), Nefersekheru and Pabasa (TT 296), Neferenepet (TT 178), Userhat (TT 51), Rai (TT 255), Nakhtamun (TT 341), Amenemopet (TT 41), Khonsu (TT 31) and Simut (TT 409), only to mention a few of them. Later on, in the iconography of the coffins of 21st Dynasty the depiction of this vignette will keep all of its former importance in tomb decoration.

[18] This gesture is specially depicted on mythological papyri produced during the 21th Dynasty. See mythological papyri of Khonsumes (Kunsthistorisches Museum, AOS 3859), Nesipakachuti (Louvre Museum, E 17401), Nesitanebetaui (Cairo Egyptian Museum, SR 40017). The same gesture is also depicted on the 21th Dynasty coffins, where this theme is very common. See coffins of Pakharu (Cairo Egyptian Museum, CG 6122/6121, now in National Museum of Alexandria), Padiamun (Cairo Egyptian Museum, CG 6233/6235), Ankhefnmut (Cairo Egyptian Museum, CG 6109), Chebet (Cairo Egyptian Museum, CG 6028), Paser (Louvre Museum, N 2570) and Amenempermut (Cairo Egyptian Museum, CG 6153).

[19] In the vignettes of the weighing of the heart, the presentation of the deceased to the god Osiris is the natural consequence of a positive outcome of that procedure.

[20] See the heart scarab among other funerary objects in U. BOURIANT, 'Tombeau de Harmhabi', *MMAF* 5 (1891), Pl. V;

[21] See Fig. 57.

[22] The vignettes of the *Book of the Dead*, especially those of chapter 26 can be an illustration of that ritual.

[23] See M. MALAISE, *Les Scarabées de Coeur*, 1957, p. 66.

[24] In the Late Period the amulet was sometimes put in the thoracic cavity of the mummy. Iufaa's mummy, found on a Late Period tomb on Abusir, revealed through radiographic analysis a heart scarab in the interior of the body. See M.-P. VANLATHEM, 'Scarabées de coeur *in situ*', *Cd'É* 76 (2001), p. 53.

[25] In fact, archaeology shows that the heart scarab and funerary statuettes were contemporary 'inventions'. Both seek to provide an alternative support that could guarantee its perennial existence in the eventuality of a physical decomposition. Just as *ushebtis* aimed to be a replica of the mummy, heart scarabs were, probably created to grant an alternative support to the cardiac organ as well.

[26] As a symbol of the god Khepri, the heart scarab has evident connotations with renewal and rebirth. See B. AFFHOLDER-GÉRARD, M.-J. CORNIC, *Angers, Musée Pincé: Collections Égyptiennes*, 1990, p. 70.

[27] See A. SHORTER, 'Notes on some funerary amulets', *JEA* 21 (1935), pp. 171-176.

in the afterlife. If chapter 30 B is clearly connected to the reanimation of the mummy, chapter 64 signals the beginning of the *peru em heru*, the 'going forth by day'. In the same way, chapter 148 stands as a turning point in the journey of the deceased in the underworld, through which he will visit the Osirian temple of the Duat in order to be reborn as the rising sun. What is important is that all these critical moments in the life of the deceased seem to be placed under the magical protection of the heart scarab. Curiosuly, once again we find no trace of any symbolic affinity between chapter 125, which, strictly speaking, deals with the weighing of the heart, and the heart scarab. Hence, we can assume that the ritual and magical function of the heart scarab may have been very closely associated with physical reanimation and rebirth, and that it was intended to signify identification between the reanimation of the heart of the deceased and the journey of the solar god.

The vignettes of chapter 30

Although the earliest versions of chapter 30 were illustrated both with the vignette of the weighing of the heart and with the representation of the sacred scarab,[28] it became more and more closely associated with the latter.[29] In these vignettes, the deceased is depicted before a scarab, which is sometimes explicitly drawn to suggest a resemblance to the heart scarab.[30] More often the scarab is simply depicted on top of a temple or over a *maetic* socle. The deceased is usually kneeling, raising one of his hands in a gesture of adoration and holding his heart in the other. This gesture is connected to the protection of the physical organ, the cardiac muscle.

The reason for the depiction of the scarab in the context of chapter 30 can be found in the rubric of the text that recommends the writing of the formula over a heart scarab: 'Words to be said facing a nephrite scarab over *electrum* and with a silver ring around the deceased's neck'.[31] It has often been written that the magical purpose of chapter 30 is related to the protection required in the weighing of the heart. However, as we have seen above, the specific vignette related to this process was connected to chapter 125 and not chapter 30. This is an important piece of information that should lead us to reconsider the magical purpose of that chapter. This formula is, in fact, concerned with the testimony of the heart in the court of Osiris. However, if we consider the *Book of the Dead* as a whole, it becomes obvious that the cardiac chapters (26-30) of the composition do not refer to the Osirian trial but to the process of reanimation of the mummy, at the moment when the physical and psychic powers of the deceased were supposed to be restored. The magical function of both the heart scarab and of chapter 30 was much more focused on the moment of reanimation of the deceased rather than on the weighing of the heart, in the strictest sense.

Of course we cannot deny that both the text and the heart scarab were intended to be of help in the court of Osiris. Nevertheless, although they did work to assist the deceased in overcoming that challenge, their main purpose was focused at an earlier moment, when the powers of life were bestowed on the deceased. Thus, when the awakening of the deceased was to happen, both the heart amulet and chapter 30 could be of help by providing the heart with the purity that would be required later in the court of Osiris.

3. The magical purpose of the heart amulet

Unlike the heart scarab, which was used exclusively in a funerary context, the heart amulet seems to have been primarily used in earthly life. Nevertheless, heart amulets were included among the deceased's funerary equipment and carried into the afterlife. As we have seen in the first chapter, the heart amulet was a very exclusive object, at least until the early 18th Dynasty.[32] Its popularity grew significantly only during the Ramessid and Third Intermediate Periods.[33] The various versions of these amulets that were created during this time, namely the human-headed amulets and the pendulum heart amulets, demonstrate that this object was closely connected to the weighing of the heart and that it was mainly used as a symbol of the justification of the deceased. Iconographic evidence from these objects also leads us to believe that, in the Ramessid Period, the object was primarily related to the justification of the deceased, which is congruent with information collected from iconographic sources. Finally, heart amulets came to be among the most common funerary apotropaic objects found in Egyptian burials from the Late Period.

The heart amulet and the word ib

We know that most Egyptian amulets can be seen as tridimensional versions of certain hieroglyphs. It seems quite obvious that the heart amulet is a three-dimensional rendering of the *ib* hieroglyph (F 34), which depicts the heart of a bull. However, we must take some care with this identification so as not to be misled into thinking that the heart amulet represents the cardiac muscle, i.e., the heart

[28] See H. MILDE, *The Vignettes in the Book of the Dead of Neferrenpet*, 1991, p. 136.

[29] The vignette of the weighing of the heart is more often associated with chapter 125 of the *Book of the Dead*.

[30] See *ibidem*, pl. 41

[31] Translated from the French in P. BARGUET, *Le Livre des Morts*, 1967, p. 76. Archaeological data show that these prescriptions were in fact followed during the funeral ritual.

[32] Although scarce, the archaeological information shows that the heart amulet was an important funerary item in royal burials in the beginning of the 18th Dynasty. See heart amulet from king Ahmose's burial (SR 9386, Cairo Egyptian Museum) and queen Ah-hotep (JE 28606/CG 52091, Cairo Egyptian Museum). The Donation Stela, from the temple of Karnak, also shows the association between the Theban royal princes with the heart amulet. See I. HARARI, "Nature de la Stéle de Donation de Fonction du roi Ahmôsis a la reine Ahmès-Nefertari", *ASAE* 56 (1956), pl. II.

[33] In the Third Intermediate Period, heart amulets were still a precious item in royal burials. An important collection of large heart amulets was found between king Psusennes's wrappings. See P. MONTET, *Les constructions et le tombeau de Psousenès à Tanis,* 1951, pl. CXIX

haty,[34] which in reality is a completely different word.[35] If we use Bardinet's anatomical definition of the cardiac words (*ib* and *haty*), the word *ib* stands for the interior of the body where the conductors *met* (such as the veins) play an important role, while the word *haty* designates the cardiac muscle itself. This is a crucial distinction, since the general shape of the amulet can lead us to interpret this object as a depiction of the cardiac organ.

This distinction helps us avoid the danger of understanding heart amulets to be no more than representations of the cardiac organ, the *haty*. Indeed, it is more likely that the vase heart amulet may have been seen as an 'artistic' or, more accurately, a 'hieroglyphic' rendering of certain key notions concerning the heart *ib*. In fact, the examples used thus far show us that the primary meaning of the heart amulet is always focused on the mental and 'psychological' sense, which is the usual understanding of the word *ib*, 'heart' in hieroglyphic writing. Nevertheless, this spiritual reading of the heart amulet does not exclude the organic notions of the heart *ib*. There is a strong possibility that such a reading may be based in anatomical notions about the heart *ib*. The side projections, so typical of heart amulets, may actually have been depicted in order to represent the conductors *met* which are an important part of the heart *ib*. According to Bardinet:

> (...) cette nature composée du *ib*, qui est à la fois l'ensemble des conduits-*met* avec ce qu'ils contiennent (liquides, air animateur), et à la fois nos viscères (simplement des endroits particuliers du *ib* pour les Égyptiens), a rendu impossible toute représentation dans l'écriture. Ainsi, le mot *ib* est écrit phonétiquement (il n'a pas d'idéogramme spécifique) et sera représenté par un signe hieroglyphique qui, en fait, est un coeur-*haty*, c'est-à-dire, la partie du corps avec laquelle il a des relations physiologiques fondamentales.[36]

So, although seeming insignificant, side projections provide the heart amulet with its real meaning, since they represent the connective function of *met* conductors which are a distinctive anatomical element of the heart *ib*.[37] Although highly un-naturalistic, the depiction of *met* conductors in a heart amulet is extremely important since they denote its life-giving connective role.[38] On the other hand, the depiction of the heart as a vase also conforms to many anatomical descriptions of the heart *ib* as the gastric cavity.[39] In Egyptian literature, there are several allusions to the heart *ib* that describe it as a container. 'To be inside the heart *ib*' meant 'to be loved' or to have someone's trust. In the *Autobiography of Uni*, for instance, the governor of Upper Egypt during the reign of Pepi I said that: 'I filled the heart *ib* of the king with my virtues'.[40] These metaphors clearly show that the emotional functions of the heart were defined by means of the depiction of the heart as a vase: something empty that has the ability to be filled with emotions and to receive knowledge. In fact, we frequently encounter the advice to 'put the books in the heart *ib*' in wisdom literature.[41] Hence, the 'psychological' definition of the heart *ib* seems to derive from the anatomical formulation of the *ra-ib*, the 'entrance of the *ib*', i.e., the stomach and not the cardiac muscle. Thus, globally speaking, the heart amulet should be seen as the symbol of the 'inner life'.

The iconographical association with the vase *nw* was perhaps the best way to describe the main function of the heart *ib*: to be receptive. Therefore, an artistic rendering of the heart amulet is highly cryptic: it writes the word *ib* combining the hieroglyphic value of the vase *nw* with that of the conductors of the heart *ib*. Through this combination, the heart amulet seems to evoke the life giving power of the blood that runs through the veins (the conducters *met*) and fills the heart *ib* with the essence of life. Although based on an anatomical view of the heart *ib*, this image could also be used to express the character of the heart *ib* on the psychological level: the mind was, like the gastric cavity, a vessel that was 'nourished' by wisdom and knowledge, the 'spiritual blood' that animated the individual with true life. In this way, the heart amulet could be fully understood as a symbol of the connective power of the heart *ib*: if the heart amulet was regarded as a symbol of life, it was no less a symbol of wisdom through which each individual could achieve social connectivity.[42] Therefore, when regarded

[34] See C. ANDREWS, *Amulets of Ancient Egypt*, 1998, p. 72.

[35] In the funerary context the heart of the sacrificial victim is usually depicted in the scenes of the opening of the mouth ceremony. In this context, the heart of the bull is inhaled by the deceased in order to give him the power of life. This could be a possible reason to use the heart amulet in the funerary context. However, this interpretation could not explain the apparent extensive use of the amulet by the living. Besides, among the heart amulets the anatomical reality may be entirely replaced by the metaphorical image of the vase, the pendulum or the inner temple which, in fact, seem to be much more important. Such replacement became sometimes so extensive that it can be very difficult to recognize some of these objects as representing a heart at all. See SR 9258/JE 27170/CG 12067 (Cairo Egyptian Museum): in G. REISNER, *Amulets*, I, 1907, pl. VIII

[36] in T. BARDINET, *Les papyrus médicaux de l'Égypte pharaonique*, 1995, pp. 71-72.

[37] About the anatomical meaning of *met* conductors see *ibidem*, p. 66-67: 'Dans les conduits-*mets* du corps passent tous les éléments essentiels à la vie, les éléments nourriciers, les différents liquides corporels ainsi que souffle vital'. In this context, the side projections depicted on the amulet are surely evocative of the blood, the bodily fluid that fills the *met* conductors and the body with the breath of life and gives to the cardiac muscle its connective role.

[38] Medical texts gives us a textual evidence of the relation betwen the cardiac muscle and the *met* conductors: 'les conduits-met de l'homme sont pour chaque endroit de son corps et il est de fait avéré qu'il (le coeur *haty*) parle devant les conduits-met appartenant à chaque endroit du corps' (Eb. 854a), in *ibidem*, p. 85.

[39] Among the many organs of the heart *ib*, the stomach is perhaps the most important. Besides, the *ra-ib*, the stomach, was understood literally as the 'entrance of the *ib*'.

[40] See H. BRUNNER, "Das Herz im ägyptischen Glauben", in: *Das hörende Herz. Kleine Schriften zur religions und Geitesgeschichte Ägyptens,* 1988, p. 17. See also A. DE BUCK, ‚Een groep dodenboekspreuken betreffende het hart', *JEOL* 9 (1944), p. 17. A pessimistic advice said: "Do not fill your heart with a brother", alerting to the danger of trusting someone. The friend was called "the great (lord) in my heart", whereas the loved one was called "the sister who is in my heart". In A. PIANKOFF, *Le 'Coeur' dans les Textes Égyptiens depuis l'Ancien jusqu'à la fin du Nouvel Empire*, 1930, p. 40.

[41] See *Ibidem*.

[42] The artistic rendering of the heart amulet is therefore highly cryptic since it combines the hieroglyphic value of the vase *nw* and the heart *ib* to deliver a religious message that had two levels of interpretation. In a bodily reading, the amulet provided purity and life but, as a symbol of

metaphorically, side projections simbolized nothing less than cosmic integration. Curiously, among the heart amulets from the Late Period on, side projections begun to be shaped as ears, providing the full image of the 'listening heart'.

4. The cardiac amulets and the cardiac words (*ib* and *haty*)

If we employ Bardinet's anatomical definition of the cardiac words (*ib* and *haty*), the word *ib* stands for the interior of the body, while the *haty* designates the cardiac muscle itself. *Haty* literally stands for 'the one who commands'. In addition to its definition as the cardiac muscle, the word *haty* is used in literary texts to suggest the driving force of the individual and is frequently seen as the seat of self-awareness.

Curiously, we encounter different connotations for these words in funerary texts, as in chapter 30 B of the *Book of the Dead*:

> Oh, my heart-*ib* of my mother, oh, my heart-*ib* of my mother! Oh, my heart-*haty* of my transformations (*kheperu*), do not stand against me as a witness, do not oppose to me in a Court of Law, do not show any hostility towards me in face of the keeper of the scales![43]

In light of the magical nature of this text, we can agree that the words *ib* and *haty* refer to cardiac amulets. Since the cardiac chapters refer to the funerary ritual, these allusions to the heart *ib* and *haty* should not be understood in either a medical or a literary context. On the contrary, we must first take into consideration the ritual context of the text and recognize it as textual evidence of a ceremony during which cardiac amulets were offered to the mummy. Other allusions to the cardiac amulets are made in the context of the cardiac chapters of the *Book of the Dead*. Mention of the 'House of Hearts' in chapter 26 seems to be related to the acquisition of hearts *ib* and *haty* that could be given to the mummy in this context.

> My heart *ib* is mine in the House of Hearts-*ibu*, my heart-*haty* is mine in the House of Hearts-*hatyw (...)*. I shall be aware (*rḫ*) in my heart (*ib*), I shall have power (*sḫm*) in my heart (*haty*), I shall have power (*sḫm*) in my arms, I shall have power (*sḫm*) in my legs, I shall have power (*sḫm*) to do whatever I desire; my soul and my corpse shall not be restrained at the portals of the West when I go in or out in peace[44]

These 'Houses of Hearts' are also mentioned in chapter 151 A of the *Book of the Dead*:

> Words spoken by Anubis (...) are upon the mummy (of Qenna), providing him with what belongs to him: (...) you will enter the House of Hearts; the place which is full of hearts; you will take the one that is yours and put it in its place without your hand being hindered.[45]

This text clearly shows us the 'House of Hearts' as a place full of hearts in which the deceased finds his heart of eternity.

It is interesting to note that these cardiac amulets can, in fact, be considered as representations of both hearts of man. Our hypothesis is that the amulet related to the heart *ib* is the heart amulet (in the exact shape of a three-dimensional *ib* hieroglyph), while the heart scarab is the amulet that allowed the deceased to gain control over his heart *haty*. This distinction provides an important clue for understanding the magical function of each of the cardiac amulets. If our assumption is correct, chapter 26 provides further explanation about the purpose of the cardiac amulets when it says *'(...). I shall be aware* (*rḫ*) *in my heart* (ib), *I shall have power* (*sḫm*) *in my heart* (haty)'. Thus, the amulet of the heart *ib* was believed to restore knowledge (*rekh*) and perhaps identity to the deceased, while the amulet of the heart *haty*, the heart scarab, allowed the deceased to have control (*sekhem*) over his bodily heart *haty*. We must not forget that the word *ib* is used explicitly in chapter 29 B to designate the heart amulet.

We can now return to the text of chapter 30 B. It is well known that this text relates the heart *ib* to the mother, while it relates the heart *haty* to the manifestations (*kheperu*). This concept has given rise to many interpretations,[46] but once again we believe that these are allusions to the symbolic meaning of the cardiac amulets and not to any anatomical or literary notions. We must bear in mind that the heart amulet derived from the vase *nw* amulet, which was the very hieroglyph used to write the name of Nut, the heavenly mother. Therefore, it is certainly possible that the heart amulet can be seen as the symbol of the wisdom and virtue required for the deceased to be united with the heavenly mother. Depictions on the inner faces of anthropoid coffins clearly show that the goddess was associated with the heart amulet.[47] The so-called 'Texts of Nut', which were sometimes inscribed in this context, also refer explicitly to the concept that the heart of the goddess belonged to the deceased:

> Tu entres en moi et j'embrasse ton image, je suis ton cercueil qui recèle ta forme secrète. Mon coeur est avec toi comme ton acte de propriété, il te parle comme 'celui qui est à l'avant du coffre de Nout'. Ma bouche est prompte à glorifier ton *ba*, ma magie est la protection de tes membres.[48]

the mind, the amulet could also recall that man should fill his mind with wisdom. In the funerary realm the mental sense of the amulet seems to be prevalent: it is used as a reminder of the value of wisdom and virtue as those qualities were measured in the weighing of the heart. Intended to fill the heart with new life (both on a physiological and on a mental sense), the heart amulet was most certainly taken as a powerful protection for earthly life and also for the afterlife.

[43] Chapter 30 B of the *Book of the Dead*. See R. FAULKNER, *The Egyptian Book of the Dead*, 1998, pl. 15.

[44] *ibidem*.

[45] J. DIJK, 'Entering the House of Hearts: An addition of chapter 151 in the Book of the Dead of Qenna', *OMRO* 75 (1995), p. 8.

[46] See, for instance, J. ASSMANN, *La Mort et l'au-delá*, 2003, p. 57.

[47] See Fig. 105.

[48] Merenptah's sarcophagus. See J. ASSMANN, *La Mort et l'au-delá*,

Thus, if the heart amulet was indeed a symbol of the deceased's wisdom and righteousness, it is possible that it may also have been seen as the required confirmation by the court of Osiris that permitted him to be received by Nut in order to be regenerated in her womb. Only a righteous and justified deceased could return to Nut's womb in order to experience a rebirth. So, magically speaking, the heart amulet could properly be seen as the 'heart of Nut', or, as chapter 30 B puts it, 'the heart of the (divine) mother', a symbol of purity and *maetic* order that was believed to be the true essence of being and that could in fact be understood as 'innate' in nature, as mentioned in the same text.[49]

We have already noted that the heart scarab must be primarily understood as a tridimensional depiction of the hieroglyph *kheper*, 'transformations'. The transformations mentioned in the text should then be understood as the result of the rebirth. Thus, the heart scarab can be seen as a symbol of the rebirth of the deceased in a new solar manifestation. The *kheperu* associated with the heart *haty* should also be understood as the individual 'manifestations' of self-awareness during his lifetime, which, once in the afterlife, will change (*kheper*) to a new form.

Futhermore, there is a strong possibility that, in addition to possessing magical attributes, each cardiac amulet was also intended to grant the connective powers of the heart *ib* or of the heart *haty*. The heart amulet, as a symbol of the connective power of wisdom, was probably destined to protect the heart *ib* as a way of assuring cosmic integration. It was, in fact, this connective power that was judged and measured during the weighing of the heart. The heart scarab, as a symbol of the newborn sun, stood for the connective powers of the physical self, which could provide a rebirth. It was the symbol of the connective powers of the cardiac muscle that assured life on the bodily level. In the funerary context, it was primarily related to the embalming ritual that transformed the aspective reality of the body into a new symbolic integrity.[50] Therefore, each cardiac amulet can be seen as a symbol of the different aspects through which the heart manifests its connective powers.

Thus, it seems that the heart scarab is closely related to the reanimation of the vital powers of the deceased, whereas the heart amulet seems to be the symbol of his wisdom. In other words, it seems that the heart scarab grants protection to the physical self of the deceased, while the heart amulet seems to be the embodiment of its social self. Ergo, the two amulets represented two distinct aspects of the connective power of the heart. As a global connective principle, the heart acted on both a physical and a social level, transforming the aspective elements of the body into a unity. In ancient Egypt, death was seen as a disaggregating principle that dissolved and isolated, while life was seen as an animating principle that created unity and wholeness.[51] In this light, life was equally the result of both social and bodily connectivity.[52] Therefore, it seems quite possible that both heart-related amulets acted to protect the heart according to the social and bodily aspects of its connective powers.

5. The symbolism of cardiac amulets

We can now return to the cardiac amulets such as Yuya's and Iui's that commingled features of the heart scarab and the heart amulet. Through additive and substitutive processes, the amulets related to the heart seem to have been coherently combined in order to express the duality of the ways by which the heart could manifest its connective powers in the afterlife. This conjunction of the two amulets allowed the entire being of the deceased to be projected into the two dimensions of eternity. The heart scarab, as a symbol of bodily connectivity, was a central part of the mummification rituals and was given to the deceased by female goddesses such as Isis and Nephtys. Above all, it had an obstetric meaning and alluded to the rebirth of the deceased in a solar manifestation, representing the integration of the deceased into the perpetual cycle of death and rebirth of the sun (*neheh*). On the other hand, the heart amulet symbolized the wisdom of the deceased, its perennial being that was to be remembered and preserved forever in the *djet* dimension of eternity. As such, the heart amulet played a central role in the weighing of the heart and in justification rituals, where male deities (such as Horsaiset) gave it to the deceased as a symbol of the triumph of purity and wisdom over death and corruption. The grouping of their features into a single object demonstrates an intention to combine the connective power of both cardiac amulets.

The symbolic trend that preferred the fusion of the cardiac amulets through a substitution process only appears in the reign of Amenhotep II and seems to reach its height during the reign of Amenhotep III. Later, during the Ramessid Period, additive processes came to take precedence: the objects are no longer completely commingled. Instead, only some features of the complementary object are selected. This trend does not seem to continue beyond this period. Beginning with the Late Period, each amulet appears as a separate entity. Curiously, while the heart scarab retained all of its importance as a central facet of mummy equipment, the heart amulet resumed its role as a small object used predominantly by the living. From this

2003, p. 253.

[49] Although each man was seen as responsible for his own behaviour and therefore, by his own salvation in the hereafter, it is possible that the virtue has largely been seen as innate, as many autobiographical texts imply: 'Straightforward, trustworthy, one free of wrong, who turns his back on crime, who does right as befits; a scribe righteous from his mother's womb, the scribe Ramosenefer, justified.', in M. LICHTHEIM, *Maat in Egyptian Autobiographies and Related Texts*, 1992, p. 40. As Miriam Lichtheim points out, the phrase "righteous from his mother's womb" makes the point that this man's virtue was born with him and it was innate. Therefore, the right behaviour was mainly seen as the result of the ability to follow the command of his heart. So, the heart was essentially equipped with innate virtue and goodness. This leads us to the idea that the heart possesses within it an essential wisdom that reflects the cosmic order. It is the sin that turns the heart crooked, removing its light and corrupting it.

[50] See J. ASSMANN, *Mort et l'au-delá*, 2003, p. 57-58.

[51] *Ibidem.*

[52] *Ibidem.*

point on, the large funerary version of the heart amulet became a thing of the past, its meaning changing so that it became a symbol of the divine children and, as such, was meant to insure protection against evil.

6. The dualistic nature of the heart

The dual nature of the heart is more commonly expressed in textual sources. Thierry Bardinet showed that, in medical texts (which clearly belong to the constelative sphere), the connective power of the heart was expressed by means of its dual formulation. The heart *ib*, the interior of the body, and the heart *haty*, the cardiac muscle, expressed the action of the blood (passive element) combined with the driving power of the cardiac muscle to insure the maintenance of life. This dual action demonstrates that, in the Egyptian view of human nature, the body is seen as a plurality of members brought together by dualistic connective elements, the blood and the cardiac muscle. In addition to physical connectivity, the dual heart was also responsible for social connectivity. The mental or psychological characterization of the heart reflects this responsibility. On the social level, the two hearts of man express the connective power of the heart by means of a parataxis: the heart *ib* stands for the inner life, just as it stood for the interior of the body on the physical level. Therefore, like the blood, the heart *ib* is a fluid mental state that is more closely related to the emotional and sensitive life and therefore highly impersonal in nature. By contrast, the heart *haty*, 'the one that commands', reflects the power of the will and better expresses personal identity, in sum, the 'earthly manifestation' of being. Curiously, it is in funerary texts, constelative in nature, that we can best see this distinction:

> Ton coeur *ib* est avec toi en vérité (lit.: Ton coeur *ib* est avec toi dans ton existence véritable), ton coeur *haty* de ton existence terrestre, tu viens dans ton aspect d'auparavant, comme le jour où tu es né.[53]

While the association between the heart *haty* and earthly existence is well documented elsewhere, the nature of the heart *ib* remains for the most part unclear. Allusions to the mother in this context must be understood in the light of ritual and myth rather than by physiological statements. As the cosmos was seen as a conjunction of heaven and earth, the heart may also have been seen as a dual entity, as can be seen in the following text:

> On t'a attaché ton coeur *ib* de ta mére, ton coeur *haty* est pour ton corps.
>
> Ton *ba* est pour le ciel et ton corps est pour être sous terre.[54]

Such texts lead us to believe that the heart *ib* was a literal representation of the *maetic* "true" nature of man, a kind of "quintessential", innate, divine power that could be equated with the *ba*. From the "psychological" point of view, one could see the truth, *maet*, via the heart *ib* while one could chose whether or not to apply it in his actions through the heart *haty*. In short, the heart *ib* and the heart *haty* recreated heaven and earth in the inner man, thus assuring his cosmic integration.

One way or the other, whether referring to the body or to social connectivity, the formulation of the two hearts appears deeply rooted in the dualistic cognitive structure of the Egyptian mind that views two things as the manifestation of a totality. The Egyptian language had no word for an all-embracing, abstract horizon of totality described by concepts such as "cosmos", "world", or "reality". Instead, we encounter not a concept but the framework of a mythical constellation. This was, most probably, the starting point of a broader religious speculation that the representation of the dualistic nature of the heart could express the Egyptian view of life and cosmic integration. We shall now return to our passage:

> On t'a attaché ton coeur *ib* de ta mére, ton coeur *haty* est pour ton corps.
>
> Ton *ba* est pour le ciel et ton corps est pour être sous terre.[55]

The allusion to the *ba* is particularly interesting in this context as it describes the manifestation of a hidden power that the text relates to heaven, while the corpse, clearly related to the heart *haty*, remains attached to the earth. This dualistic formulation of the heart corresponds to the dualistic definition of human nature as the *ba* and the corpse that are re-united at night. In a manner of speaking, this image recalls the union of Re and Osiris.[56] The Egyptians imagined the constellation in which Re and Osiris worked together as embodiments of the two antinomic or complementary aspects of time, as a *ba* and a corpse. The deceased led an eternal life, "going in" and "going out", as a *ba* in the *neheh*-time of the sun, and "enduring", as a corpse, in the *djet*-time of Osiris. In the ultimate abstraction, this life was conceived as a union of *ba* and corpse, or a union of the heart *ib* and heart *haty*.[57]

This dualistic reading of the heart seems to have a parallel in the production of large cardiac amulets that commingle the features of the heart scarab and the heart amulet in a single object. We must also bear in mind that the concept of the tomb changed in the New Kingdom in order to express the double nature of man. The tomb became a place where the deceased had contact not only with posterity, but also with the divine, this latter aspect gaining ever more significance.[58] From this point on, tomb and temple seem to be combined in funerary architecture in a way that appears to correspond to the combination of the heart scarab with the heart amulet. In fact, each amulet was seen as a symbol of an entire set of rituals. The heart scarab symbolized the mummification rituals and depicted the

[53] A. PIANKOFF, *Le Coeur dans les Textes Égyptiéns*, 1930, p. 66.
[54] *Ibidem.*

[55] In *ibidem.*
[56] J. ASSMANN, *The Search for God in Ancient Egypt*, 1984, p. 78-79
[57] *Ibidem.*
[58] *Idem*, p. 166

solar rebirth of the deceased that was supposed to occur in the hidden funeral chamber of the tomb. On the other hand, the heart amulet symbolized the justification rituals, a role that demonstrated an identification with Osiris, and the ability of the deceased to perform the Osirian cult that was supposed to occur in the superstructure of the tomb, planned as a temple. Furthermore, while the heart scarab was associated with the power of love to restore the integrity of the corpse, the heart amulet was mainly associated with the power of wisdom and knowledge to insure the manifestation of the *ba*.[59]

Interestingly, this double nature of the heart seems to have been explored largely in iconography, particularly in 21st Dynasty depictions of the heart amulet and the solar scarab in the decoration of coffins. The heart amulet is usually black (or dark blue) and is inscribed with the Osirian name of the deceased.[60] Osirian symbols such as the *ta uer* emerge from it in certain examples.[61] In other depictions, the amulet is shown surrounded by other associated symbols: the *benu* bird,[62] the word *djet*, the sign of the West (*Amentet*), the sign of the starry sky (*pet*) and even the name or effigy of Nut. By means of these symbols, the heart amulet is represented as the Osirian aspect of the deceased and it could be interpreted as the deceased's identification with Osiris, the chthonic principle that rejuvenated the universe. On the other hand, the solar scarab was seen as the image of the identification of the deceased with Re, the solar principle that ruled the universe. Thus, in the context of 21st Dynasty theological beliefs, the two funerary symbols of the heart seemed to be fully identified with the two principles of the universe, Osiris and Re, following a long tradition of religious speculation. The two cardiac amulets, the heart scarab and the heart amulet, interpreted the duality of the heart in light of the dual constellation of Re and Osiris. The cosmos existed through the combined effectiveness of these gods, as did life. In the ultimate abstraction, this life was conceived of as a union of *ba* and corpse, or as a union of the heart *ib* and the heart *haty*.[63]

Before we conclude, we should bear in mind that dualism in Egypt is not only a matter of totality: it also reflects a ritual 'cosmogonic' purpose. Whatever contexts they were applied to, the dualistic categories tend to view reality as unfinished: the Two Lands need to be unified by the Pharaoh; heaven and earth need to be kept together; the Two Maet need to be put into practice. Dualistic categories create constellations where the meaning of the cosmic order, *maet*, needs to be reasserted in face of its opposite principle, *isfet*. If *maet* designates the idea of a meaningful, all-pervasive order that embraces the world of humankind, objects and nature, *isfet*, "lack", corresponds to sickness, death, scarcity, injustice, falsehood, theft, violence, war, and enmity. Dualism viewed cosmic reality as an incomplete process, forever at risk. Thus, through its dualistic formulation, the human body shares the same nature as the universe or Egypt. Life means connectivity and cohesion, while death means aspectivity and disintegration. The contrast between life and death generally reflects the struggle for the maintenance of the cosmic order. Thus, death is a manifestation of "lack" in a world that has fallen into disorder through the loss of its original plenitude of meaning. The meaning of creation, as it was planned by the creator, lies in its plenitude, which yields order and justice. [64] Suffering, crime and death had no meaning *per se*. They were symptoms of an emptying or estrangement of meaning from the world, which had distanced itself from its origins over the course of history. Through the dualistic formulation of the heart, mind and cosmos were intrinsically identified with each other and the cardiac symbols were seen as the embodiment of the cosmic principles that rule the universe, the body and the mind. Thus, through the dualistic expression of the heart, a new beginning was intended, which was largely the equivalent of cosmic recreation.

[59] See Fig. 64 - statue of the *ba* bird of Yuya depicting the heart amulet: JE 95312 (Cairo Egyptian Museum). It was probably this association between the cardiac amulets and both tomb structures that perhaps explains why this particular category of objects were produced during a short period of time, mainly during the reign of Amen-hotep III. Although highly significant, these double amulets did not allow a distinct use in the rituals celebrated in the superstructure and within the funeral chamber, thus being out of use very rapidly.

[60] See Fig. 65.

[61] See anthropoid coffin CG 6153, Cairo Egyptian Museum.

[62] Sometimes, through an additive process, the *benu* bird, a typical feature of the heart amulet, can be depicted on a heart scarab. See C. MÜLLER-WINKLER, *Die Ägyptischen Objekt-Amulette*, 1987, p. 217.

[63] J. ASSMANN, *The Search for God in Ancient Egypt*, 1984, p. 79

[64] See *ibidem*, p. 3

CONCLUSION

THE "IMPLICIT THEORY" OF THE HEART

To understand the Egyptian iconography of the heart we must consider it within the broader context of Egyptian religion. As Jan Assmann pointed out, the Egyptian concept of religion can be concisely defined as the realization of *maet*. This is the domain of explicit theology which deals with the problem of theodicy, the justification of god in the singular and speculation about *maet*.[1]

The evolution traced by Jan Assmann in the 'theory of the heart' is a typical phenomenon derived from the context of explicit theology. It deals with a complex set of beliefs that are expressed through a discourse with its own history. The discourse about the heart in ancient Egypt has a history and, from the beginning it has nothing to do with mythology: it is clearly a process that evolved through three stages of development, as Assmann pointed out. As such, we encounter reflection about the heart in the context of autobiographies, wisdom texts and religious hymns. Interestingly, the notion of the heart that is conveyed through these discoursive sources mirrors the formulation of god as a singular entity: although the two words, *ib* and *haty*, are used, they are employed mainly as synonyms and express the formulation of the heart as a singular entity as well.

However, in the narrower sense, religion was primarily related to the cult and ritual.[2] This was the domain of implicit theology where constelative interactions of the gods became manifest in rituals and symbols. In the sources emanating from the context of implicit theology a very different picture of the heart emerges. Ritual is the main concern of these sources: an "implicit theory" of the heart is present in medical texts, funerary texts, amulets and symbols. While the discoursive sources "enunciate" in an explicit way, these implicit ideas and symbols of the heart are enunciated so as to be effective. They do not require explanation. The characterization of the heart provided by these sources is magical and constelative in nature, i.e., the ideas and symbols about the heart emanate from a mythical context, where they become the objects of an action with a magical or ritual purpose performed by a particular god.

Obviously, all notions related to the heart amulet emanate from implicit theology. There are distinct mythical interpretations of its meaning in each of the subtle variations of its depiction. The challenge we face at this point, like a coiled cobra, is similar to the one we encountered at the beginning of this book. We will now re-examine the various uses of the heart amulet, but now we will attempt to identify the mythical constellation that lies behind its use.

1. The heart amulet of illumination and the mythic cycle of Horus

The struggle to return to the original plenitude of the world is mythically rendered in the combat of Horus and Seth.[3] If Seth embodies the principle of death, isolation and disintegration, Horus is the agent of life, the guarantee of connectivity, cohesion and unity. In the political sphere, cosmic order was insured anew by the re-enactment of the triumph of Horus, through the coronation of the Pharaoh. However, in medical practice, doctors also entered into combat with Seth in order to re-establish the *maetic* order in the body of the sick person. Thus, in every realm of Egyptian life in need of cosmic reassurance, the mythic cycle of Horus provided the ritual context through which the connective power of the world could be reaffirmed.

In this mythic context, Horus acted as a connective principle in many of his manifestations: as a solar god he insured the cosmic union of heaven and earth, but as the personification of the Pharaoh he also insured the union of the Two Lands on earth. The representation of the heart as a connective element is therefore rooted in the mythic cycle that explained the foundation of the cosmic order. Thus, it is no wonder that we can also see the manifestation of the connective powers of Horus in the heart of man through its characterization as a dual entity, as noted in the previous chapter.

The solar heart amulet[4] provides the best illustration of the victory of Horus over Seth and expresses perfectly the identification of the heart with the connective power of Horus that imbues both the body and the mind of its user with life and *maet*. Framed within this mythical context, use of the golden heart amulet may have occurred in a largely political context. Originally, the solar heart amulet seems to have been a royal object that signified the illuminated heart of the Pharaoh. Such an object should be understood as a depiction of the heart of Horus and as a symbol of his victory over Seth, or, in other words, as a symbol of Horus' connective powers.[5] This power explains the Pharaoh's

[1] *Ibidem*, p. 12

[2] *Ibidem*.

[3] See E. HORNUNG, *Les Dieux de l'Égypte:l'Un et le Multiple*, 1986, p. 158.

[4] Such are the depictions of Thutmosis III/Hatshepsut and the golden heart amulets inscribed with a royal cartouche. See Fig. 45. We group under this ritual context the depictions of the heart amulet that we have named in the first chapter under the designations of 'heart of illumination' and 'heart of wisdom'.

[5] Curiously enough, the connective power of Horus was expressed in royal inscriptions by means of vital powers such as *ankh* ("life"), *was* ("power"), *seneb* ("health") and *aut-ib* ("joy"). Joy, the 'expansion of the heart', was symbolically related to the rebirth of the sun and to its

ability to guide his subjects wisely. It is possible that, in divine iconography, the depiction of the solar heart in the avian statues of Horus might be a symbol of the "solar" heart of Horus, thus expressing the connective power of his heart.

From the reign of Hatshepsut on, at least, the 'heart of wisdom', the golden heart amulet inscribed with the royal cartouche, was used as a royal decoration, as a symbol of (inner) obedience to the king.[6] In fact, from the reign of Tuthmosis III to the reign of Amenhotep III, the golden heart amulet seems to have been used as a royal decoration that could be understood as the earlier political ideal of 'being in the king's heart'. In this way, a high official in possession of this decoration could be seen as an ally of Horus in his combat with Seth, thus signifying both his obedience to the king and his wisdom. This loyalty would be understood as the ability to follow the command of the heart. Obviously, this mythical reading of the connective power of the heart amulet is predominant in the context of earthly life.

2. The heart amulet of justification and the mythic cycle of Osiris

The reconstruction of the physical integrity of Osiris was guaranteed by the work of the female deities, as a matter of "love". The next stage in the full reanimation of Osiris was insured by Horus and Thoth, who then played a paramount role in the reestablishment of his social identity, his dignity and his social status. Male deities would restore the connectivity of life on the social level and complete the work begun by Isis by means of a "moral mummification".[7] If the restoration of the body refers to the constellation "man-woman" and was a phenomenon of a sexual nature, the restoration of social identity refers to the constellation "father-son".[8] It is certainly not by chance that the "moral mummification" was insured by means of the weighing of the heart. In order to be fully invested with divine status, the deceased would be evaluated in his own heart, understood as the seat of his identity. Once his *maetic* value was proved, the deceased was provided with an Osirian (divine) identity.

Iconographical evidence, largely from the Theban area, suggests that the heart amulet came to be closely associated with the imagery of the weighing of the heart, especially from the Ramessid Period on. This association was so strong that, during the 21st Dynasty, the heart amulet seems to have been used as the central piece in an entire set of funerary rituals performed in the context of the Theban necropolis, particularly in the collective burials of the priests of Amun found at Deir el-Bahari, as is suggested in the iconographical programme of the papyrus of Nesipautitaui and related documents.[9] It seems highly plausible that a consecration ceremony for the heart amulet could have occurred in the context of the funeral rituals in order to signify the justification of the deceased, i.e., his victory over Seth. In earlier depictions, such a ritual is presented as a lustral purification ceremony, as in the lustration scene in the tomb of Ramose (TT 55). In this context, the amulet embodied the purity and knowledge of the deceased and was seen literally as the *maetic* heart of Osiris that Horus gave back to his father in order to restore his identity and his dignity. Hence, the heart amulet was the symbol of the knowledge and purity required to overcome the perils of the transition to the next life and to gain admission to the community of the netherworld as a member in good standing.

The development of beliefs related to the weighing of the heart inspired the creation of particular types of heart amulets, such as the human-headed heart amulets and pendulum heart amulets.

The heart amulet and the slaughter of Seth

As a symbol of purity the heart amulet was a sign of the victory of Osiris over Seth.[10] As such, the heart amulet can be depicted above the chests of enemies of Egypt to illustrate the punishment of Seth.[11] Now justified, the deceased was invested with the attributes of royalty and was required to demonstrate his dominion over the forces of chaos by destroying them. Therefore, the removal of the hearts of enemies was a vehicle for the reaffirmation of the cosmic order. The heart of the enemy was removed since it was the critical point from which the evil powers of Seth could threaten the cosmic order. Certain scenes in tombs in the Valley of the Kings show the corpses of the enemies of Egypt without their hearts.[12] This is the visual and literal translation of the act of "cut[ting] off the heart" as mentioned in funerary texts, an act which guaranteed the final death of royal enemies. In other representations,

vital powers. Joy was seen as the full expression of the power of the sun to irradiate life and light, the same power that assured triumph over the enemies of the cosmic order. It is perhaps the better statement of the Egyptian view of the connective power of the heart of Horus, which expanded itself to all the living beings of creation. See royal inscription of Sneferu from Sinai, JE 38568 (Cairo Egyptian Museum). In M. SALEH, H. SOUROUZIAN, *Official Catalogue of the Egyptian Museum Cairo*, 1987, n° 24.

[6] The first stage of the "Theory of the Heart" described by Jan Assmann must therefore be entirely understood in the light of the constelative nature of the myth. Since the heart of the Pharaoh is linked to the heart of Horus, the "king-guided man" follows the command of Horus, whose heart is the only one to be able to fully perform the connective responsibility of keeping *maet* in motion. This notion not only explains the desire of the Old Kingdom subjects to 'be in the king's heart' but it also explains the first known occurrences of the heart amulet, as golden objects inscribed with royal cartouches.

[7] J. ASSMANN, *Mort et au-delà dans l'Égypte ancienne*, 2003, p. 74-80.

[8] *Ibidem.*

[9] A. NIWINSKI, '*The Book of the Dead on the Coffins of the 21st Dynasty*', in H. Backes, I. Munro, S. Stor (eds.), *Totenbuch-Forschungen*, 2006, pp. 245-264.

[10] See Figs. 87.and 88.

[11] The punishment of Seth took the form of an animal slaughter, in which the heart of Seth was removed to assure his final annihilation. This sacrifice was made in the ritual of opening the mouth. The heart of the victim was placed before the mummy to provide the reanimation of the deceased. This gesture reflected both the ritual annihilation of Seth and the final victory of Osiris over death. J. ASSMANN, *Mort e au-delà dans l'Égypte ancienne*, 2003, p. 119.

[12] See E. HORNUNG, *The Ancient Egyptian Books of the Afterlife*, 1999, p. 92.

the enemies are killed and torn apart, and their heads and hearts are incinerated.[13] This act typically belongs to the constellation of Osiris and Seth and celebrates the triumph of life over death.

3. The heart amulet of divine birth and the mythic cycle of the Sun god

Documents such as the papyrus of Nasipautitaui reveal a strong influence of the solar beliefs related to the afterlife: in such documents the journey of the deceased mirrors the journey of the Sun god through the underworld. Among the solar cycle the heart amulet is still a symbol of the justification of the deceased but it is now supposed to open the way to the womb of the cosmic goddess, following the myth of the rebirth of the Sun god.

The heart amulet and rebirth

In the solar cycle, the heart amulet leads leads the way to a journey of change and rebirth. In the first place, the heart amulet protects the deceased during his journey *to* through the Duat. It identifies the deceased to the gods of the hereafter and lends him power over the demons that could present a danger. When this meaning is intended, the deceased may be depicted with the heart in his hands before the gods of the beyond[14]. This gesture is intended to demonstrate the purity of his heart (which was measured in the weighing of the heart) in order for him to be admitted into the company of the other gods. Knowledge of the netherworld conferred on the deceased a netherwordly identity as a "holy god in the following of Thoth", the god who was both the deceased's guide and the learned one.[15] When in possession of the heart amulet, the deceased could enter the most mysterious regions of the underworld so as to be regenerated. It is most assuredly with this meaning that the heart amulet is depicted in the chest of the Aker sphinx in the 5th hour of the *Book of the Amduat*.[16]

In this context, the heart amulet was the symbol of the deceased's wisdom and righteousness, and thus of his pure 'quintessential' being fully restored to the *maetic* primordial order. On occasion, this connection between the heart amulet and cosmic purity is expressed by means of the association of the Wedjat eye with the heart amulet.[17] Although rare, iconographic evidence shows that the heart amulet opened the way to cosmic integration. The depiction of the divine scale beside the primordial couple Geb and Nut,[18] and the depiction of the heart amulet on the hest of the god Shu, in a similar context,[19] clearly show that the justification symbolized by the heart amulet was seen as a prerequisite for regeneration and rebirth.

In the journey of the deceased through the underworld, the magical purpose of the heart amulet is understood as preceding the solar rebirth, which is illustrated by the heart scarab. This interpretation of the heart amulet within the belief system of the solar cycle is iconographically expressed in documents such as the papyrus of Nesipautitaui. In this sense, the heart amulet could have been seen as a 'key' which allowed the deceased to open the gates of the underworld and to come out into the light. This is the reason why the object is depicted in the context of the "going forth by day", or even in the context of the solar journey. The depictions of the solar lustrations of the deceased, such as the one depicted in the tomb of Sennefer (TT 96), should also be understood as having this same meaning. By means of this ritual,[20] the deceased, identified with the sun, is seen to rise from the tomb. Depicted in this context, the heart amulet appears once again as a symbol of the power of wisdom and of purity to open the way into the light.

The heart amulet and the mother goddess

The funerary significance of the solar cycle is largely connected to the solar rebirth that occurred as a return to the beginning of time, to the womb of the great cosmic mother. The divinity that presided over this cycle was Nut, the celestial goddess who welcomed the deceased onto her lap:

> Tu entres en moi et j'embrasse ton image,
> Je suis ton cercueil qui recèle ta forme secrète.
> Mon coeur est avec toi comme ton acte de propriété,
> Il te parle comme 'celui qui est à l'avant du coffre de Nout'.
> Ma bouche est prompte à glorifier ton *ba*,
> Ma magie est la protection de tes membres.[21]

Solar rebirth was only available to those who had triumphed over Seth. Therefore, the possibility of entering the womb of the cosmic goddess depended on the justification achieved in the court of Osiris:

> Bienvenue, Thotemheb, justifié,
> Toi le calme, le silencieux de Karnak (...)
> Mon coeur est pénétré de ton être,
> J'ai fait une large place pour ta momie,

---

13 See H. FRANKFORT, *The Cenotaph of Seti I*, 1933, E.W. VII

14 See Fig. 54 - funerary papyrus of Nesipautitaui (SR 1025, Cairo Egyptian Museum) in A. PIANKOFF, *Mythological Papyri*, Pl. 77. See also Fig. 52 - Funerary Papyrus of Userhatmose (SR 10249, Cairo Egyptian Museum), 21st Dynasty.

15 J. ASSMANN, *The Search for God in Ancient Egypt*, 1984, p. 67

16 See Fig. 89.

17 See the depiction of the heart amulet suspended on a winged Wedjat eye in the coffin A. 228 kept in the Victoria Museum of Egyptian Antiquities, Uppsala - Fig. 111.

18 See Fig. 101 - the depiction of a divine scale next to the primordial couple: in A. NIWINSKI, *Studies on the Illustrated Theban Funerary Papyri*, pl. 29 c-d.

19 See the depiction of a heart amulet on the chest of Shu, in Leiden Papyrus AMS 34 (T.7). See Fig. 102

20 See lustral ceremonies from tomb of Sennefer (Fig. 74) and Ramose (Fig. 75). In both tombs the depiction faces the east and the entrance of the tomb. Similar lustral rituals are depicted among other Theban tombs, such as the tomb of Duauneheh (TT 125) and the tomb of Userhat (Fig. 76) and Khaemhat (TT 57). Note that the lustration depicted on Ramose seems to be performed on the statue of the *ka* but nevertheless with association to the going forth by day. Lustrations cerimonies performed on Sennefer, Userhat and Khaemhat are clearly seen as an event supposed to occur in the Duat and not merely as funerary rituals.

21 .In J. ASSMANN, *Mort et au-delà dans l'Égypte ancienne*, 2003, p. 253.

J'ai sanctifié l'emplacement de ton corps.
Je t'annoncerais auprès du grand dieu,
Pour qu'il te souhaite la bienvenue.
Je te confierai à Harakhty,
Pour qu'il t'accueille parmi ses adorateurs.
Je te recommanderai au maître d'Hermopolis,
Pour qu'il fixe tes offrandres (...)[22]

Therefore, the solar rebirth was the *summum bonum*: only the righteous could be rejuvenated in the womb of the great mother goddess. [23] Within the body of Nut, the deceased merged with the waters of the Nun in order to be purified and completely regenerated.[24] This set of beliefs was deeply rooted in ancestral royal prerogatives and already exists in the *Pyramid Texts*:

> Be pure! Your mother Nut the Great Protectress purifies you, she protects you.[25]

Symbolized by the coffin, the goddess enveloped the deceased and nourished him with her own heart, word and magic. The expression "my heart is with you as yours" indicates that it was the heart of the goddess that could give life to the dead.

It is using this meaning that we must understand the heart amulets depicted on the chests of later depictions of the goddess Nut or Isis.[26] The heart amulet is still a symbol of the justification of the deceased, but now it is supposed to open the way to the womb of the cosmic goddess as well. This regeneration would be followed by the rebirth of the deceased in the guise of Khepri, the rising sun. The triumph of life over death would then be complete.

The cornice heart amulet and the solar child

From the Late Period on the heart amulet seems to be used almost exclusively in the context of the "child-mother goddess" constellation. Although it may be difficult to identify a precise set of rituals, the heart amulet is primarily used as an attribute of the divine children. Later, as mother of the Horus child, Isis is identified as the bestower of legitimate kingship. Having a special significance, the ritual of royal suckling seems to better illustrate the meaning of the heart amulet in this context since it alludes to the goddess as the one who heals. [27] We know for a fact that, during later periods, the heart amulet was primarily used in earthly life. In a particular category of heart amulets, the cornice amulets, the "patient" could be identified with Horus and thus included in a constellation and a mythic situation in which Horus, the embodiment of the helpless child, was bitten by a serpent or a scorpion and healed by his mother Isis through her magical power. [28]

More generally, the Horus child was the figure with whom the sick were identified. The helplessness of the Horus child made him the archetype of all patients, and Isis' magical and protective power was the archetype of medical help. Once interpreted in light of myths about mother and child, the heart amulet was invested with a new meaning. It most probably became a symbol of the all-embracing protection of Isis (or another mother goddess such as Hathor or Neit), a reflection of the growing influence of the concept of "god" in the singular in ritual and magical practices.

Curiously, this later female sacred imagery seems to have always been implicit from the first occurrences of the heart amulet (thus in the context of the *heart of Horus*), since it seems to have been derived from the vase *nw*, the symbol of the mother goddess Nut. This becomes less intriguing if we remember that the royal significance of the later ritual context is not at all diminished. When the mother goddess suckles the divine child, she plays the role of "kingmaker".[29] The later use of the heart amulet in the monumental locks of temple gateways also reaffirms the role of the great goddess as the mother who reveals the hidden cosmic mysteries to the Pharaoh. Thus, the cornice heart amulet should be seen as a symbol of the protective concealment of Horus in Khemmis, the mythic place in the Delta where Isis raised her child Horus in total seclusion, in order to "make him strong".[30] In the same way, once he had reached the beyond, the deceased used the amulet in order to be "suckled" by Nut and to be reborn as a living god.[31]

4. The heart scarab and the mummification

The dismemberment of the body of Osiris means, at first, the momentary triumph of Seth and the failure of the connective principle of life. The lethargy and inertia of the dead Osiris were expressed in his famous epithet "He whose heart no longer beats" or in the expression "still of heart", *wredj ib*.[32] Therefore, the first step in insuring the reanimation of the dead Osiris was to restore the heart to the body, a gesture intended to be performed by female goddesses such as Nut, Isis or Nephtys:

> Recitation by Nut: O King, I have given to you your sister Isis, that she may lay hold of you and give to you your heart for your body. [33]

This gesture was, in fact, re-enacted during mummification and it is possible that it may have been followed by the placement of a cardiac amulet that could be viewed as a heart of eternity. Although the first known archaeological instances of the use of a cardiac amulet such as the heart

[22] In *idem*, p. 261.
[23] *Idem*, p. 267.
[24] In L. SPELLEERS, 'La résurrection et la toilette du mort selon les Textes des Pyramides', *RdE* 3 (1938), pp. 37-67.
[25] Spell 843, in R. FAULKNER, *The Ancient Egyptian Pyramid Texts*, 1969, p. 150.
[26] See Figs. 105 and 106.
[27] J. ASSMANN, *The Search for God in Ancient Egypt*, 1984, p. 134
[28] *Ibidem*, p. 69. See Fig. 98. See also Fig. 99.
[29] See Fig. 95 and 107.
[30] See *ibidem*, p. 133.
[31] The strong connection between the amulet ant the mother goddess can be seen in Fig. 109 and 110.
[32] See A. BLACKMAN, 'The significance of incense and libations in funerary and temple ritual', *ZÄS* 50 (1912), p. 71.
[33] Spell 4 in R. FAULKNER, *The Ancient Egyptian Pyramid Texts*, 1969, p. 2.

scarab occur no earlier than the 13th Dynasty, this practice seems to be described in the *Pyramid Texts*:

> My father has remade his heart, the other having been removed for him because it objected to (?) his ascending to the sky when he had waded in the waters of the Winding Waterway.[34]

The restoration of the heart was a highly symbolic act in that it summarizes the entire process of mummification. This gesture, performed by female deities, was the symbol of the connective power of love. It was the love of Isis that filled the heart of Osiris with life.[35] Thus, the large heart scarab can be seen as a symbol of the connective power of the love of Isis, which was able to reintroduce life to the dismembered, aspective body of Osiris.[36] As a result of the restoration of the heart, a new bodily connectivity could be set in motion. The vital powers of the deceased were recovered and other anthropological elements were assembled:

> C'est profitable pour moi, c'est efficace (?) pour moi. Mon *ba* est avec moi, mon coeur est dans mon corps; mon cadavre est dans la terre, je ne l'ai pas pleuré. La puissance magique est dans mon corps, elle n'a pas été dérobée. J'ai mon pouvoir magique, j'ai mes modes de manifestation, de sorte que je peux manger mes repas avec mon *ka*. Habitant de la terre, je passe la nuit à être renouvelée, à être rajeuni. [37]

The meaningfulness of this gesture explains why it was so often depicted in so many different funerary contexts. Sometimes this gesture is followed by the restoration of other anthropological elements, such as the body, the *ka* and the *ba*, in this way expressing the connective power of the heart to re-unite the multiple elements of life.[38]

The placement of a cardiac amulet within the wrappings of the mummy, or even within the corpse itself, was done in the context of the constellation of Isis, Nephtys and Osiris. It would seem that the heart scarab was the object most closely associated with this ritual that was intended to restore the bodily connectivity of Osiris. Notwithstanding this closer association of the heart scarab with mummification rituals, the heart amulet is also used on occasion to illustrate vignettes of the *Book of the Dead* dedicated to this theme.[39] In this context, we must bear in mind that a phenomenon of magical convergence occurred in funerary cardiac amulets, thus leading to the creation of hybrid objects displaying their dual articulation. Heart amulets depicted in these contexts are the result of an additive, or even a substitutive, integration of the features of the heart scarab. In addition to the depiction of heart amulets, many other depictions may allude to the restoration of the heart to the deceased as a symbolic gesture intended to restore the connective powers of his body. In this context, it may be depicted together with the offering of the *ba*, the *ka* and the corpse.[40] Unlike the heart amulet, the heart scarab retained all of its ritual significance associated with the mummification rituals and also with solar rebirth until the Greco-Roman Period.

*

* *

Integrated within a constelative context, the cardiac amulets were necessarily seen as the result of an interaction between gods and its use seems to be largely interpreted in the timeless light of myth, even when a political and well-defined historical background appears to justify its use.

The ritual contexts of cardiac amulets suggest that, although harkening back to timeless mythical constellations, their meaning did not remain static over time. The contrast between the stability of the ritual use of the heart scarab and the continual reinterpretation of the mythical context of the heart amulet is particularly striking. An explanation for this stems from the close relationship of the heart amulet to the concept of the 'social connectivity', i.e., cosmic integration. Since cosmic integration was the main focus of thinking about explicit theology, it is therefore logical to assume some kind of "contamination" of ritual practices of implicit theology by ideas formulated on the discoursive level of explicit theology. Therefore, the ritual use of the heart amulet as a symbol of justification reflects a significant shift in the use of the object that, much later than the point at which the textual sources formulated it, becomes a symbol of the 'heart-guided man'. Later, when another change in the ritual occurred, once again we witness the clear influence of ideas that sprang up in the context of explicit theology. Although expressed through the imagery of the mother goddess, the use of the heart amulet, from the Late Period on, reflects the 'god-guided man' and the theological formulation of the all-encompassing role of Isis as mother goddess.

Although 'contaminated' by ideas that emerged on the discoursive level, mythic readings of the heart amulet are timeless and should not be interpreted in the context of a chronological framework. Unlike the "theory of the heart", it is virtually impossible to position the "implicit theory of the heart" on the historical continuum. Their differing

[34] Pir 512, § 1162, R. FAULKNER, *The Ancient Egyptian Pyramid Texts*, 1969, p. 188.

[35] See *Idem.*, pp. 65-70.

[36] See J. ASSMANN; *Mort et l'au-delà dans l'Égypte ancienne*, 2003, p. 58-72.

[37] TdS 304, in P. BARGUET, *Les Textes des Sarcophages*, 1986, pp. 230-231.

[38] See block from the tomb of Amenemhat (TT 163). Also in the tomb of Petosiris a similar depiction can be seen. See G. LEFEBVRE, *Le Tombeau de Petosiris*, 1924, pl. XXXII-XXXIII.

[39] See Fig. 58.

[40] The vignette most frequently related to chapter 26 consists in the representation of the deceased kneeling in front of his own *ba* bird. See Fig. 63. The reason for the representation of the *ba* bird in the context of a cardiac spell is related to the magical function of chapter 26, which is a spell that aims to give to the deceased his vital powers back and, among them, the freedom of movements required to the *ba*. See Chapter 26 of the Book of the Dead: 'j'ai de nouveau connaissance grâce à mon coeur (...) on ne retiendra pas prisionners mon âme (*ba*) et mon corps aux portes de l'Occident', in P. BARGUET, *Le Livre des Morts*, 1967, p. 72.

structures and categories are always evident although their valuation may vary over time.

It is curious to note that, in explicit theology, the heart is represented primarily as a single entity: it was first formulated as the seat from which the will of the Pharaoh could reveal itself to his subjects and later as the seat of god in the singular. The heart was then seen as the inner temple from which, once the voice of the self had been silenced, the voice and guidance of the divine could be heard and heeded. In this context, any distinction between cardiac terms assumed a secondary importance. The term *haty* is physically well defined, and it is most closely connected to the idea of the divine, which was central to the concept of personal piety. It was almost certainly because of this that it was ultimately chosen as "the" heart in the singular, an idea that conformed better to the manifestation of the will of the great transcendent god. As a result, this word became the sole cardiac term used in later periods.

On the other hand, in the sources that emerged from the context of implicit theology we are presented with a very different picture of the representation of the heart. This is the realm of images, symbols and iconography. In this context, the heart is primarily viewed as a dualistic entity. As with many other dual instances, including the Two Lands and the Two Maet, this dualistic formulation was intended to express the heart as the all-encompassing seat of life. The two hearts supposed the connective power of Horus, bestower of life and *maet* in the cosmos (through the unification of the Two Lands) and in the microcosmos (the human life). Therefore, the dual definition of the heart was first formulated in light of the mythic combat between Horus and Seth and, at a later point, in light of the mythical union of Re and Osiris. Through the dual heart, understood as both body and mind, a complex mythologisation of human nature which posited the depiction of man as a microcosm where life was seen as a reflection of the *maetic* order was achieved. We view this as a significant and inspiring legacy that has been handed down to us from the Egyptian mind.

DOCUMENTAL CORPUS

A – HEART SCARABS

Cairo Egyptian Museum	SR 9385 SR 9957 SR 9959 SR 10105 CG 12207 CG 85799 JE 41829 CG 13403 SR 95301 CG 12204 JE 61884 JE 72172
Bristish Museum	EA 38073 BM 7925
Reijksmuseum van Oudheden	AO 1a L. II.6
Louvre Museum	E 14005 AF 6981 N 2780 N 2780a N 2780b 2781 AF 6981
Musée Pincée	MTC 719-1
Metropolitan Museum of Art	36.3.2
Kunsthistorisches Museum	5025
Sammlung Ägyptischer Kunst	1595

B – HEART AMULETS

Petrie Museum	UC 8451 UC 52177 UC 38418 UC 38438 UC 28181 UC 28737 UC 38759 UC 38427 UC 38426 UC 38425 UC 38424 UC 38433 UC 38441 UC 38430 UC 38437 UC 38442 UC 38432 UC 28207 UC 28205 UC 28208 UC 38431 UC 38434 UC 38445 UC 38423 UC 22239 UC 38451 UC 1959 UC 61462 UC 38422 UC 58020 UC 22885 UC 22884 UC 22883 UC 22882 i,iii UC 38439 UC 38417 UC 38436 UC 38449 UC 38435 UC 38443 UC 71972 UC 38440 UC 28204 UC 38419 UC 22527 UC 38429 UC 38428 UC 22526 UC 22524 UC 22525 UC 38447 UC 52194 UC 38420 UC 12811 UC 52051 UC 38446 UC 69861 UC 52609 UC 52606 UC 52607 UC 52608 UC 52612 UC 52605 UC 13212 UC 52611 UC 52616 UC 52618 UC 52620 UC 52613 UC 22526 A
Cairo Egyptian Museum	SR 9222 SR 9228

SR 9276
CG 12051
SR 9386
SR 9202
SR 9208
SR 9218
SR 9198
CG 53436
SR 9195
JE 28734
CG 12958
CG 12960
JE 54922
JE 68509
JE 68510
JE 67209
JE 67210
JE 67211
SR 9254
CG 13041
JE 67212
SR 9243
CG 13026
CG 5240
CG 5257
SR 9238
JE 54027
JE 67208
CG 13002
JE 68508
SR 9273
CG 5239
CG 12957
JE 54920
JE 54919
JE 54924
CG 5255
SR 9271
JE 85726
SR 9249
CG 5221
CG 62067
SR 9220
SR 9197
SR 9201
CG 12056
SR 9259
CG 5233
SR 9219
SR 9194
JE 85801
CG 12069
SR 5047
CG 52683
JE 35375
SR 9227
SR 9224
JE 46352b
SR 9225

SR 9203
SR 9199
SR 9258
SR 9252
SR 9230
SR 9229
SR 9236
SR 9231
SR 9211
SR 9256
CG 12137
JE 85802
SR 9260
SR 9280
SR 9226
CG 53191
SR 9246
SR 9245
JE 85727
SR 9248
CG 13151
CG 13216
CG 13146
SR 9266
JE 46352a
CG 53212
CG 13233
CG 13299
SR 9274
SR 9232
SR 9267
CG 5254
JE 85728
JE 45460
CG 12062
SR 9282
CG 13152
CG 13232
CG 13302
CG 13301
CG 13297
CG 12060
SR 9265
CG 13300
SR 9264
CG 5251
SR 9272
JE 85806-85812
JE 85804
JE 85803
JE 86044
SR 9217
JE 92634
CG 53221
CG 53220
SR 9262
SR 9239
JE 68016
SR 9205

SR 9213
JE 92635
SR 10813
JE 86043
SR 9210
SR 9215
SR 9221
SR 9200
SR 9196
JE 86976
SR 9204
SR 10824
JE 92638
SR 9261
SR 9279
SR 9269
SR 9263
SR 9214
JE 86045
CG 5230
CG 34415
CG 12127269a.3 (CIV)
256.uuu (CIV)
256.qqq (CIV)
JE 92638
JE 85777
JE 28606
JE 98783
CG 52956

Nubian Museum, Aswan

1034

Louvre Museum

E 18243
E 18248
E 2267
AF 8837
AEO 24749
E 2770
AF 11552
AF 9901
E 18223
AF 9900
AEO 30354
E 13709
AF 11534
N 4619
AEO 09644
AEO 10167
AEO 10248
AF 2589
E 14708
E 3573
E 4960
N 551
AF 9101
AE028135
AE028134
AE028133
E 3577
AE0096587
AEO 23346
AF 11543
AF 11543
AEO 09652
AEO 23440
AF 11526
AEO 30788
AF 8826
AF 9902
AF 9903
AEO 23441
AF 11559
E 18245
AF 8828
AF 11547
AEO 23345
AEO 23442
E 18242
AEO 23347
AF 8822
AEO 35074
AF 11531
AF 11561
ALO 31504
AEO 23438
E 18237
AEO 09660
AF 11553
AEO 10284
AF 6968
AF 10855E 1688
AE 028353
AF 11523
E 2309
AF 2333
E 16221
AF 2578
AEO 30798
AEO 30053
AF 11524
AF 10447
AF 12141
N 4622
E 1107
AE O10164
E 11682
AEO10414
AEO31622
AEO3148

British Museum

64201
EA50742
6261
64181
65544

3624
64292
8128
5600
15598
89.10-14-207
26807
EA29440
EA 48978
EA 35412

Allard Pierson Museum 12994

Turin Egyptian Museum n. Cat. 6862
Inv. Prov. 1315

Kunsthistorisches Museum Inv. Nr. 4367

Museum of Fine Arts of Budapest N Inv. 512656
N. Inv. 50.353

Metropolitam Museum of Art 22.2.24/54831
10.130.1771
26.7.743
10.130.1806
10.130.1795
10.130.2538
38.8/115512 tf

Rijksmuseum van Oudheden B326

Kestner Museum, Hannover Inv. Nr 1951,5

Roemer & Pelizaeus Museum, Hildesheim Inv. Nr. 195

Michael C. Carlos Museum, Atlanta 192172

Museu Nacional de Arqueologia, Lisboa Cat. 191, E 57

C – MEASUREMENT INSTRUMENTS

Cairo Egyptian Museum

SR 39473CG
1930JE
27258CG
2005

Louvre Museum E 18224

Pelizaeus Museum, Hildesheim 5115

Museu da Farmácia, Lisboa Nº Catálogo 53

D – HEART AMULETS ON MONUMENTAL LOCKS

Cairo Egyptian Museum CG 37765

Berlin Egyptian Museum N 15424

E – HEART SHAPPED VASES

Cairo Egyptian Museum JE 57203
829
JE 86848

Musée Champollion, Figéac E 21801

Museu da Farmácia, Lisboa Nº de catálogo 34

F – DEPICTIONS OF THE HEART/HEART AMULET

Cairo Egyptian Museum-

Coffin (29651)
Coffin (CG 6044)
Coffin of a man (CG 6153)
Coffin of a man (17432 A)
Coffin of Amenempermut (CG 6153)
Coffin of Ankhefenmut (CG 6109)
Coffin of Chebeti (CG 6028)
Outer coffin of Direpu (JE 29771)
Inner coffin of Direpu (J.E. 29669/CG 6084)
Coffin of Djedmaetiuesankh
Coffin of Duasahotep (21/11/16/11
Inner coffin of Maherpa - JE 31378
Outer coffin of Nesikhonsu (JE 26199/SR 10325)Inner coffin of Nesikhonsu (SR 10325)
Coffin of Nesitanebet-taui (JE 29716)
Coffin of Padiamun (CG 6233/6235)
Mummy cover of Padiamun (CG 6235)
Coffin of Pamechem (CG 6009-6011)
Inner coffin of Pakharu (CG 6122/6121)
Mummy cover of Pakharu (CG 6122/6121)
Outer coffin of Pakharu (CG 6122/6121)
Outer coffin of Pinedjem II (JE 26197)
Inner coffin of Pindejem II (J.E. 26197)
Coffin of Senu (JE 29651)
Coffin of Tauheret (C.G. 61032)
Cartonage of Tenkeret (JE 35055)
Coffin of Tjenetethatnetjeru (CG 6191Sarcophagus of Pekheti (14/11/24/3)
Sarcophagus (JE 34632)
Sarcophagus of Setueret (23/1/21/9)
Shawabty of Yuya (SR 95368)
Statuette of a *ba* bird of Yuya (JE 95312)
Avian statuette of Horus (JE 30335)
Statuette of a bird *akhem* (SR 6850
Group sculpture of Sennefer (JE 36574)
Statue (JE 58508)
Statue of Kahep (?) (SR 6311)
Group sculpture of princes and nanny (JE 98831)
Statue of a divine child (SR 46380)

Statue of Ísis and Horpakhered (JE 91326)
Statuette of Horpakhered (CG 38182)Statuette of Horpakhered (CG 38176
Cippus of Horpakhered (CG 9402)

Tomb relief from the tomb of Siesi (SR 13459)
Funerary stela (SR 7270)
Funerary papyrus (SR 10236)
Funerary papyrus (SR 10229)
Funerary papyrus of Isitemakhbit (JE 95657)
Funerary papyrus of Nesipatiutaui (SR 1025)
Funerary papyrus of Nisitanebet-taui (SR 40017)

Funerary papyrus (SR IV 982)
Funerary papyrus (JE 95652)
Funerary papyrus Djedkhonsuiefankh (s/n)
Funerary papyrus Tawedjatré (s/n)
Funerary papyrus Tabaketenkhonsu (SR 10223)
Funerary papyrus (SR 10232)
Funerary papyrus of Padiamun (SR 10236)
Funerary papyrus of Nesitanebet-taui (SR 40017)
Book of the Dead of Yuya
Book of the Dead of Userhatmés (SR 10249)
Book of the Dead of Maherpa (CG 24095)
Book of the Dead of Pinedjem I (SR 11488)

Louvre Museum

Funerary mask (N 28676)
Funerary mask (E 26834)
Coffin (E 13028)Mummy cartonage (E 32634)
Coffin of Amen-hotep (E 13028)
Coffin of Amenemopet (E 3864)
Coffin of Besenmut (E 10374)
Coffin of Kaahapi (N 2566)
Coffin of Irethor (E 11296)
Coffin of Itnedjés (N 2564)
Inner coffin of Paser (N 2570)
Coffin of Udjarenés (N 2626)
Coffin of Unet (AF 9593)
Mummy cover of Unet (AF 9593)
Coffin of Tanutamon (N 2562)
Inner coffin of Tanethereret (E 13034)
Funerary chest of Tjauen-hui (N 4124)
Corn mummy (E 12183)
Ram's coffin (number unknown)
Stela of Mesu and Api (C 280)
Ostracon (N 1562)
Ostracon (E 25309Statue of Isis and Horpakhered (E 3637)
Ave *akhem* (E 5844)

Painted linen (N 3076)
Painted linen (AF 6486)
Jumilhac Papyrus (E 17110)
Funerary Papyrus (N 3128)
Funerary Papyrus (E 8079)
Funerary Papyrus (6335)
Funerary Papyrus of Ahmose (N 3281)
Funerary Papyrus of Amenemsaef (N 3292)
Funerary Papyrus of Pacheri and Achakhet (N 3126)
Funerary Papyrus of Nesipakachuti (E 17401)
Funerary papyrus of Tabaketenkhonsu (N 3287)
Funerary papyrus of Takhibiat (N 3248)
Funerary Papyrus of Usiruer (N 3125)
Funerary Papyrus of Usiruer (N 3284)
Book of the Dead (N 3099)
Book of the Dead (N 3073)
Book of the Dead (E 7716)
Book of the Dead (N 3198)
Book of the Dead (AEO 23825)
Book of the Dead of Ahmose (N 3086)
Book of the Dead of Amenet (N 3151)
Book of the Dead of Amenemheb Mahu (N 3097)
Book of the Dead of Asetirchet (E 6130)
Book of the Dead of Chachanuk (N 3089)
Book of the Dead of Chechonk (N 3152)
Book of the Dead of Djedhor (N 3079)
Book of the Dead of Horsaiset (N 3082)
Book of the Dead of Horsaiset (N 3144)
Book of the Dead of Hornedjitef (N 3081)
Book of the Dead of Imhotep (N 3142)
Book of the Dead of Khnumibré (SN 173)
Book of the Dead of Nebked (N 3068)
Book of the Dead of Nedjemet (E 6258)
Book of the Dead of Neferibré (N 3084)
Book of the Dead of Neferuebenef (N 3092)
Book of the Dead of Nehemesrataui (N 3087)
Book of the Dead of Nesiptah (N 3100)
Book of the Dead of Nesipameduchepsés (N 3153)
Book of the Dead of Nesmin (N 3096)
Book of the Dead of Padihorparé (N 3249)
Book of the Dead of Padipep (E 3233)
Book of the Dead of Pebereré and Pediamenopet (N 3090)
Book of the Dead of Serusir (N 3129)
Book of the Dead of Takhonsu (N 3207)
Book of the Dead of Takheben (N 3272)
Book of the Dead of Tjahapiamon (N 3094)
Book of the Dead of Uennefer (N 5450)
Book of the Dead of Usiruer (N 3143)
Book of the Dead of Usiruer (N 3296)

Gregorian Museum, Vatican

Coffin of Ikhi (N. Inv. 2503533)
Mummy cover of Ikhi (N. Inv. 2503532)
Coffin of Hetep-heres (N. Inv. 3807321)

Bristish Museum

Block from the tomb of Amenemhat (TT 163)
Coffin (BM 24793)
Outter coffin of Amenemopet
Coffin of Irthoreru (20045)
Coffin of Itineb (BM 6693)
Coffin of Pasen-hor (BM 24906)
Funerary mask (29472)
Funerary Papyrus (BM 9932)
Funerary Papyrus (N° 9900)
Funerary Papyrus of Keracher (BM 9995)
Funerary Papyrus of Nedjemet (EA 10541)
Funerary Papyrus of Nesitanebetacheru (BM 10554)
Funerary Papyrus of Padikhonsu (BM 10004)
Book of the Dead of Ani (N 10407)
Book of the Dead of An-hai (BM 10472/4)
Book of the Dead of Hor
Book of the Dead of Hunefer (N° 9901)
Book of the Dead of Nebseni (EA 9900/32)
Book of the Dead of Tameniu

Turin Egyptian Museum

Coffin of Nebankh
Book of the Dead of Kha and Merit

Berlin Egyptian Museum

Ostracon(N 728Shawabty (N. Inv. 4401)
Menat collar
Funerary mask (N. Inv. 1258)
Cippus of Horpakhered (N. Inv. 4434)
Statuette of Horpakhered (Inv. N. 7559)
Statuette of Horpakhered (Inv.N. 8794)
Funerary Papyrus of Amenemuia (Inv. Nr. P 3127)
Book of the Dead of Nakhtamon (N° Inv. 22)

Kunsthistorisches Museum

Group sculpture of Meriptah (N. Inv. 48).
Book of the Dead of Nebseni (N. Inv. AOS 3859)
Book of the Dead of Khonsui (N. Inv. 3862)
Funerary Papyrus of Khonsumés (N. Inv. AOS 3859)

Metropolitan Museum of Art

Relief of Menkheper (41.160.104)
Corn Mummy (5898 A-D)
Book of the Dead of Nani (0.3.31)

Aswan Museum

Sarcophagus of Khai (2686)

Cleveland Museum of Art

Shawabty of Tacheri (1914.597)
Shawabty of Djehutimés (1914.589)
Shawabty of Djehutimés (1914.590)
Book of the Dead of Hori (1921.1032).
Coffin of Bakenmut (1914.561.a-b)
Eton College, Windsor
Coffin of Amen-hotep (ECM 1876)

Museu Nacional de Arqueologia, Lisboa

Inner coffin of Pabasa (E 332)

Château-Musée de Boulogne-sur-mer

Coffin of Nehemsimontu

Museu Kestner, Hannover

Funerary mask (N 1976.68)

Oriental Institut Museum, Chicago

Papyrus Ryerson (OIM 9787)
Papyrus Milbank (OIM 10486)

Museum of Fine Arts, Boston

Plaquete (S 23-M-591)

Rijksmuseum van Oudheden, Leiden

Book of the Dead of Tauheret (N. Inv. MAS 40)
Book of the Dead (N° 11)
Book of the Dead (N° 1)

Roemer Pelizaeus Museum

Second coffin of Penniu (Inv 1902b)
Third coffin of Penniu (Inv 1902c)
Michael Carlos Museum, Atlanta
Inner coffin of Iautaicheret (1999.I.A-D)
Coffin of Tanakhtentahat (1999.I.17 A-D)

Ny Carlsberg Glypotek

Coffin of Sesekhneferu (1908 E 118)
Coffin of Gautsechenu (1930 A 583),

TEMPLE DECORATION

Deir el-Bahari, temple of Hatshepsut, second terrace, south colonnade: Hatshepsut/Thutmosis III wears the solar amulet

Abido, cenotaph's temple of Seti I: Lustration ceremony of the Pharaoh Merenptah. Slaughter of the enemies

Karnak, Gate of Ptolemy III, South façade: offering of a double heart amulet

Karnak, Temple of Ptah: depiction of a divine child with the amulet

Musauarat es-Sufra, Temple of Apedemak: depiction of Arnekhanami

Ermant, Ptolemaic *mammisi*: Depiction of Nefertum Philae, Temple of Isis: Horpakhered wears the amulet in many of the scenes depicted on the temple

Philae, *mammisi:* Horpakhered wears the amulet in many of the scenes depicted on the temple. Depiction of a god with a vase and a heart on the top of his head
Gate of Adrian, South wall: depiction of the heart amulet on a monumental lock
Dendera, temple of Hathor: Ihi wears the amulet in many of the scenes depicted on the temple

Medinet Habu, Funerary chapel of Amenirdis: Scene of the opening of the mouth cerimony

Deir el-Medina, temple of Hathor: s

TOMB DECORATION

Valley of the Kings
Tomb of Ramses IX (KV 6): Slaughter of the enemies
Tomb of Ramses VI (KV 9),
Book of the Night: Osiris wears the heart amulet.
Book of the Amduat: The Aker sphinx wears the heart amulet
Theban necropolis
Tomb of Khakhebenet (TT 2)
Tomb of Neferabu (TT 5)
Tomb of Khonsu (TT 31)
Tomb of Amenemopet (TT 41)
Tomb of Userhat (TT 51)
Tomb of Ramose (TT 55)
Tomb of Khaemhat (TT 57)
Tomb of Menna (TT 69)
Tomb of Sennefer (TT 96)
Tomb of Duauneheh (TT 125)
Tomb of Amenemuia (TT 178)
Tomb of Neferenpet (TT 178)
Tomb of Ipuki and Nebamon (TT 181)
Tomb of Nebenmaet (TT 219)
Tomb of Rai (TT 255)
Tomb of Irinefer (TT 290)
Tomb of Nefersekheru and Pabasa (TT 296)
Tomb of Nakhtamon (TT 341)
Tomb of Inherkhaui (TT 359)
Tomb of Simut (TT 409)

Tuna el-Gebel
Tomb of Petosiris

Tanis, royal necropolis
Tomb of Osorkon II
Tomb of Osorkon III

Aswan
Tomb of Kagumu (n° 15)

Bahariya oasis
Tomb of BannentiuTomb of Taneferetebastet

Dakhla oasis
Tomb of Petubastis
Tomb of Petosíris

Aniba
Tomb of Penniut

ILLUSTRATIONS

1. HEART AMULETS

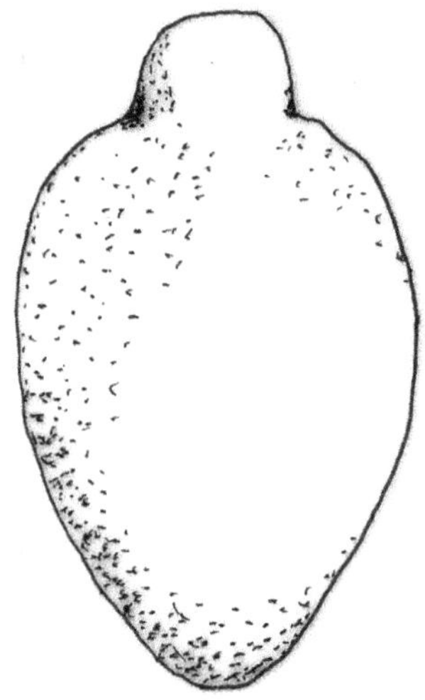

1. Pendulum heart amulet
(UC 52194, Petrie Museum)

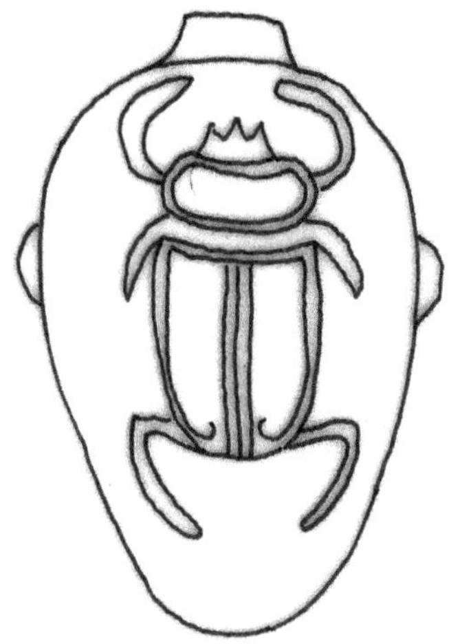

2. Pendulum heart amulet
(SR 9205/CG 12127, Cairo
Egyptian Museum), from Bab
el-Gasus, 21st Dynasty

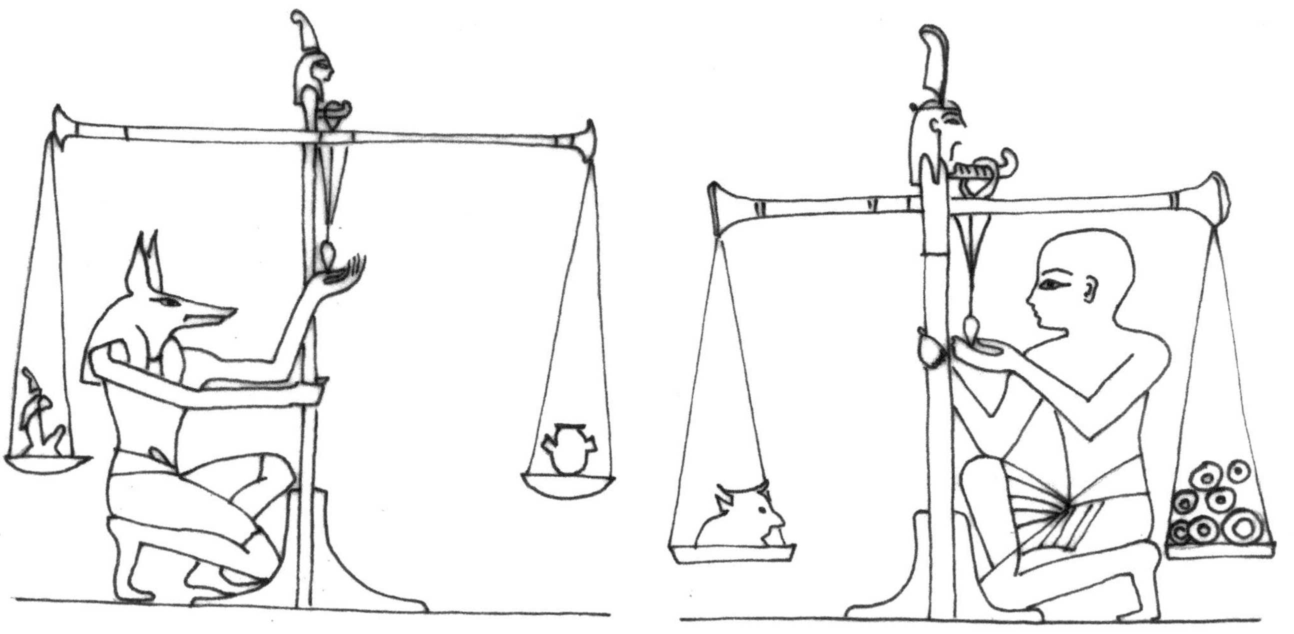

3. Depictions of scales
Left: Scale depicted in the scene of the weighing of the heart of the papyrus of Neferuebenef
(N 3092, Louvre Museum)
Right: Scale used in earthly activities depicted in the tomb of Ipuki (TT 181). New Kingdom

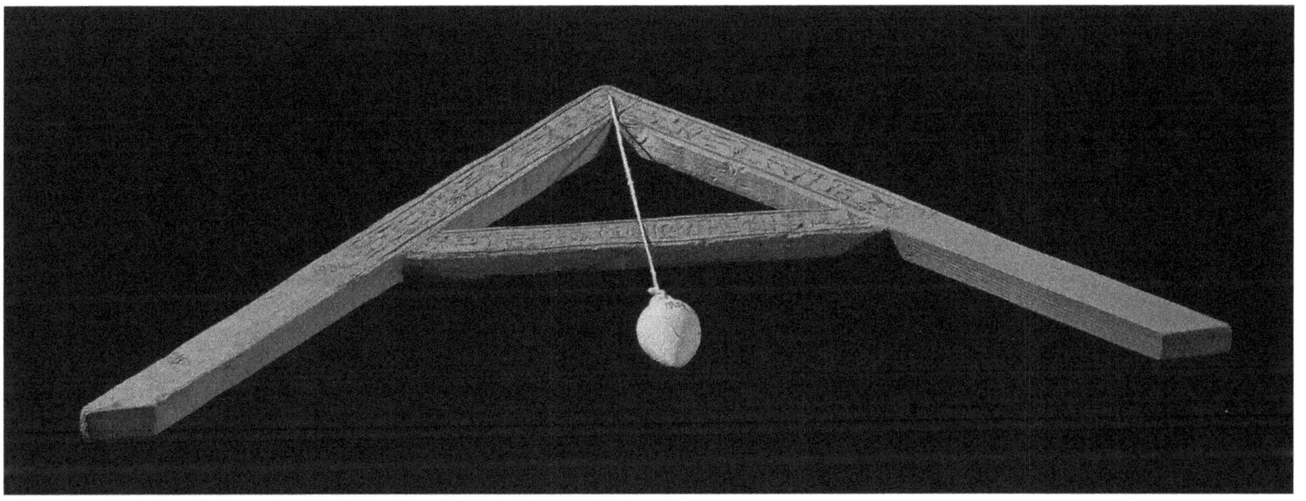

3.a. Horizontal level. (JE 27258, Cairo Egyptian Museum), from the tomb of Sennedjem (TT 1), Ramessid Period. Photo in E. HORNUNG, B. BRYAN, *The Quest of Immortality: Treasures of Ancient Egypt*, 2002, p. 148

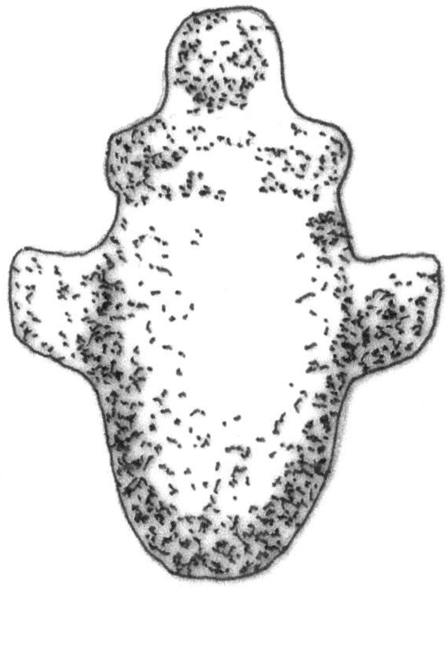

4. Pendulum of a scale shaped as a heart amulet (E 18224, Louvre Museum), Late Period

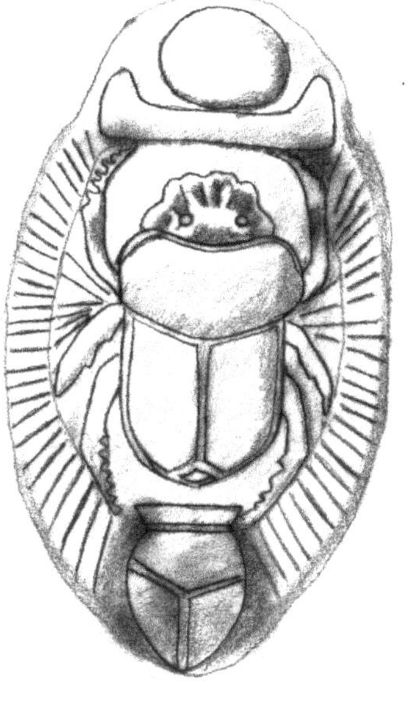

5. Pendulum heart amulet of Khaemwaset (Collection Hoffmann), Ramessid Period

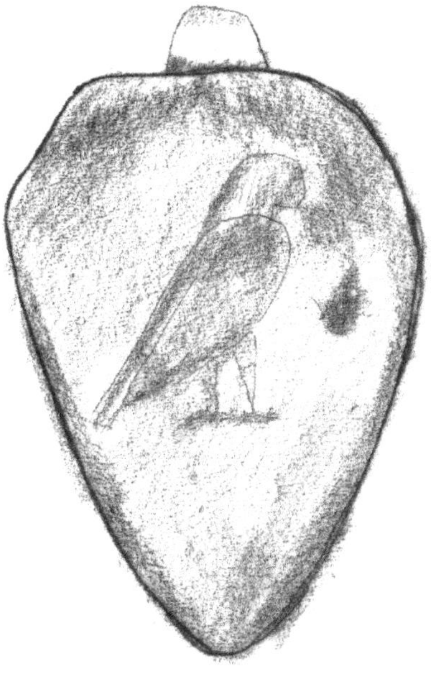

6. Pendulum heart amulet with the depiction of a *ba* bird (JE 41826, Cairo Egyptian Museum), from Aniba, Ramessid Period

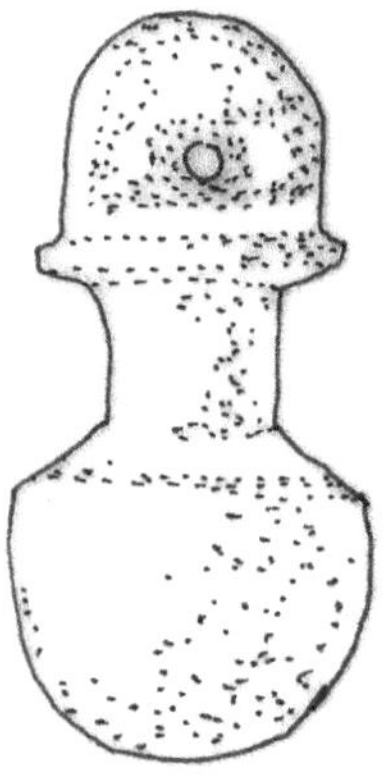

7. Vase amulet, from mastaba of Imapepi (Dakhla Oasis), Old Kingdom. Drawing after MINAULT-GOUT, *Balat II: Le mastaba d'Ima-Pepi*, 1992, p. 90

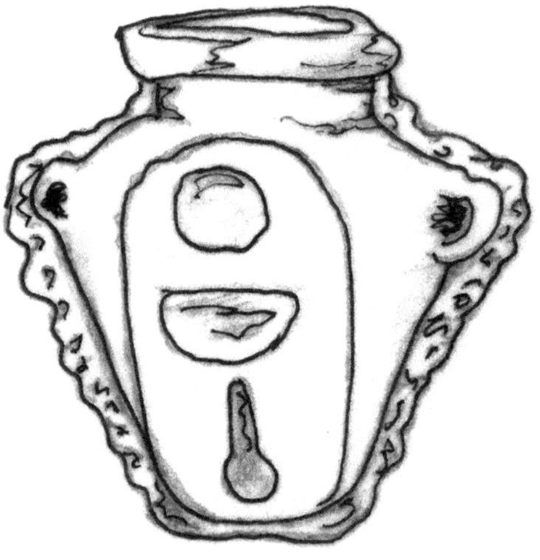

8. Vase heart amulet Louvre Museum (N 551), from Theban necropolis (?), reign of Mentuhotep II

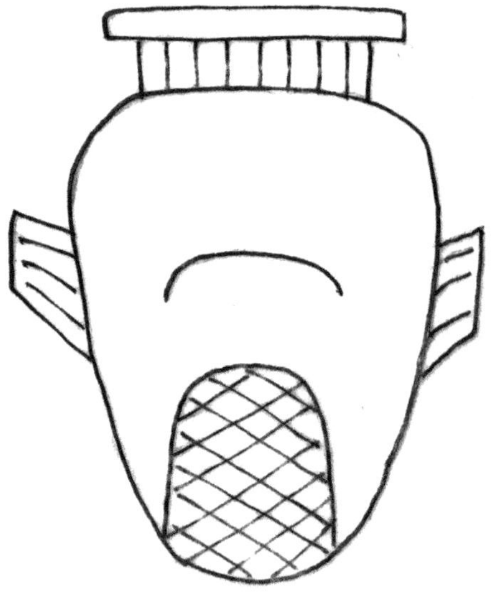

9. Vase heart amulet (SR 9199/JE 28490/CG 12053, Cairo Egyptian Museum), from Mit Rahina, Late Period (?). Hollow object

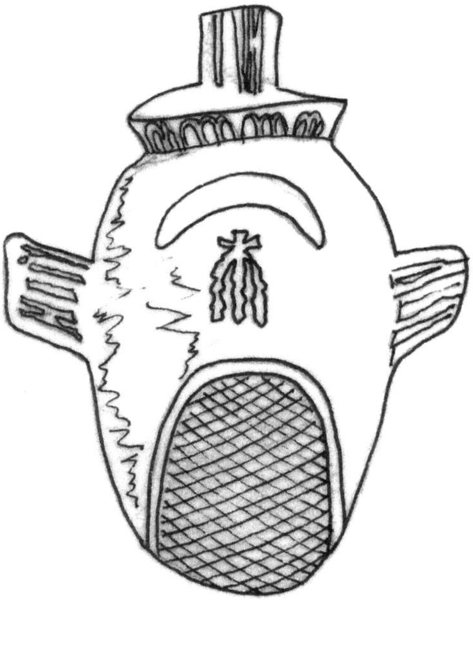

10. Vase heart amulet (E 14708, Louvre Museum), Late Period (?)

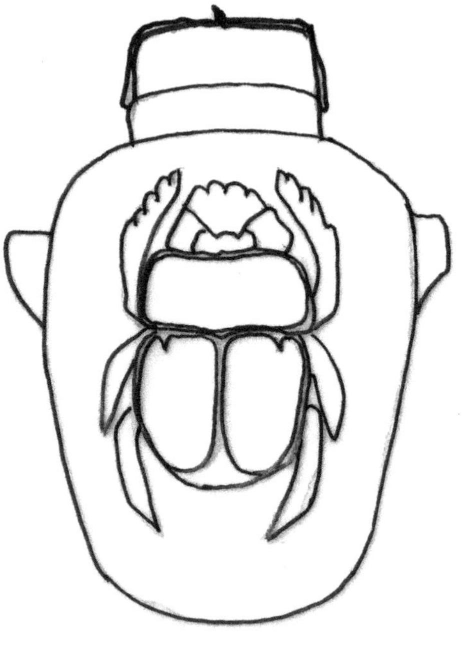

11. Vase heart amulet (SR 9203/CG 12914, Cairo Egyptian Museum). Hollow object

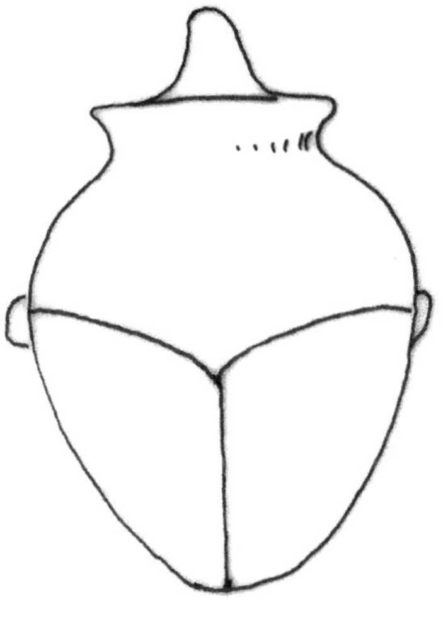

12. Vase heart amulet (CG 5233, Cairo Egyptian Museum), Third Intermediate Period. Drawing after G. REISNER, *Amulets*, I, pl. I

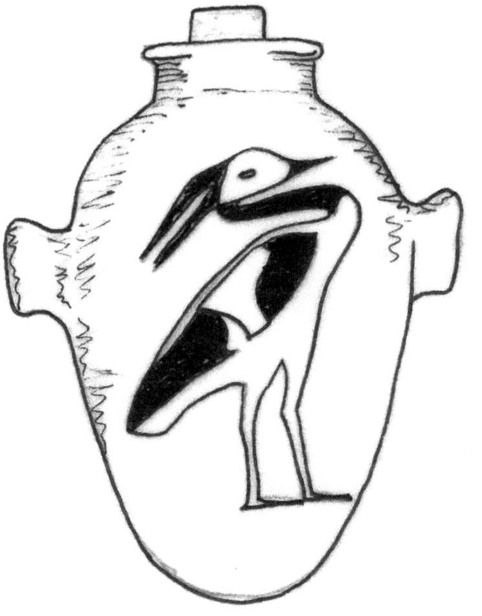

13. Vase heart amulet (CG 62067, Cairo Egyptian Museum), from the tomb of Tutankhamun (KV 62)

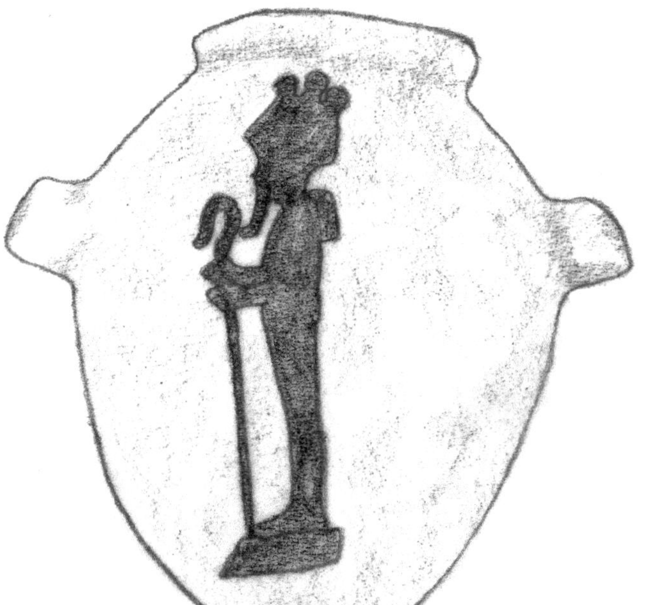

14. Vase heart amulet with the depiction of a standing Osiris (JE 34409, Cairo Egyptian Museum)

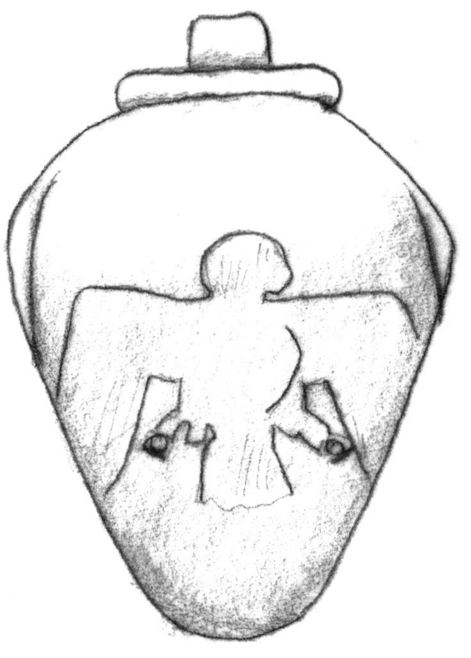

15. Vase heart amulet with the depiction of a *ba* bird (1034, Nubian Museum)

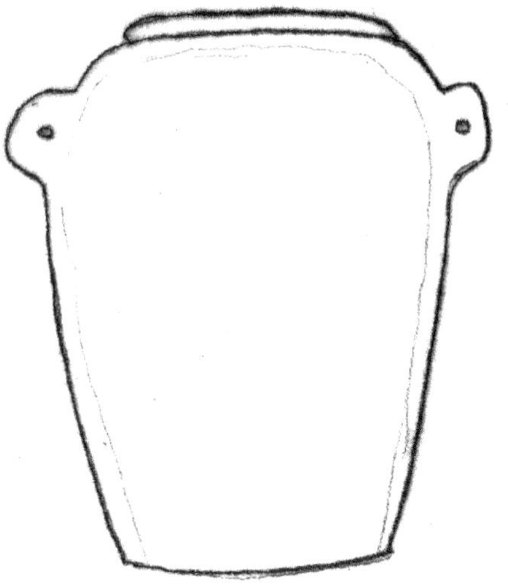

16. Heart-shaped vase inscribed with the cartouches of Apries (CG 829, Cairo Egyptian Museum), Late Period

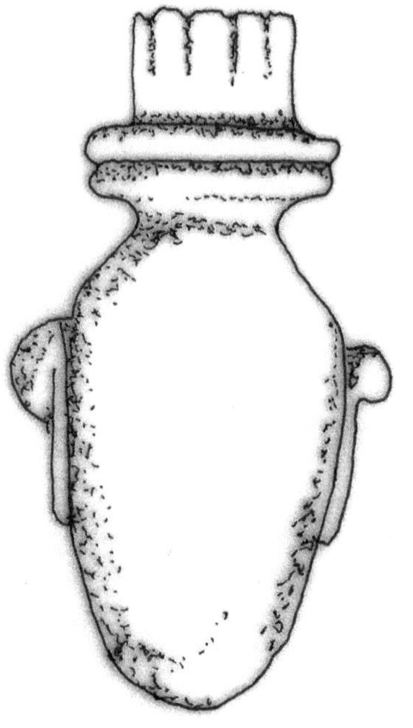

17. Cornice heart amulet (AF 11531, Louvre Museum)

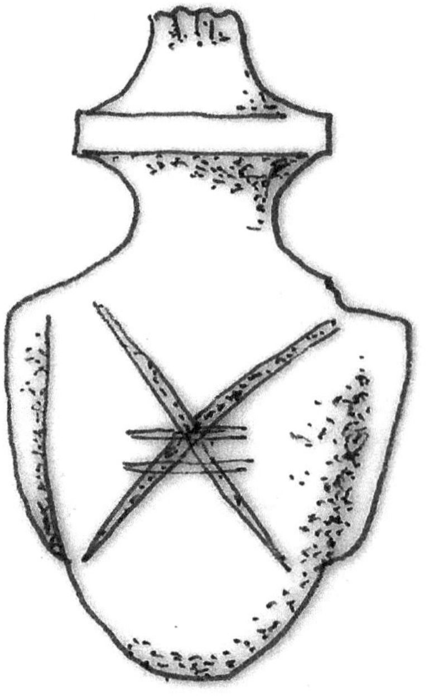

18. Cornice heart amulet (UC 38428, Petrie Museum)

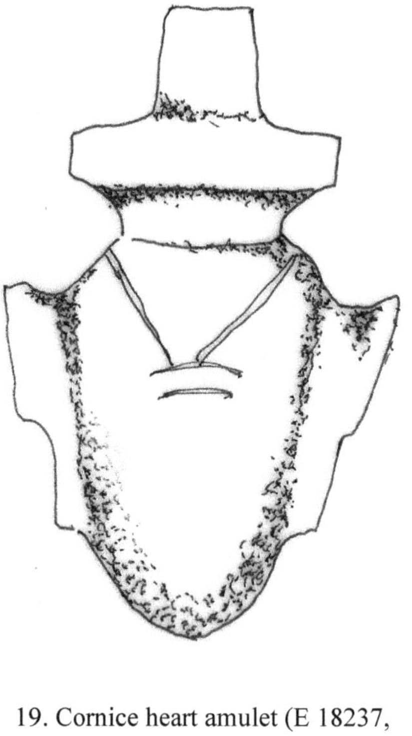

19. Cornice heart amulet (E 18237, Louvre Museum)

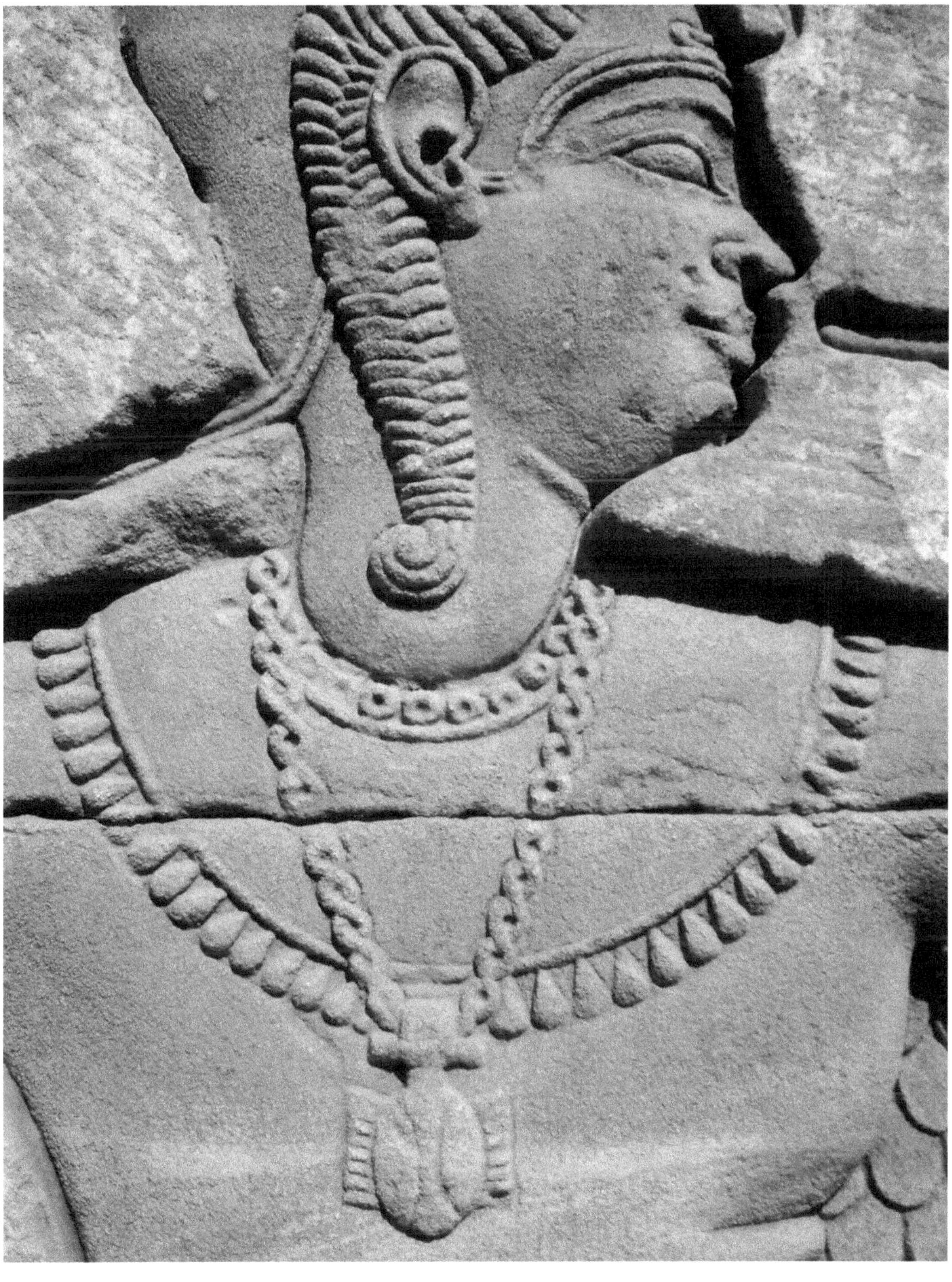

20. Dendera, precinct of Hathor, Roman *mammisi*

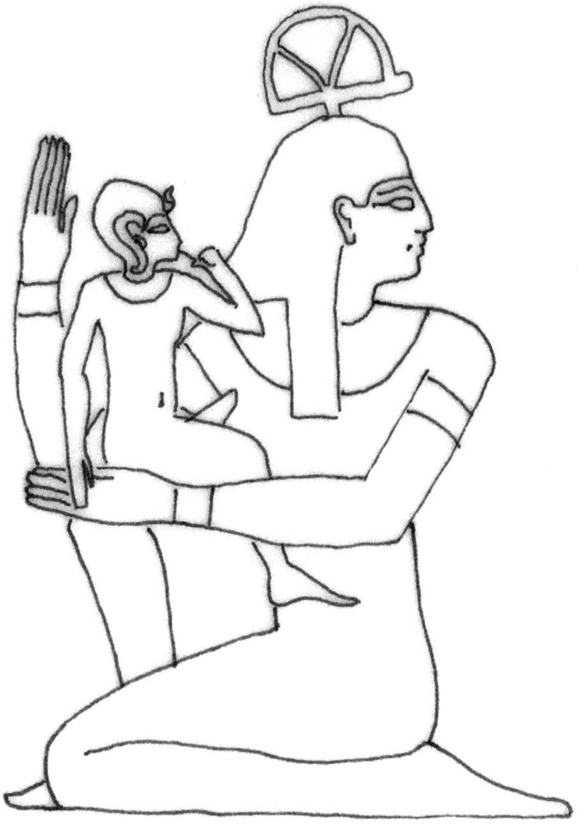

21. Ermant, Greco-Roman *mammisi* (now lost). Drawing after R. LEPSIUS, *Denkmäler,* Abth.IV.Bl.59

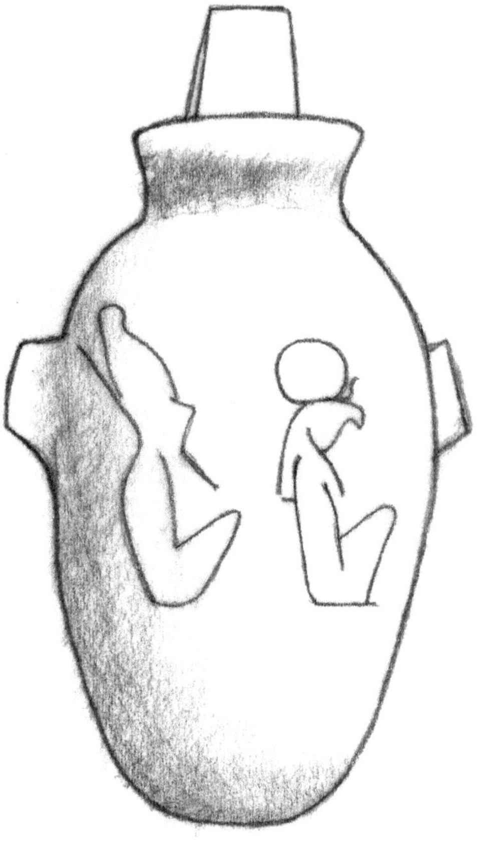

22. Cornice heart amulet (AE0 28353, Louvre Museum)

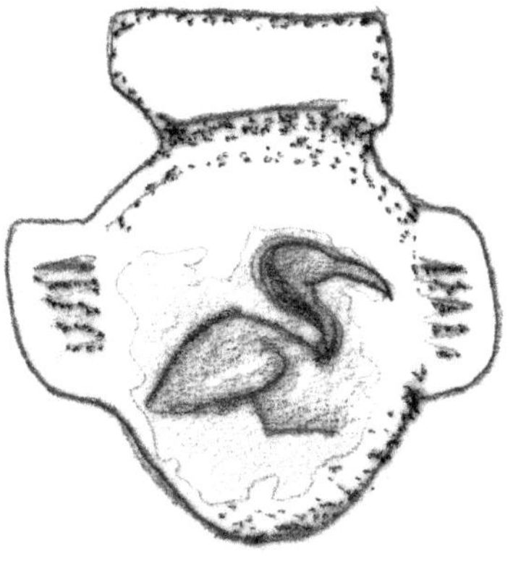

23. Cornice heart amulet with the depiction of an ibis (UC 38447, Petrie Museum), from Dendera, Greco-Roman Period

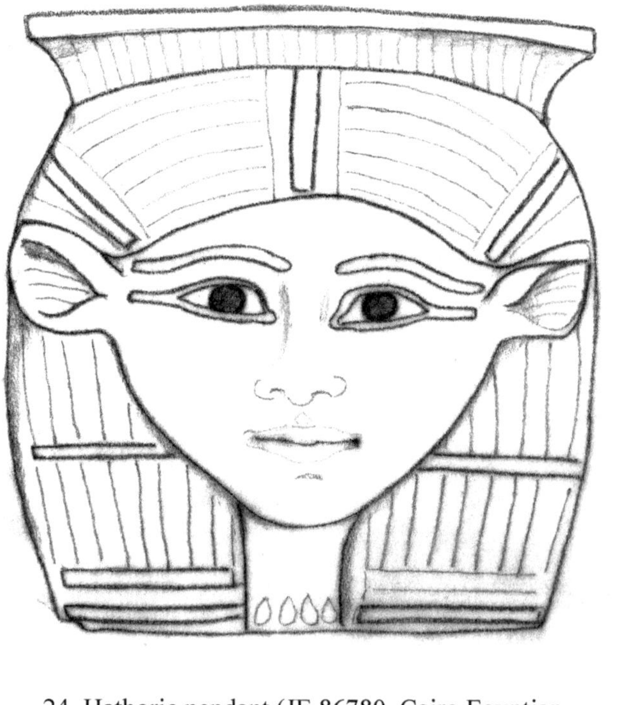

24. Hathoric pendant (JE 86780, Cairo Egyptian Museum), from Mit Rahina, Third Intermediate Period

2. COMPOSITE FORMS OF THE HEART AMULET

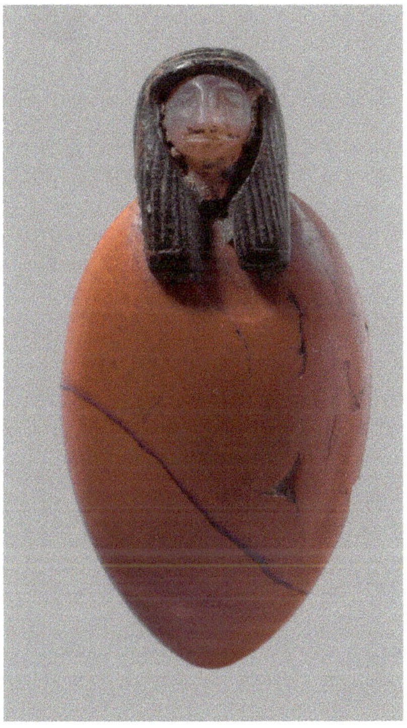

25. Human-headed heart amulet (DP136533, Metropolitan Museum of Art). Gift of Miss A. M. Hegemann, 1938 (38.8).Copyright: The Metropolitan Museum of Art

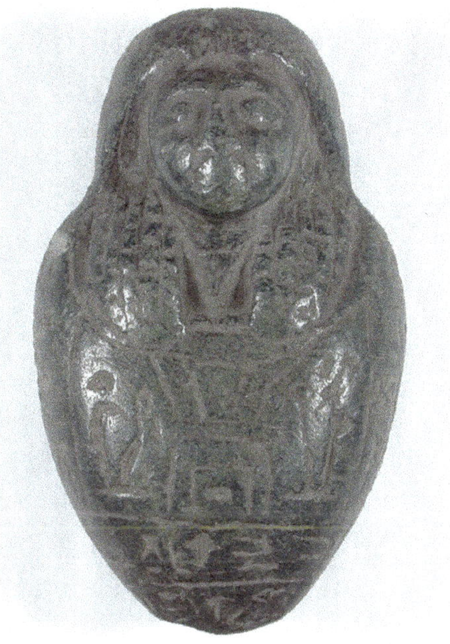

26. Human-headed heart amulet (UC 52605, Petrie Museum). Copyright: Petrie Museum of Egyptian Archaeology, University College London

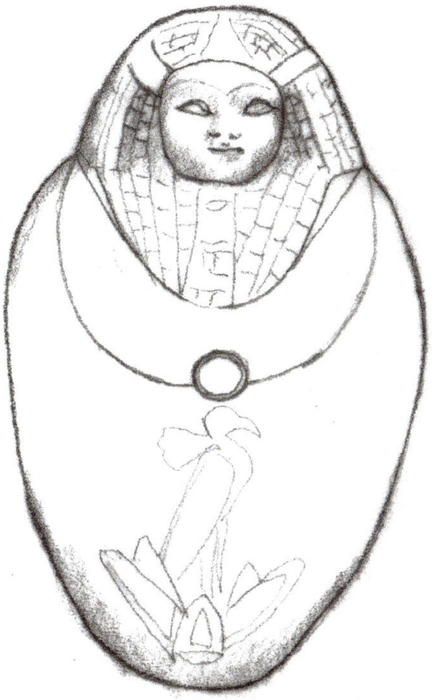

27. Human-headed heart amulet (Inv. B326, Rijksmuseum van Oudheden)

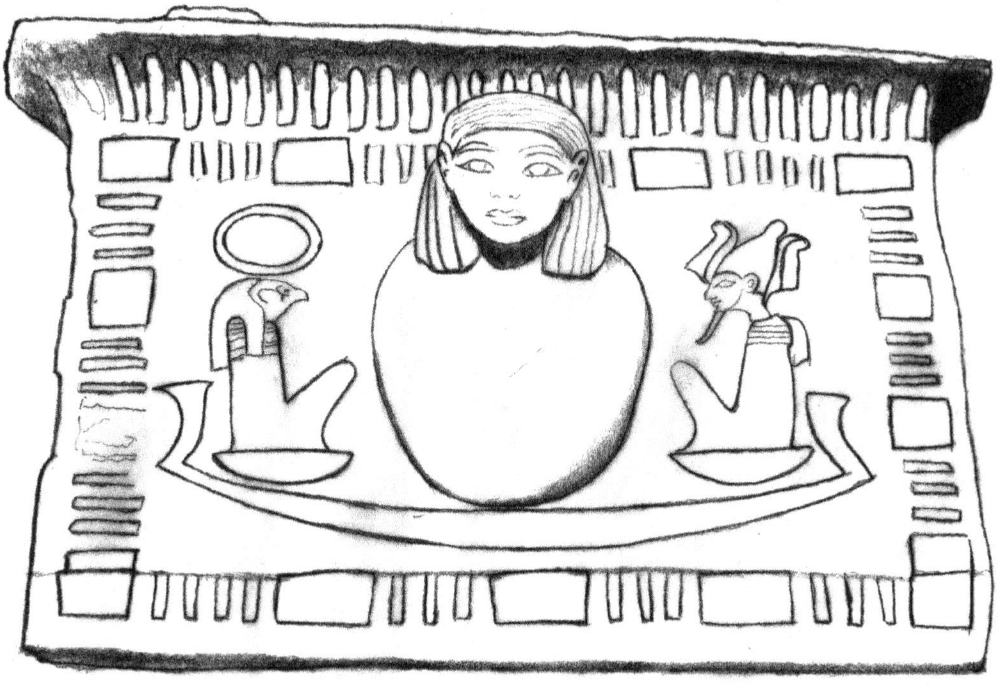

28. Pectoral of the lady Kiemneferwy (JE 92638, Cairo Egyptian Museum), from the funerary complex of Sekhemkhet (Sakara), Ramessid Period

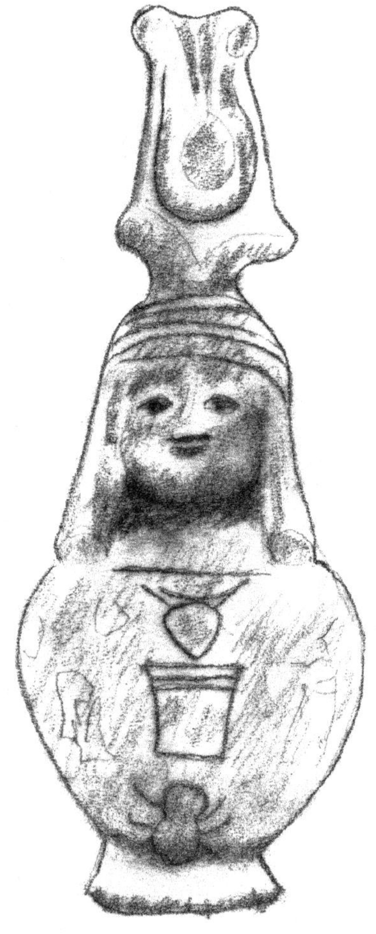

29. Miniature statuette of Osiris Canopus, Greco-Roman Period. Drawing after W. PETRIE, *Amulets*, 1914, p. 36

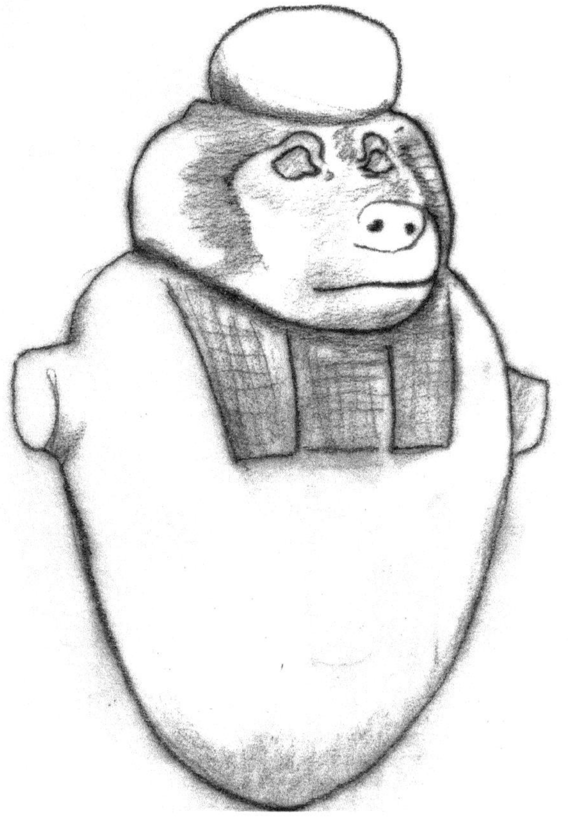

30. Animal-headed heart amulet (JE 86045, Cairo Egyptian Museum), from the burial of Psusennes I (Tanis), 21st Dynasty

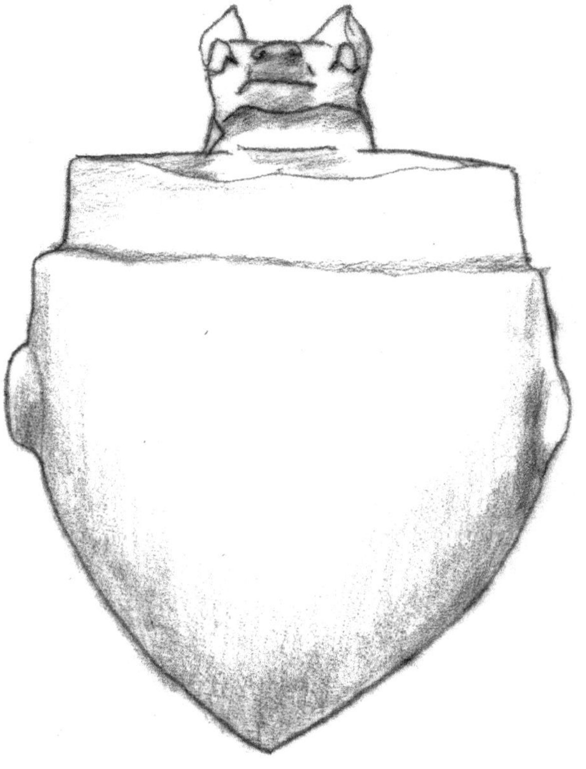

31. Animal-headed heart amulet
(E 11682, Louvre Museum)

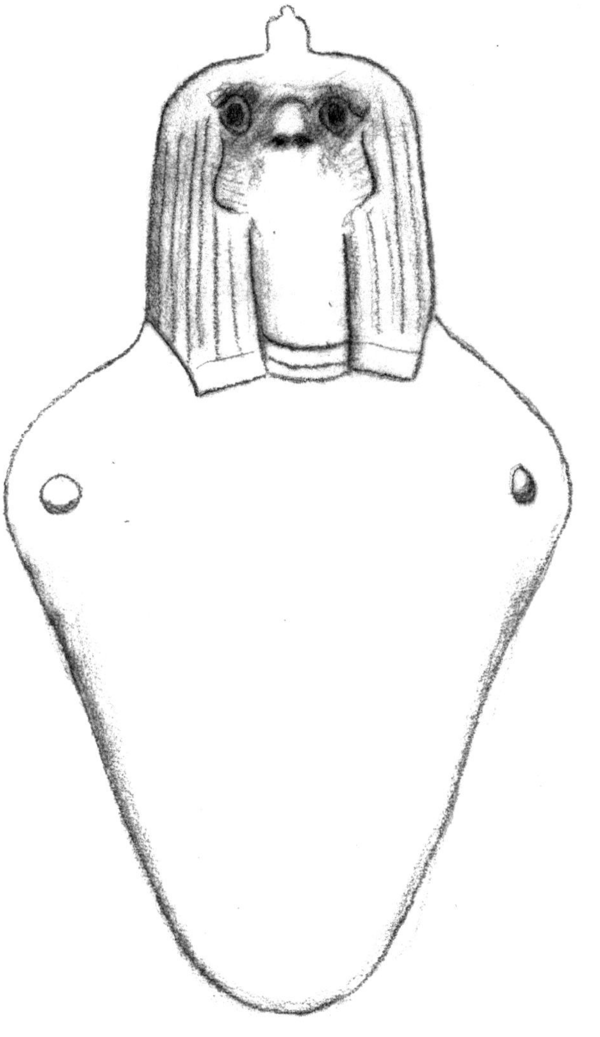

32. Animal-headed heart amulet
(35412, Bristish Museum)

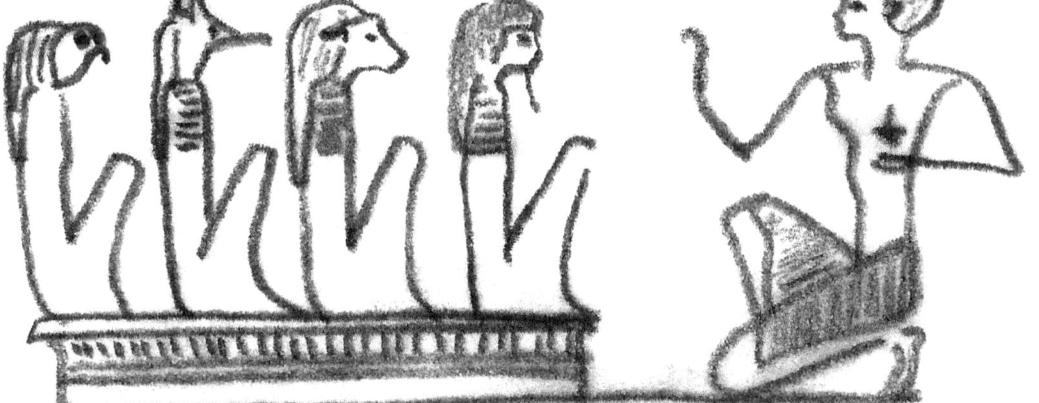

33. Vignette of chapter 27 from the *Book of the Dead* of Ahmose (N 3086, Louvre Museum), Ptolemaic Period (?)

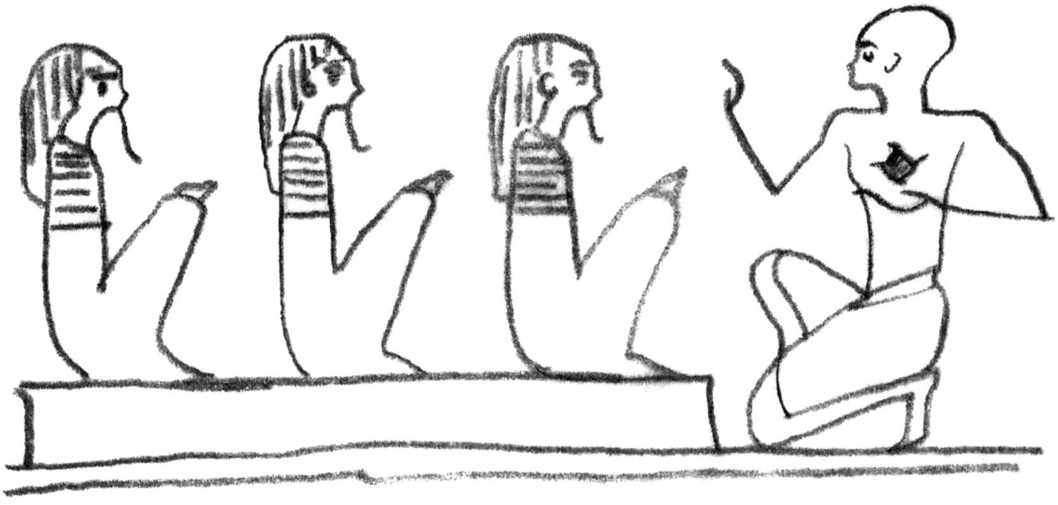

34. Vignette of chapter 27 from the *Book of the Dead* of Horsaiset (N 3082, Louvre Museum), Ptolemaic Period (?)

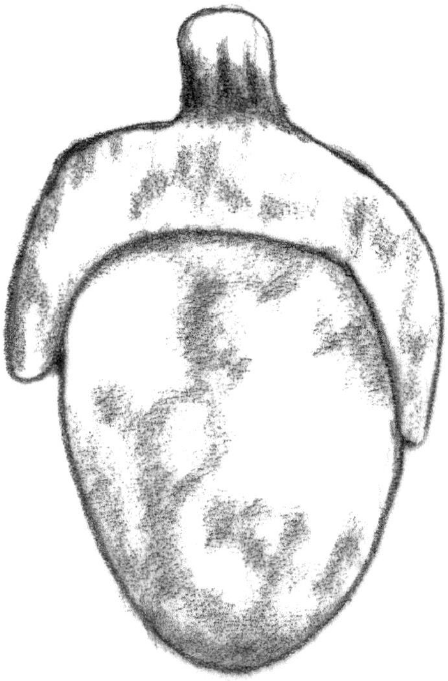

35. Flower heart amulet (AEO 30053, Louvre Museum)

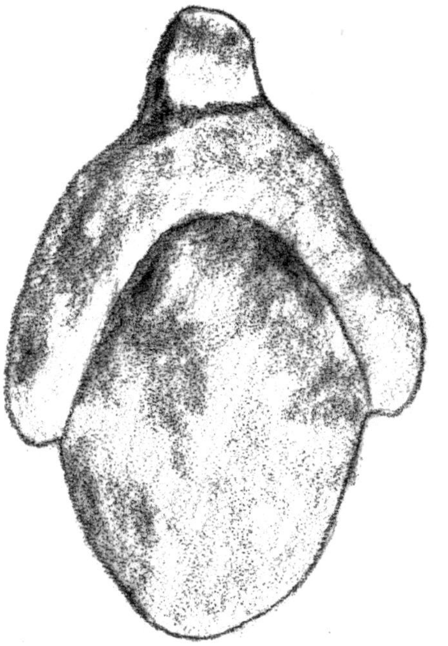

36. Flower heart amulet (AF 11524, Louvre Museum)

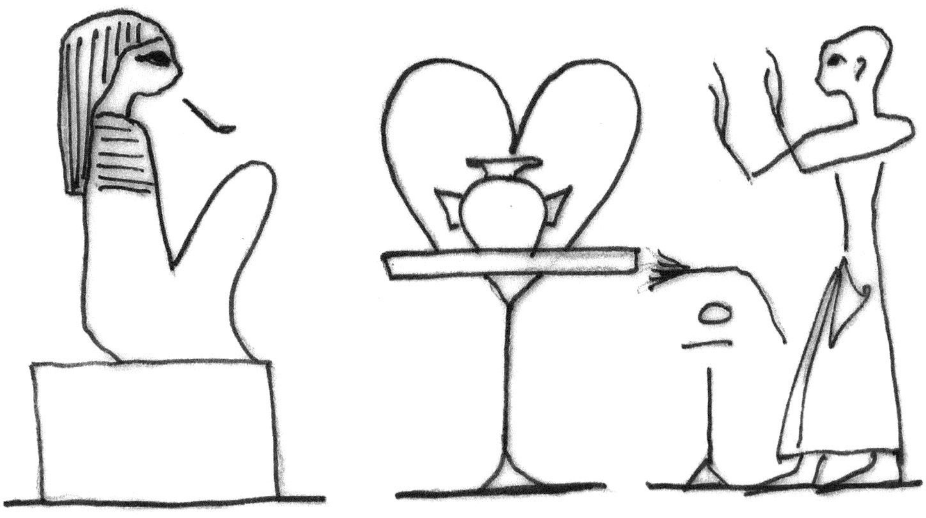

37. Vignette of chapter 28 from the *Book of the Dead* of Djedhor (N 3079, Louvre Museum), Late Period

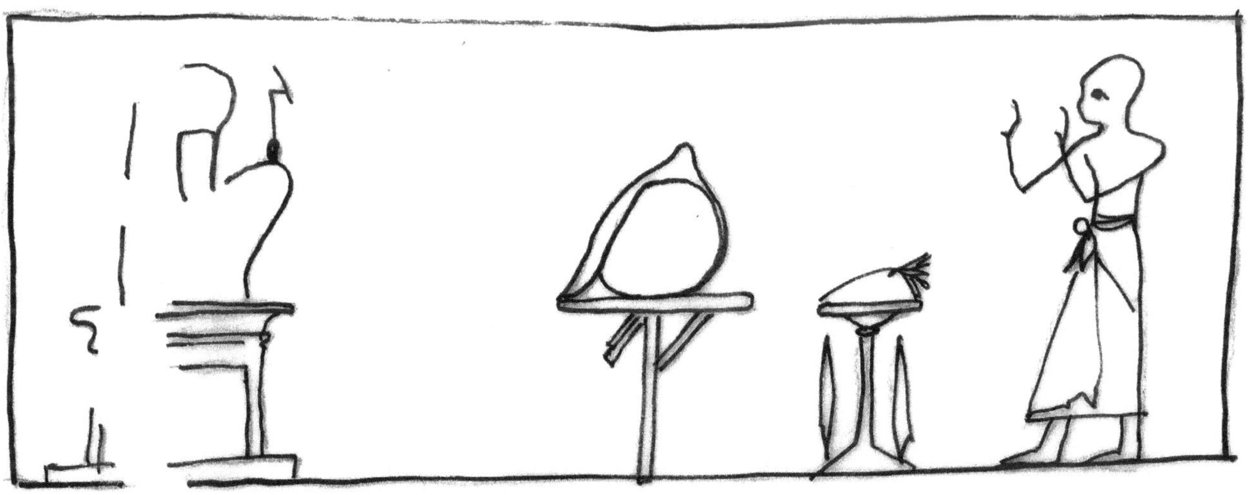

38. Vignette of chapter 28 from the *Book of the Dead* of Hornedjitef (N 3081, Louvre Museum), Ptolemaic Period

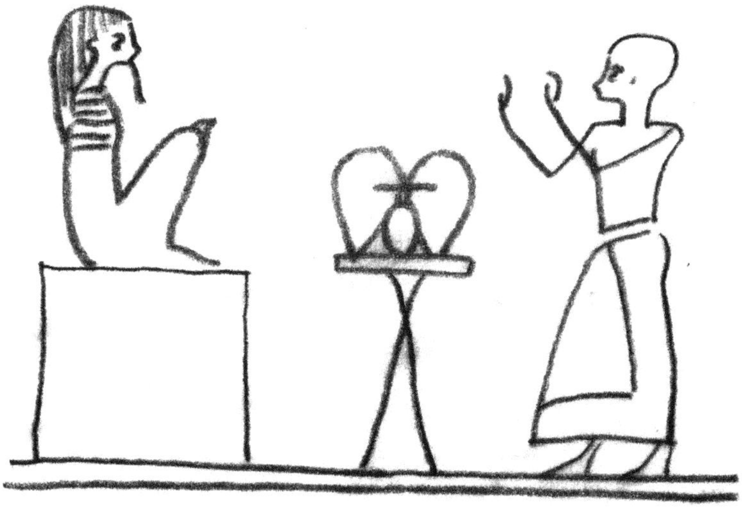

39. Vignette of chapter 28 from the *Book of the Dead* of Horsaiset (N 3082, Louvre Museum), Ptolemaic Period (?)

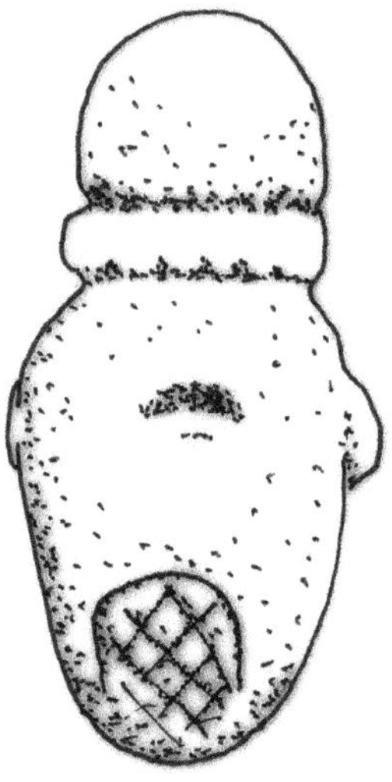

40. Solar heart amulet (UC 22526 A, Petrie Museum)

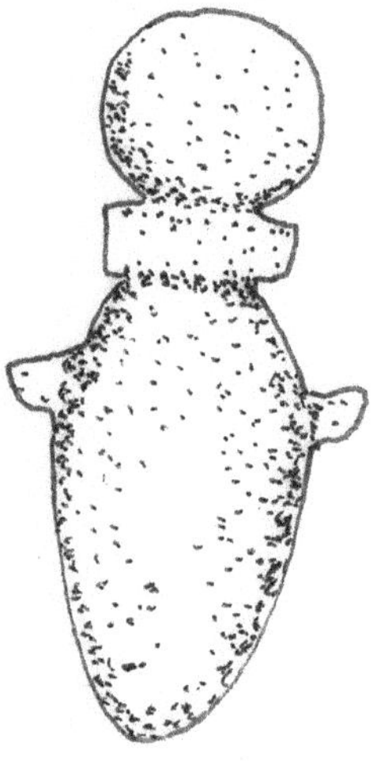

41. Solar heart amulet (SR 9279/CG 5223, Cairo Egyptian Museum)

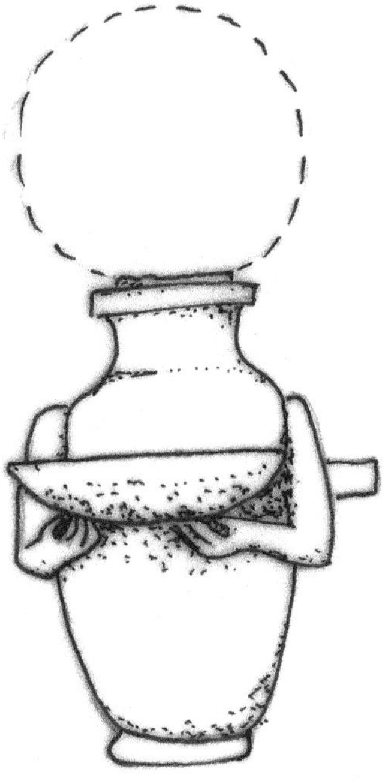

42. Votive heart amulet (N. Inv. 50.353, Museum of Fine Arts of Budapest)

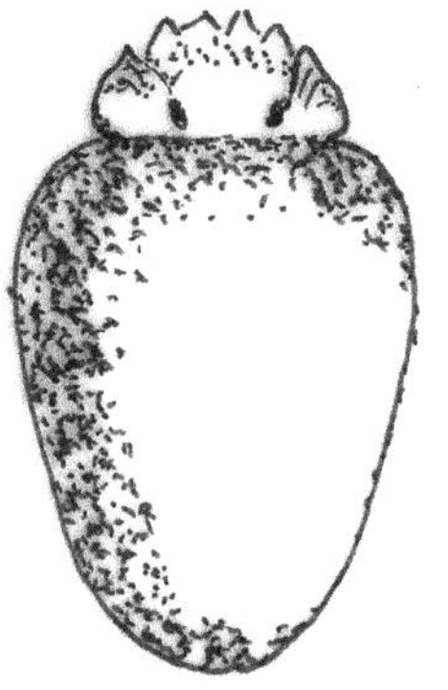

43. Heart amulet with the head of a scarab (37.492E, Brooklyn Museum)

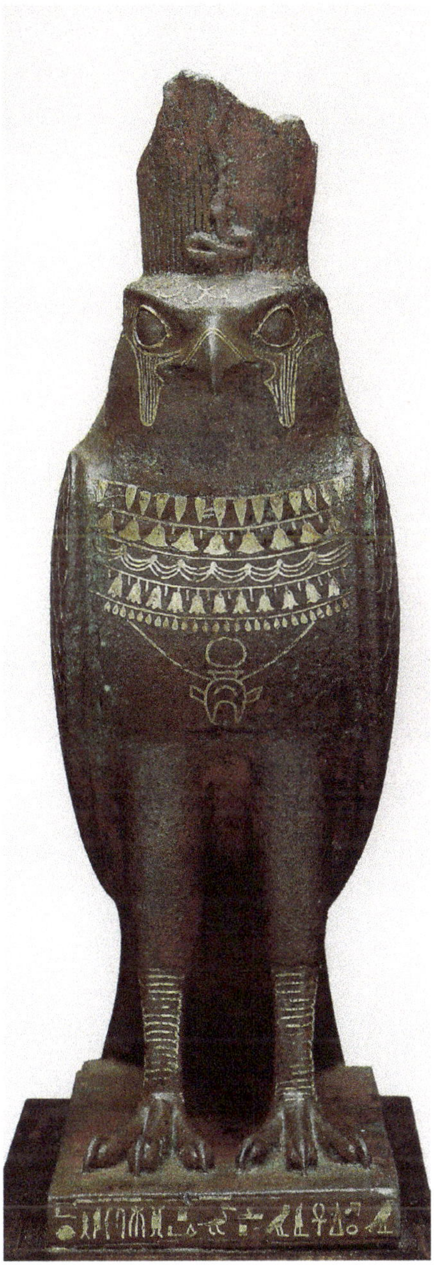

44. Avian statue of Horus (JE 30335, Cairo Egyptian Museum), Third Intermediate Period. Photo in J.P. CORTEGGIANI, *L'Égypte des Pharaons au Musée du Caire*, 1986, p. 160

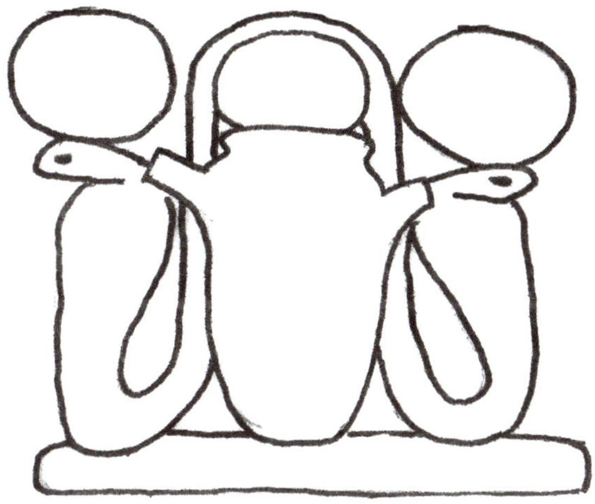

45. Solar heart amulet. Detail from fig. 70

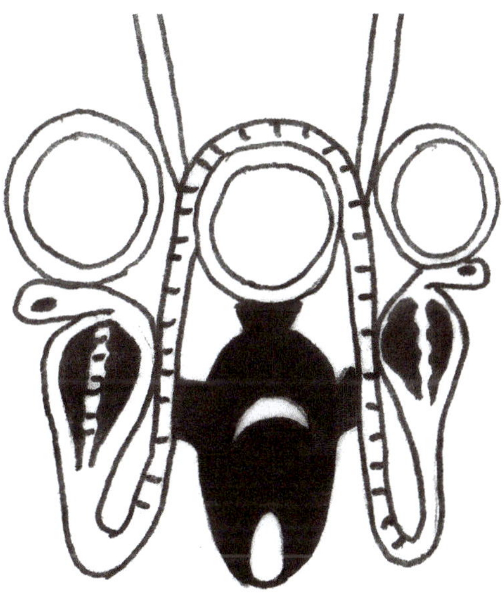

46. Coffin of the lady Unet (AF 9593, Louvre Museum), 21st Dynasty. Detail of the lid

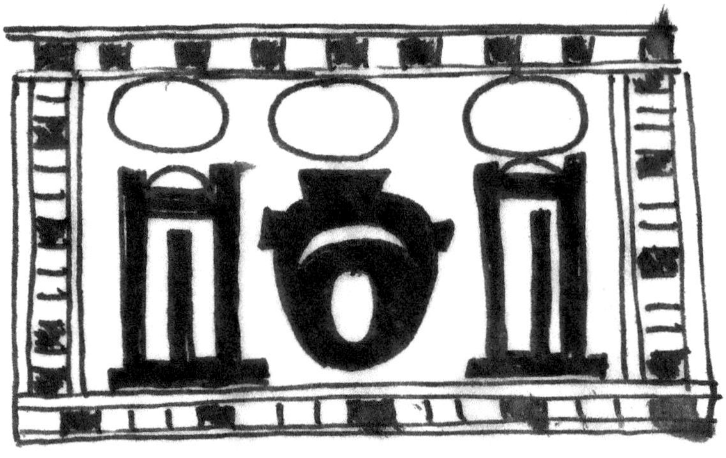

47. Outer coffin of the lady Direpu (J.E. 29669/CG 6028, Cairo Egyptian Museum), 21st Dynasty. Detail of the lid

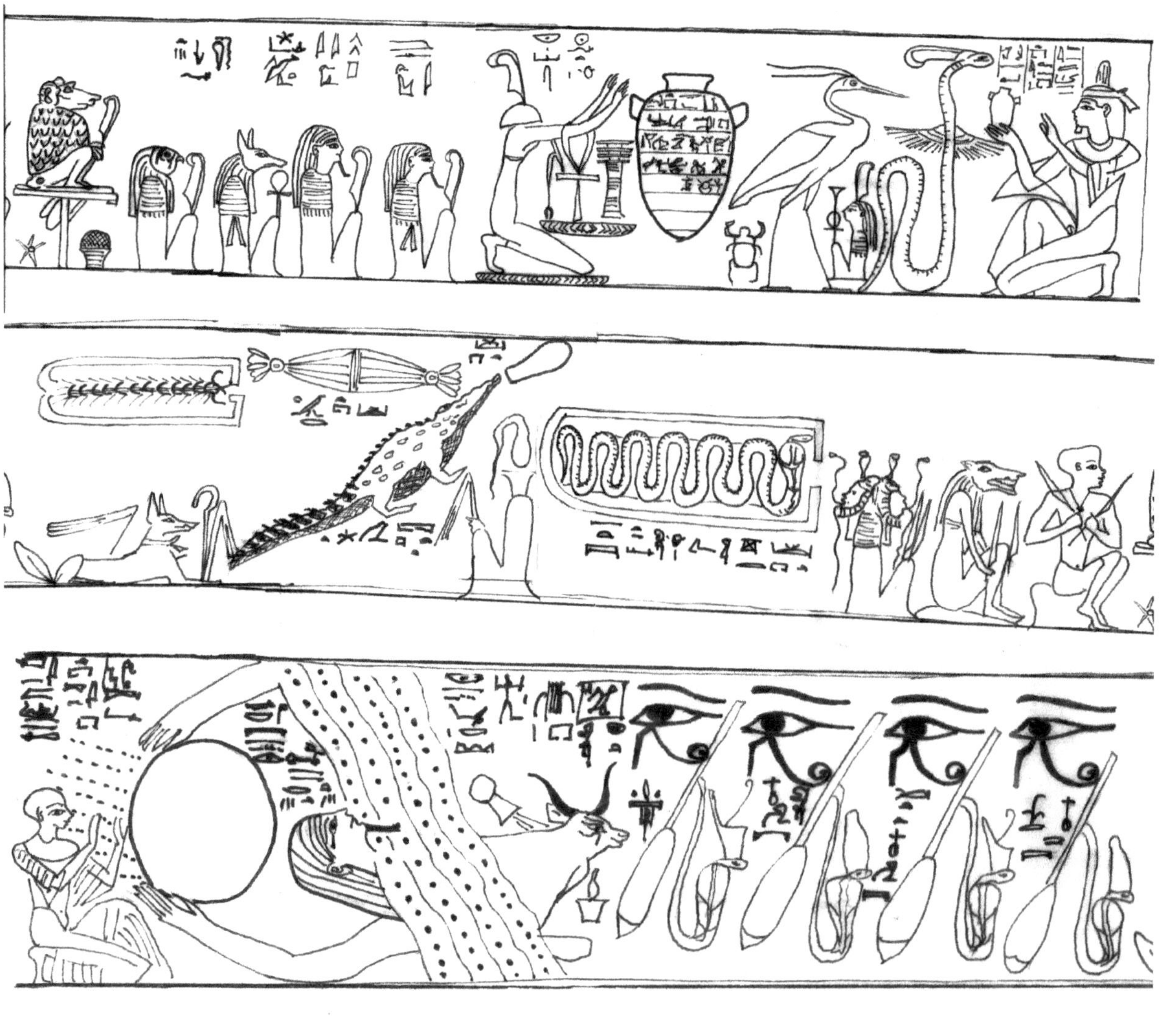

48. Funerary papyrus of Amenemwya (nº P 3127, Berlin Egyptian Museum), Ramessid Period

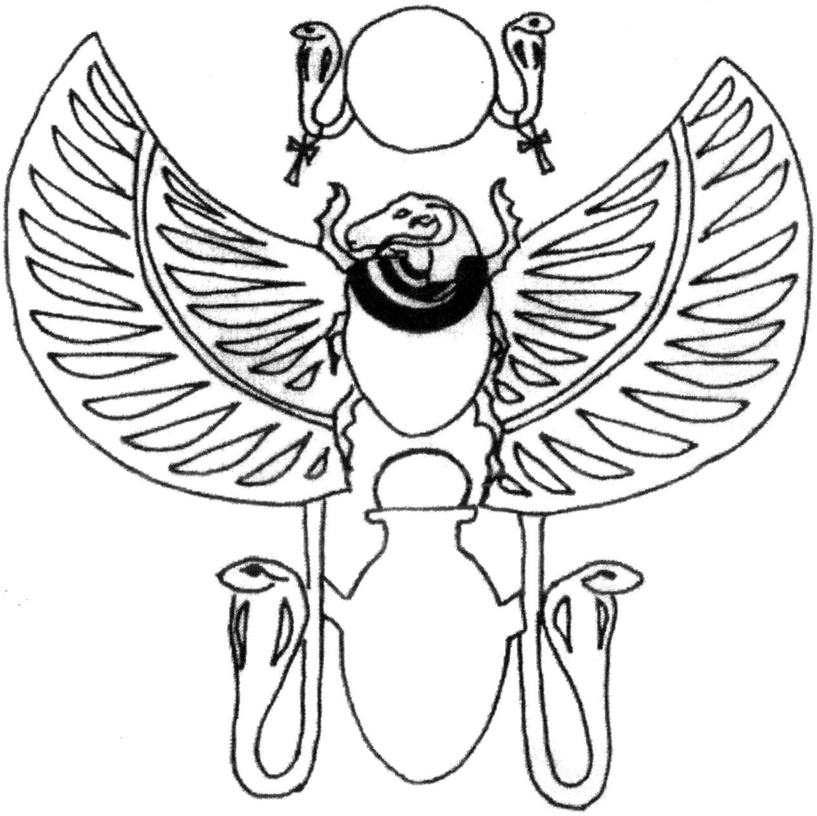

49. Mummy-cover of Padiamun, (CG 6235, Cairo Egyptian Museum). Detail. Drawing after E. HORNUNG, B. BRYAN, *The Quest for immortality*, 2002, p. 158.

3. HEART AMULETS AND SACRED LOCKS

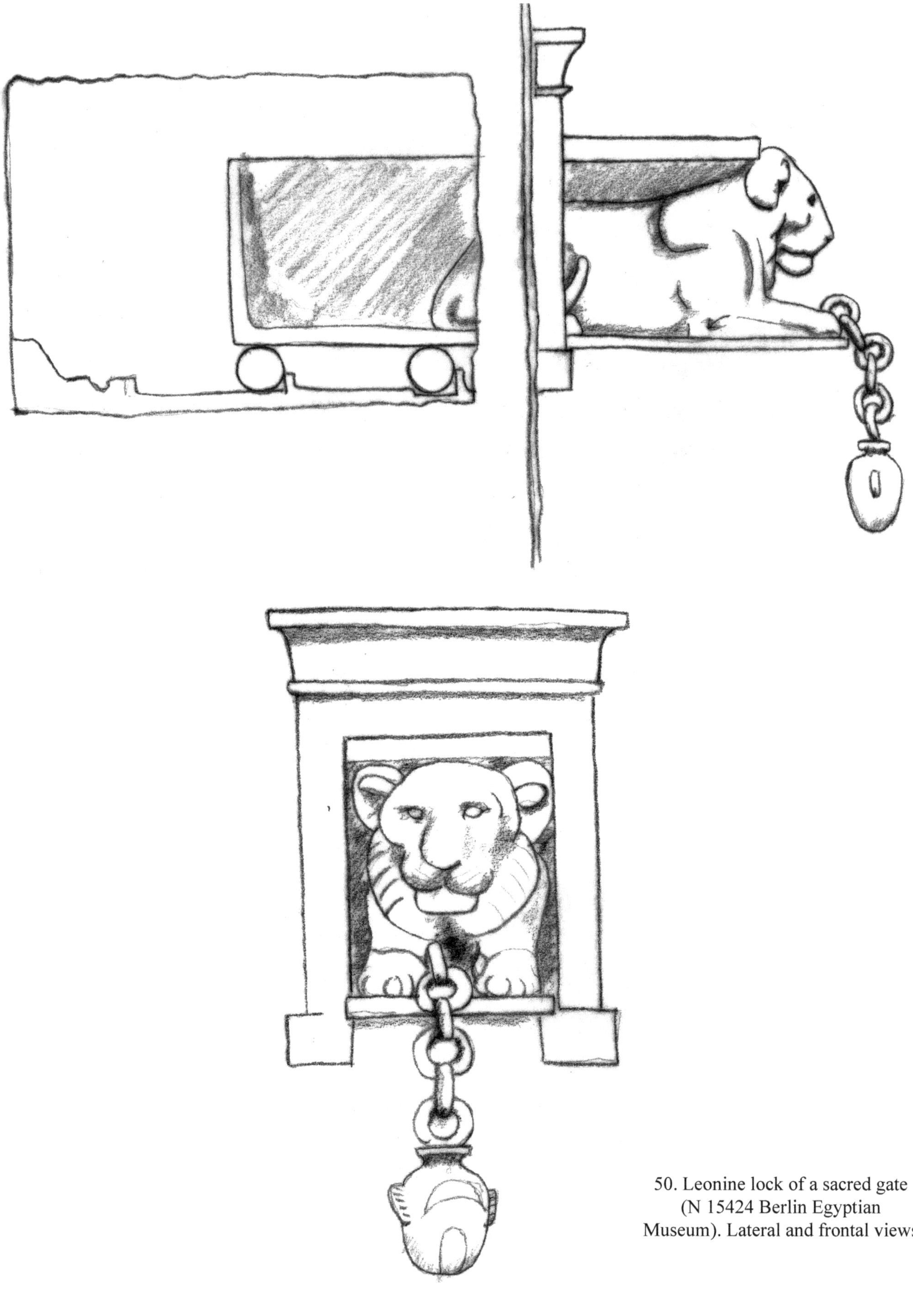

50. Leonine lock of a sacred gate (N 15424 Berlin Egyptian Museum). Lateral and frontal views

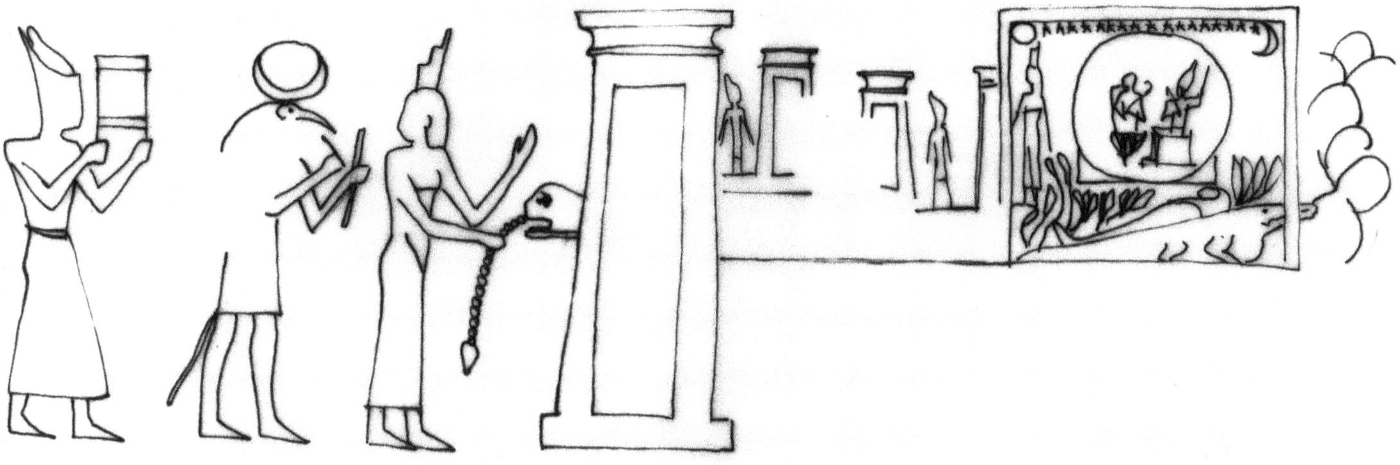

51. Philae, Gate of Adrian, south wall

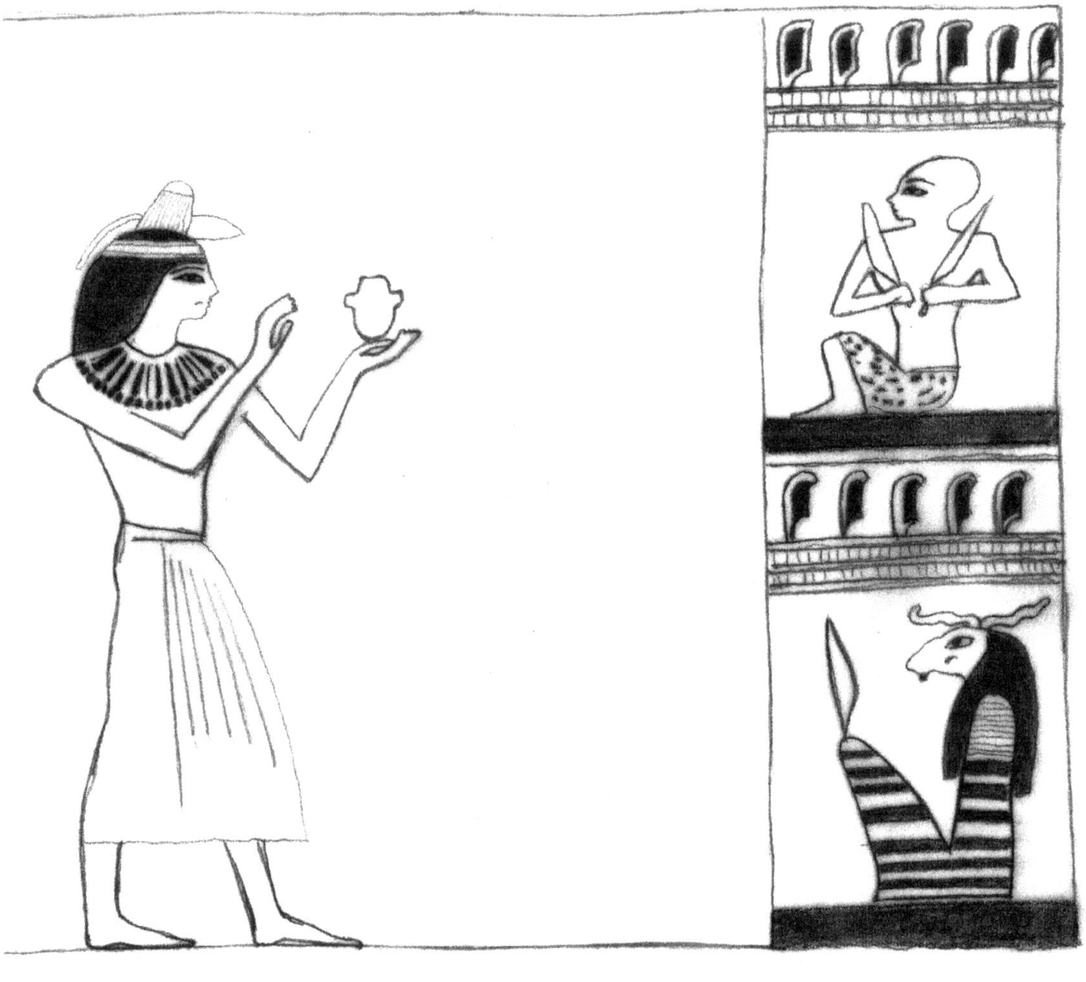

52. Funerary papyrus of Userhatmose (SR 10249, Cairo Egyptian Museum), 21st Dynasty

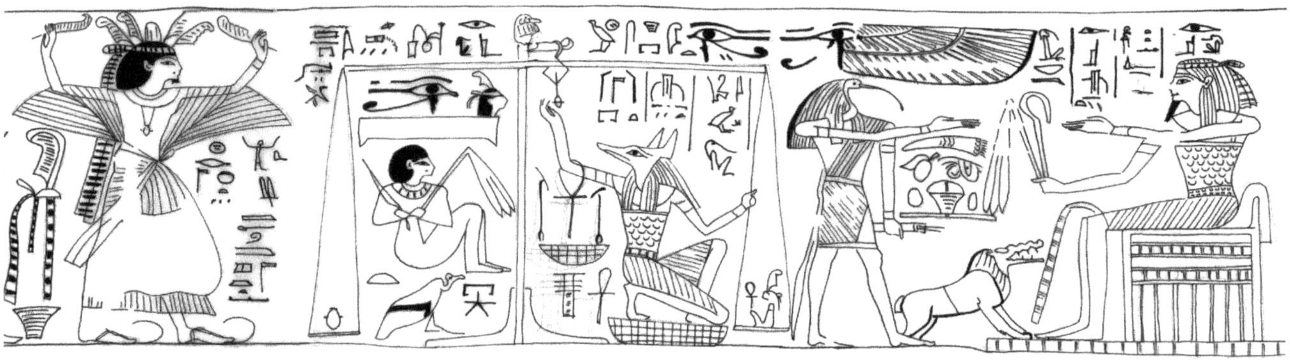

53. Funerary papyrus of Nesipakachuti (E 17401, Louvre Museum), vignette of the weighing of the heart

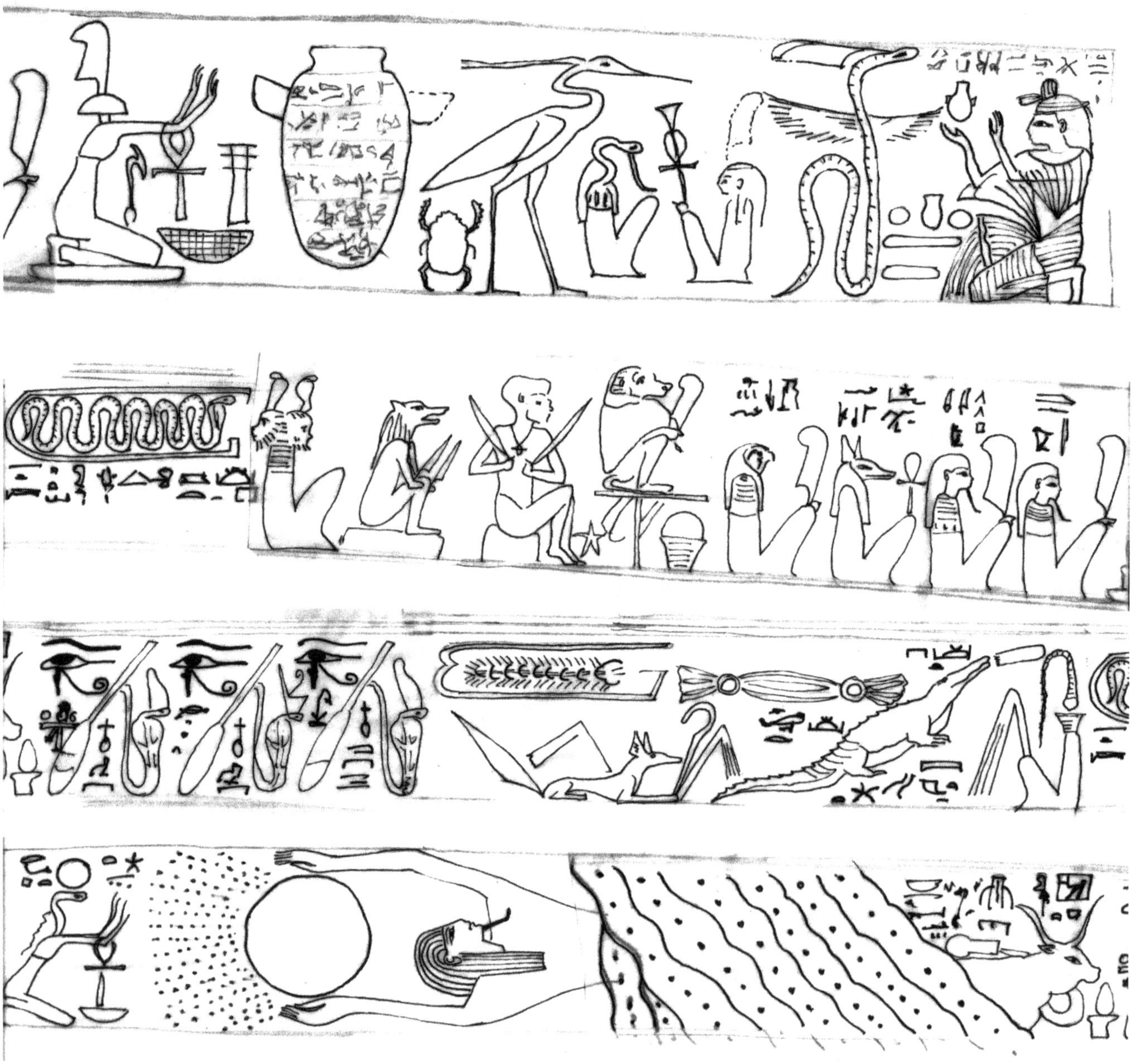

54. Funerary papyrus of Nesipautitaui, (SR 1025, Cairo Egyptian Museum), 21st Dynasty

4. CARDIAC AMULETS AND DUALISTIC SYMBOLISM OF THE HEART

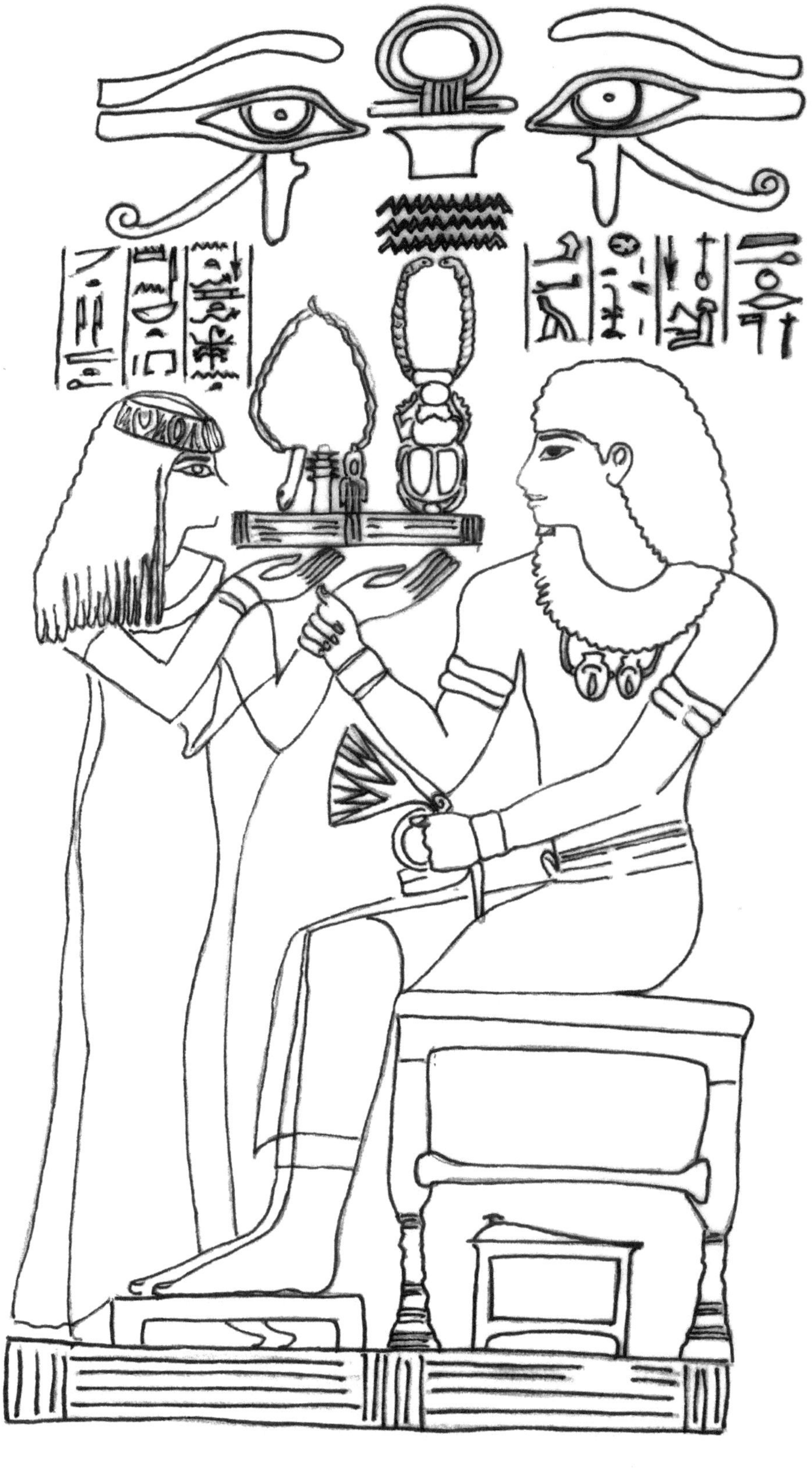

55. Sheikh Abd el-Gurnah, tomb of Sennefer (TT 96)

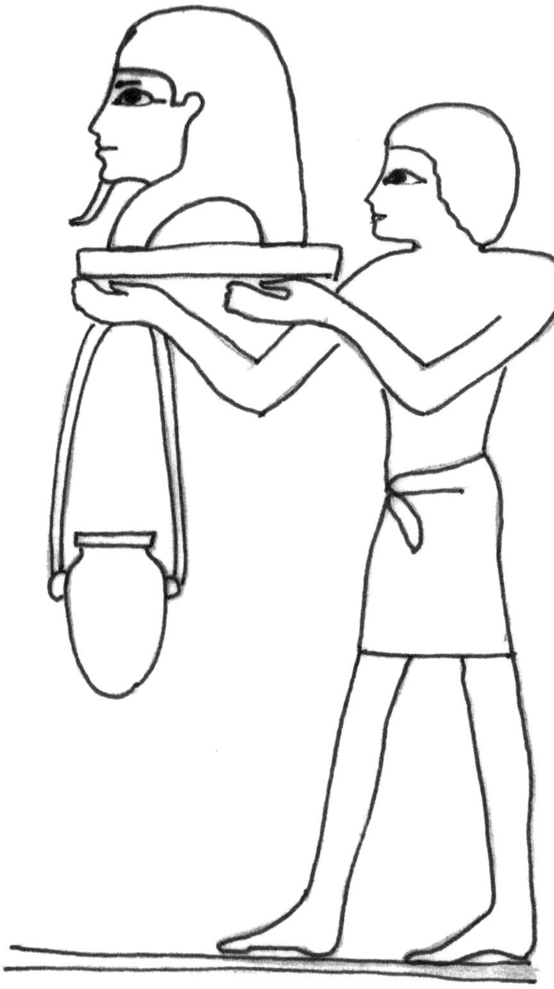

56. Sheikh Abd el-Gurnah, tomb of Sennefer (TT 96)

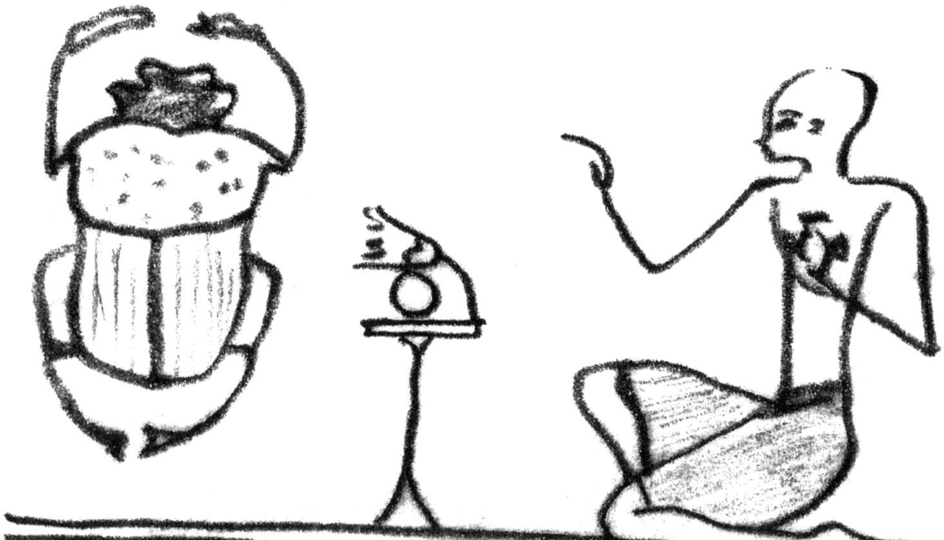

57. Vignette of chapter 30 B of the *Book of the Dead* of Usirwer
(N 3143, Louvre Museum)

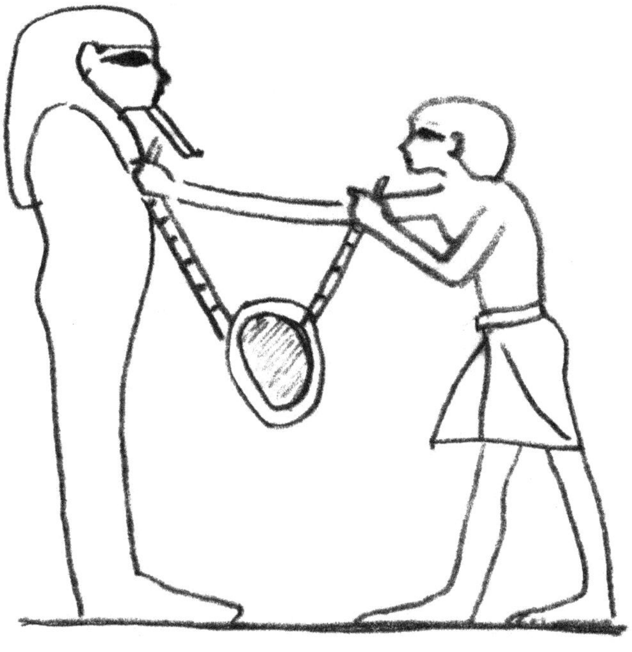

58. Vignette of the *Book of the Dead* of Nebked, (N 3082, Louvre Museum)

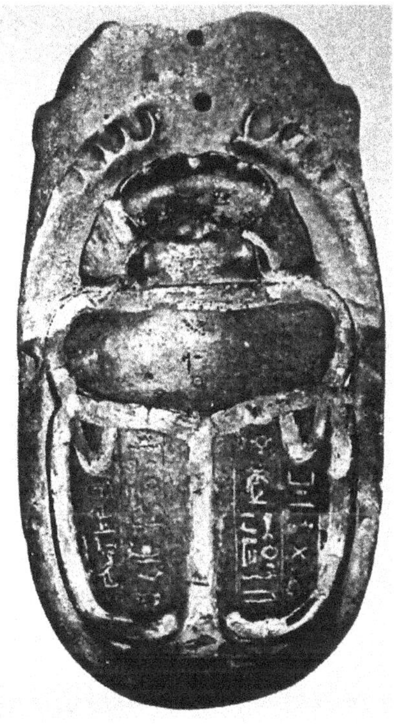

59. Cardiac amulet of Yuya (SR 9530/CG 51165, Cairo Egyptian Museum), from KV 46, 18th Dynasty. Photo in J. QUIBELL, *The Tomb of Yuaa and Thuiu*, 1908, PL. XLIX

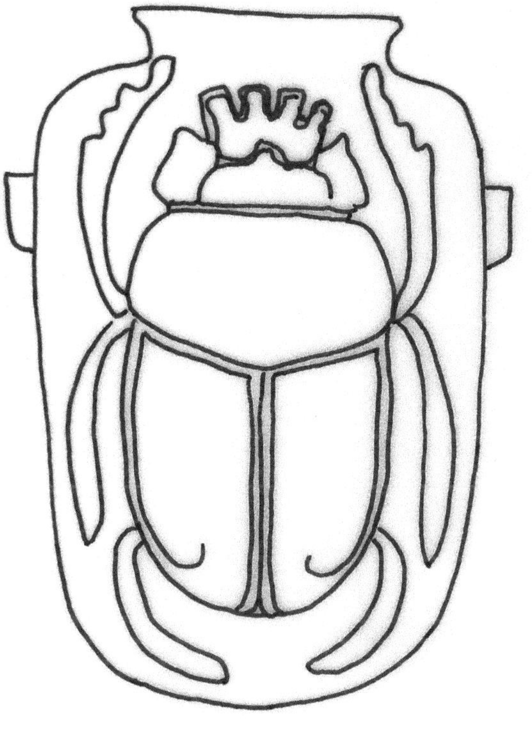

60. Heart amulet (CG 12056, Cairo Egyptian Museum). Drawing after M. REISNER, *Amulets*, I, pl. VII.

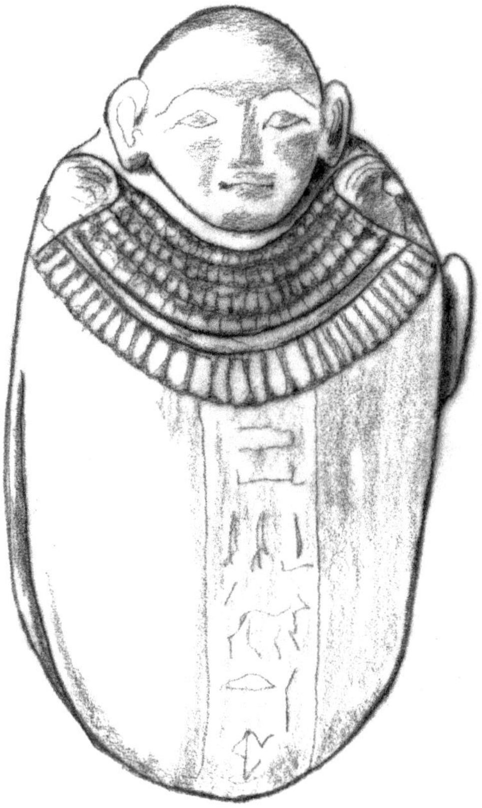

61. Heart scarab (?) of Mayré (Inv. Nr 1951,5; Kestner Museum), Ramessid Period

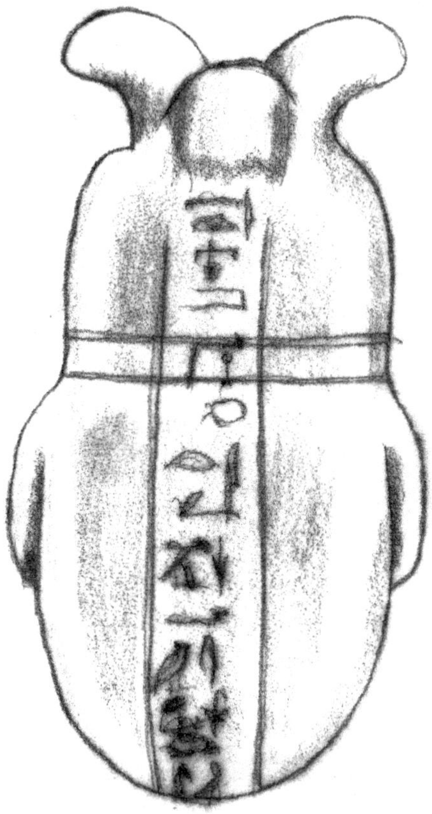

62. Heart amulet of Khaemwaset (AF 2333, Louvre Museum), from Sakara (Serapeum), Ramessid Period

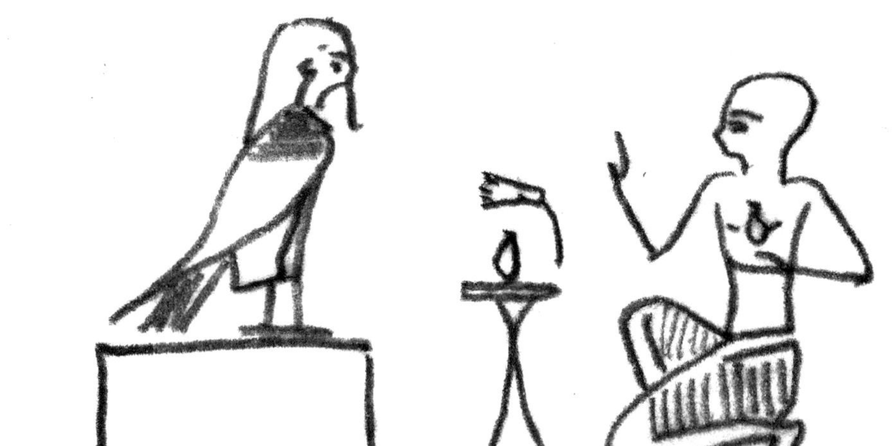

63. Vignette of chapter 26 of the *Book of the Dead* of Horsaiset (N 3082, Louvre Museum), Greco-Roman Period

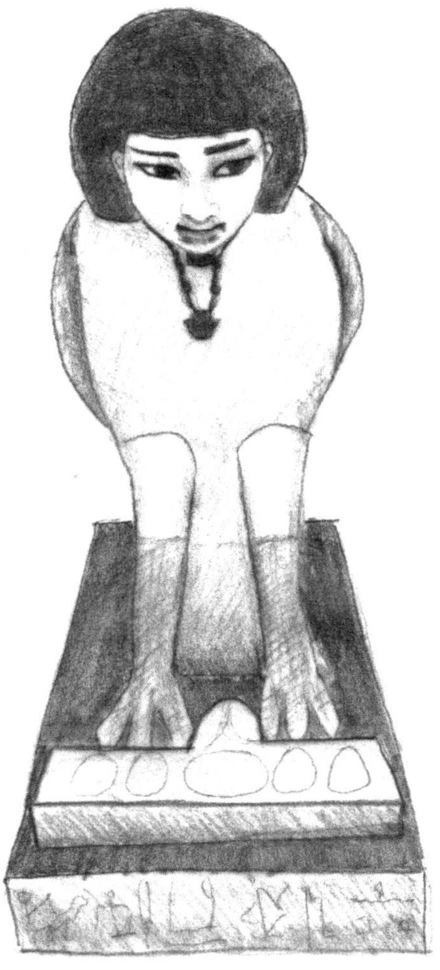

64. *Ba* bird statuette of Yuiya (JE 95312, Cairo Egyptian Museum) from KV 46, 18th Dynasty

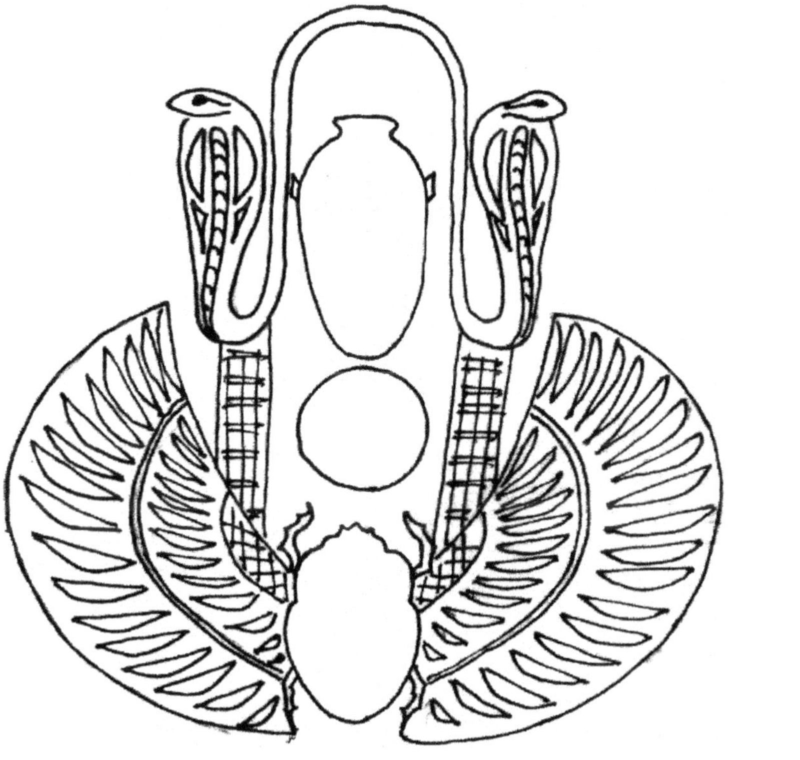

65. Coffin of Nebankh (Turin Egyptian Museum), Third Intermediate Period, detail of the lid

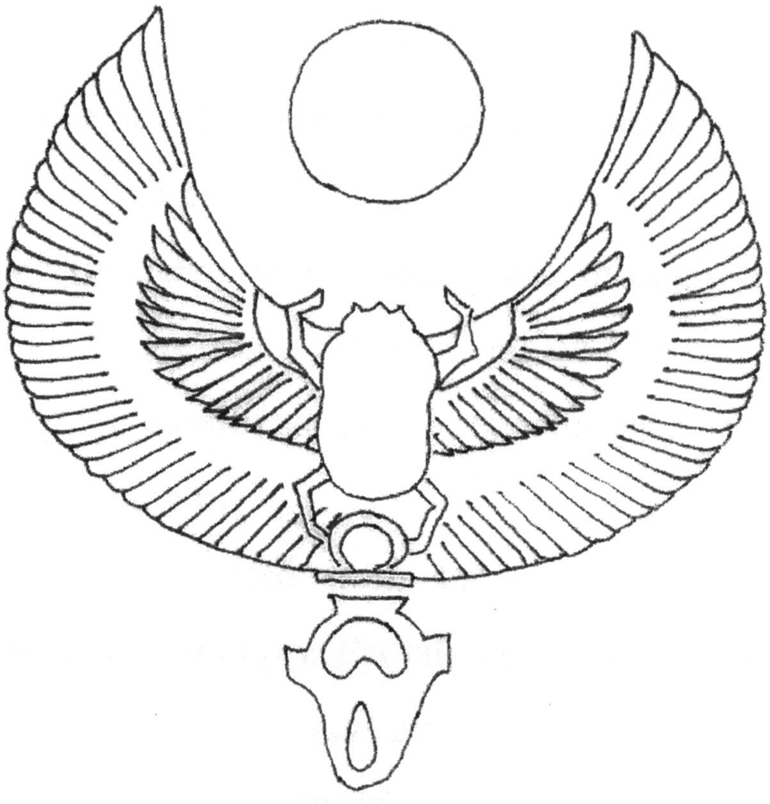

66. Outer coffin of Pinedjem II (JE 26197/CG 61029C, Cairo Egyptian Museum), 21st Dynasty, detail of the lid

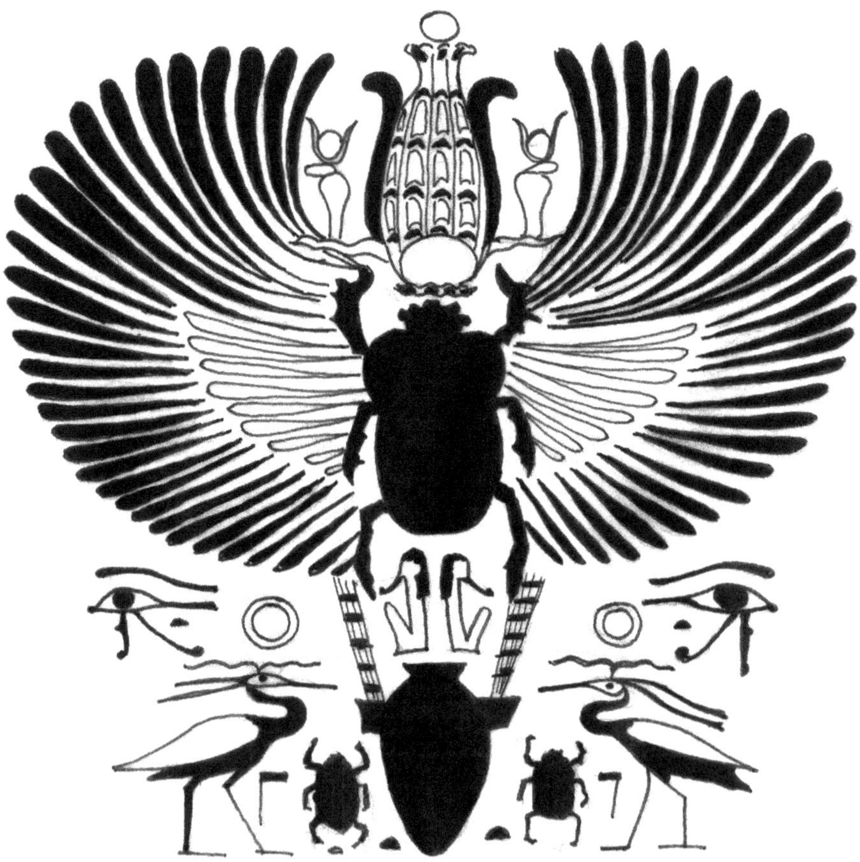

67. Mummy-cover from Bab el-Gasus's burial A.87 (JE 29668, Cairo Egyptian Museum), 21st Dynasty, detail

5. DEPICTIONS OF THE HEART AMULET IN EGYPTIAN ART

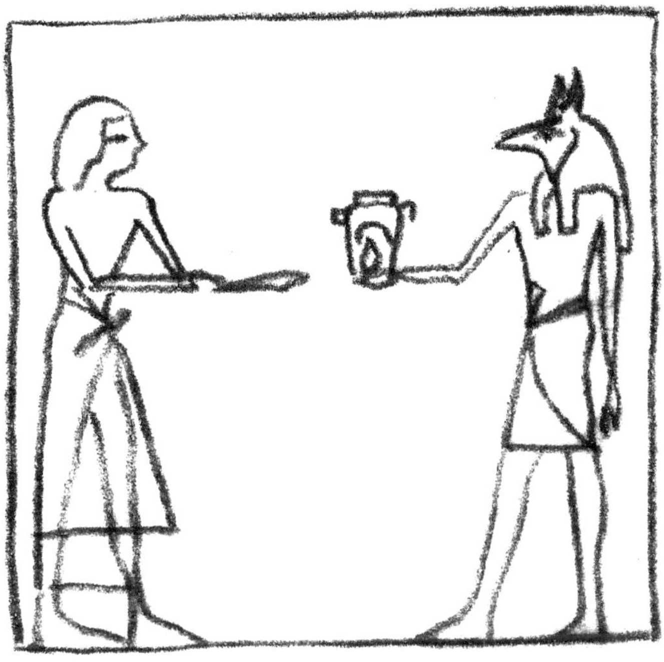

68. Vignette of chapter 26 (n° 9900, British Museum)

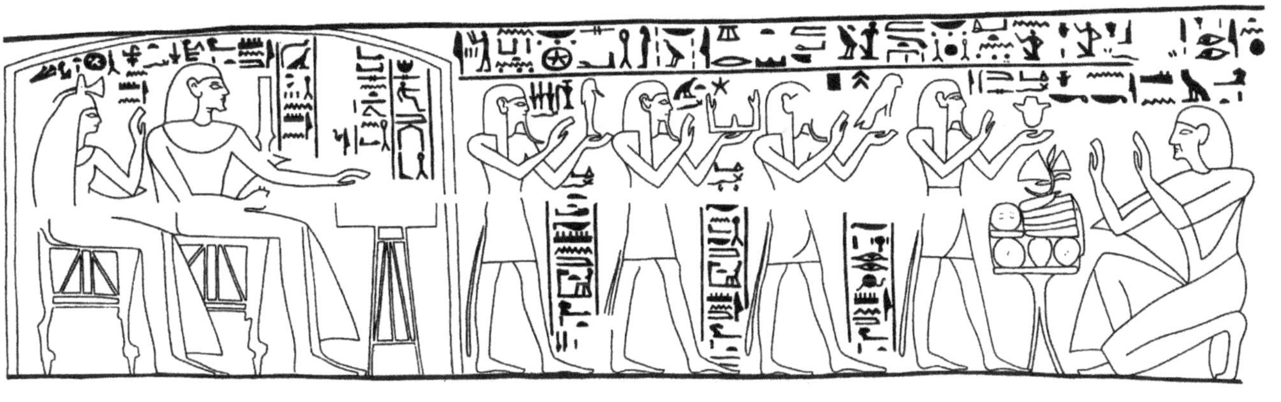

69. Block fragment from the tomb of Amenemhat (TT 163), Ramessid Period. Drawing in J. ASSMANN, *Mort et l'au-delà dans l'Égypte ancienne*, 2003, p. 142

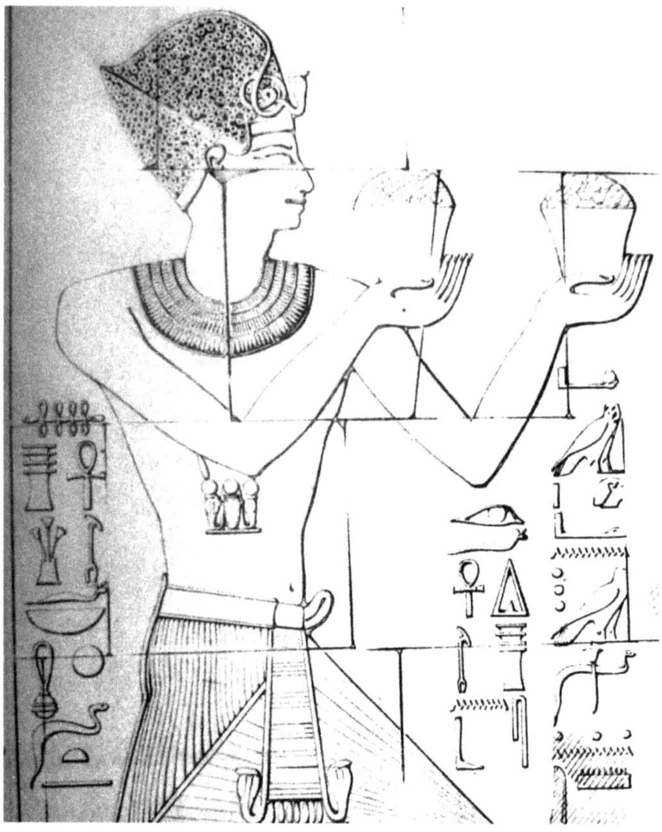

70. Deir el-Bahari, funerary temple of Hatshepsut, second terrace, south colonnade. Drawing in E. NAVILLE, *The Temple of Deir el-Bahari*, Part III, 1898, Pl. LXXXII

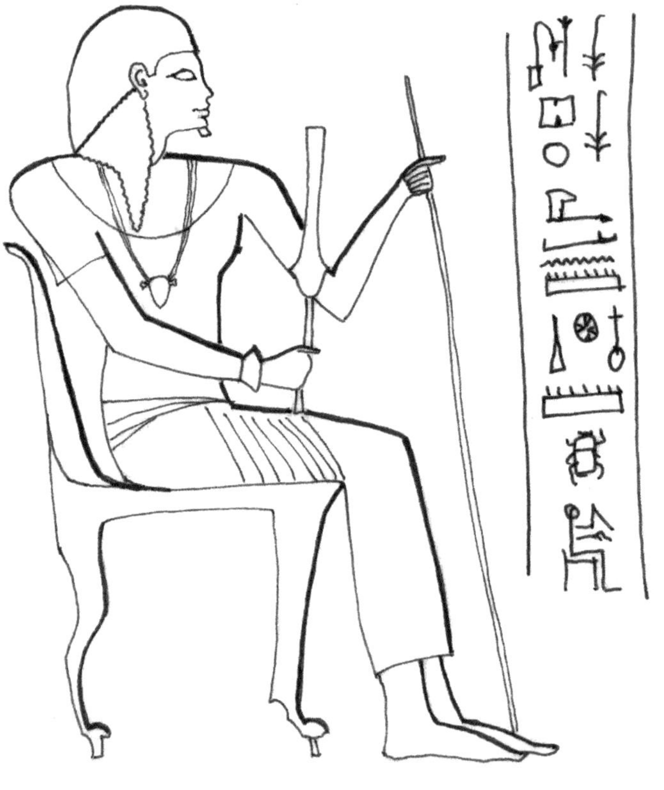

71. Fragment of a door jamb from Theban tomb of Menkheper (41.160.104, Metropolitan Museum of Art)

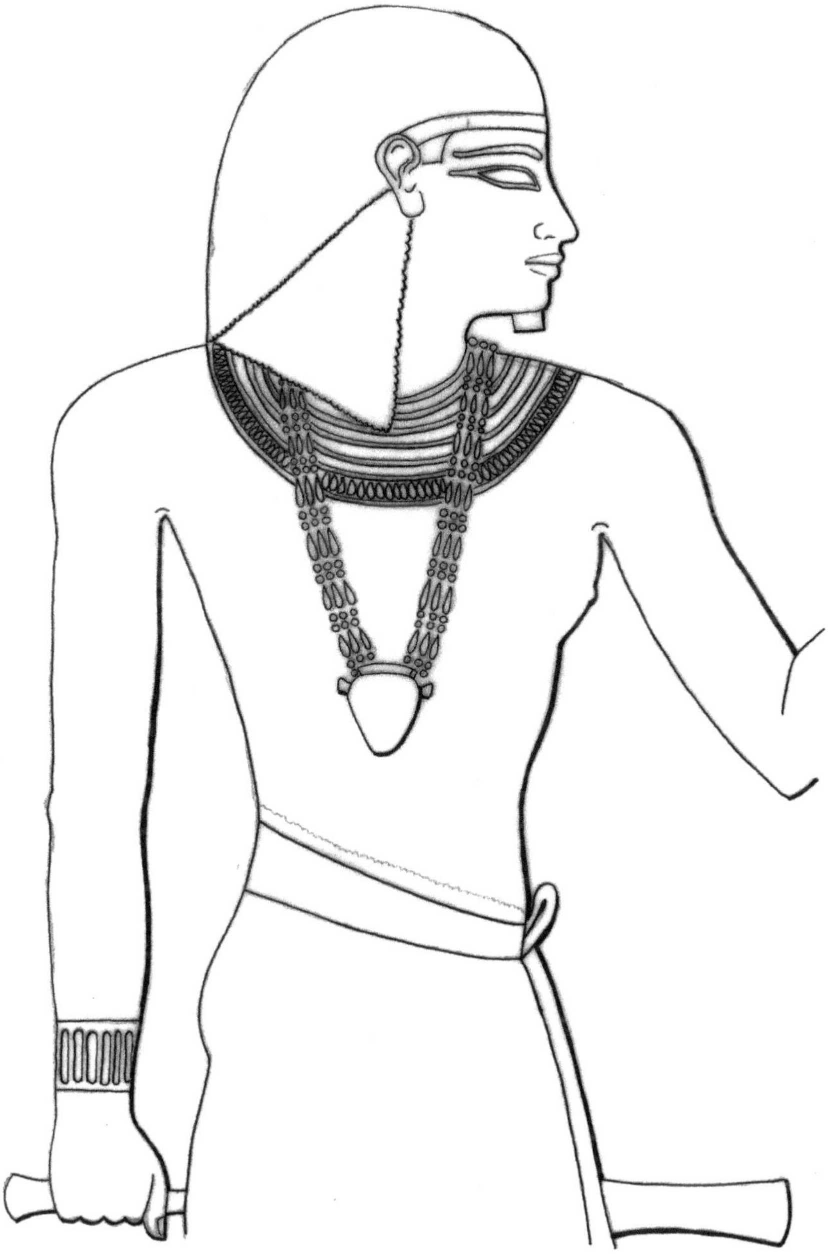

72. Sheikh Abd el-Gurnah, tomb of Khaemhat (TT 57)

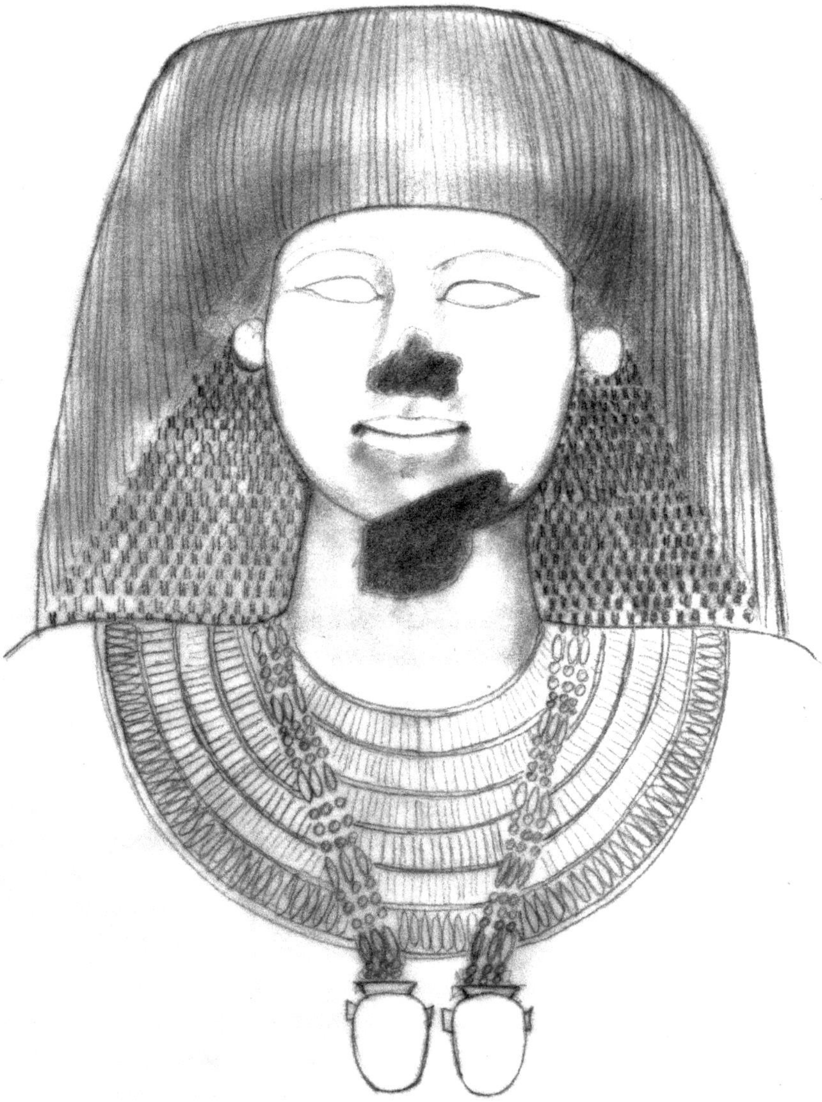

73. Sheikh Abd el-Gurnah, tomb of Khaemhat (TT 57)

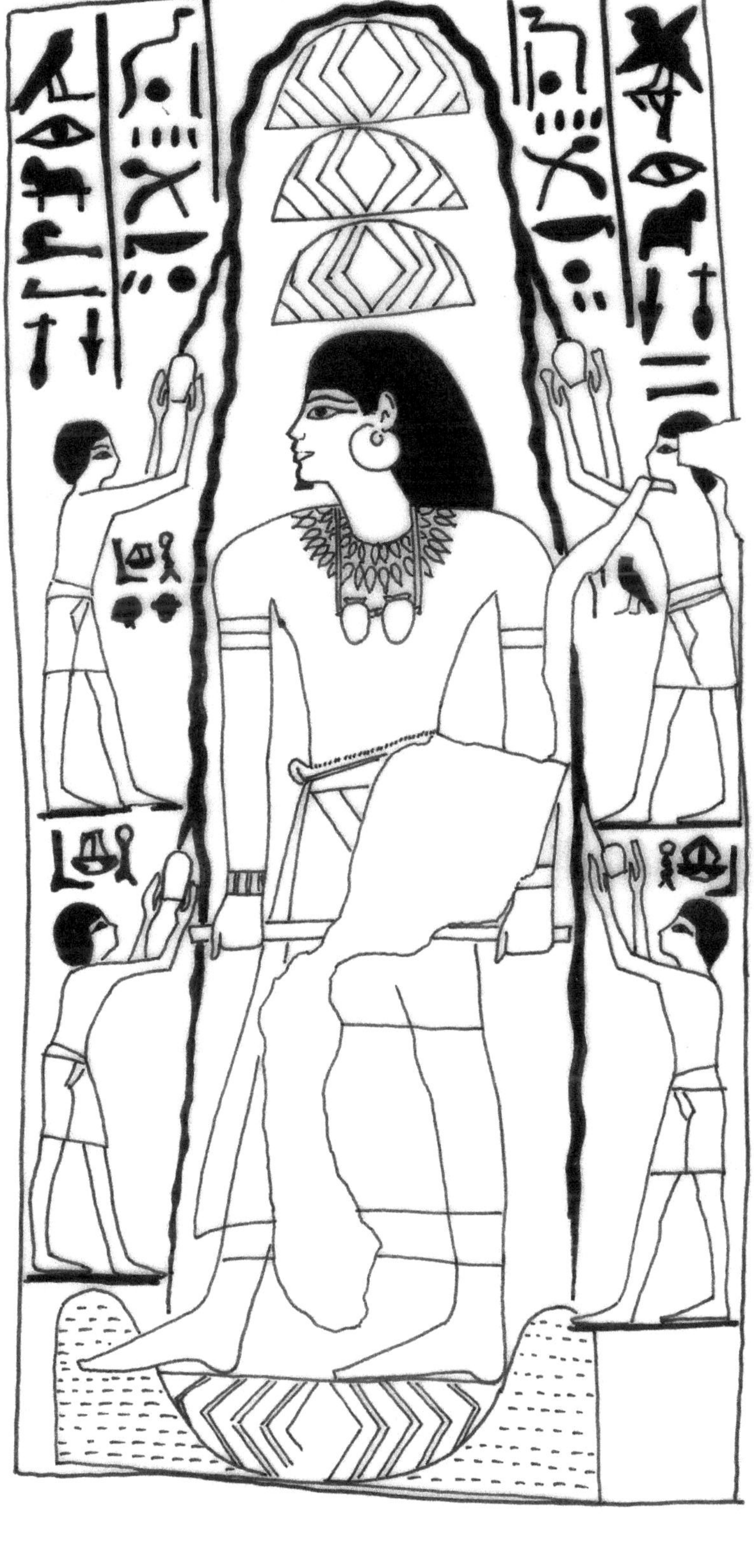

74. Sheikh Abd el-Gurnah, tomb of Sennefer (TT 96)

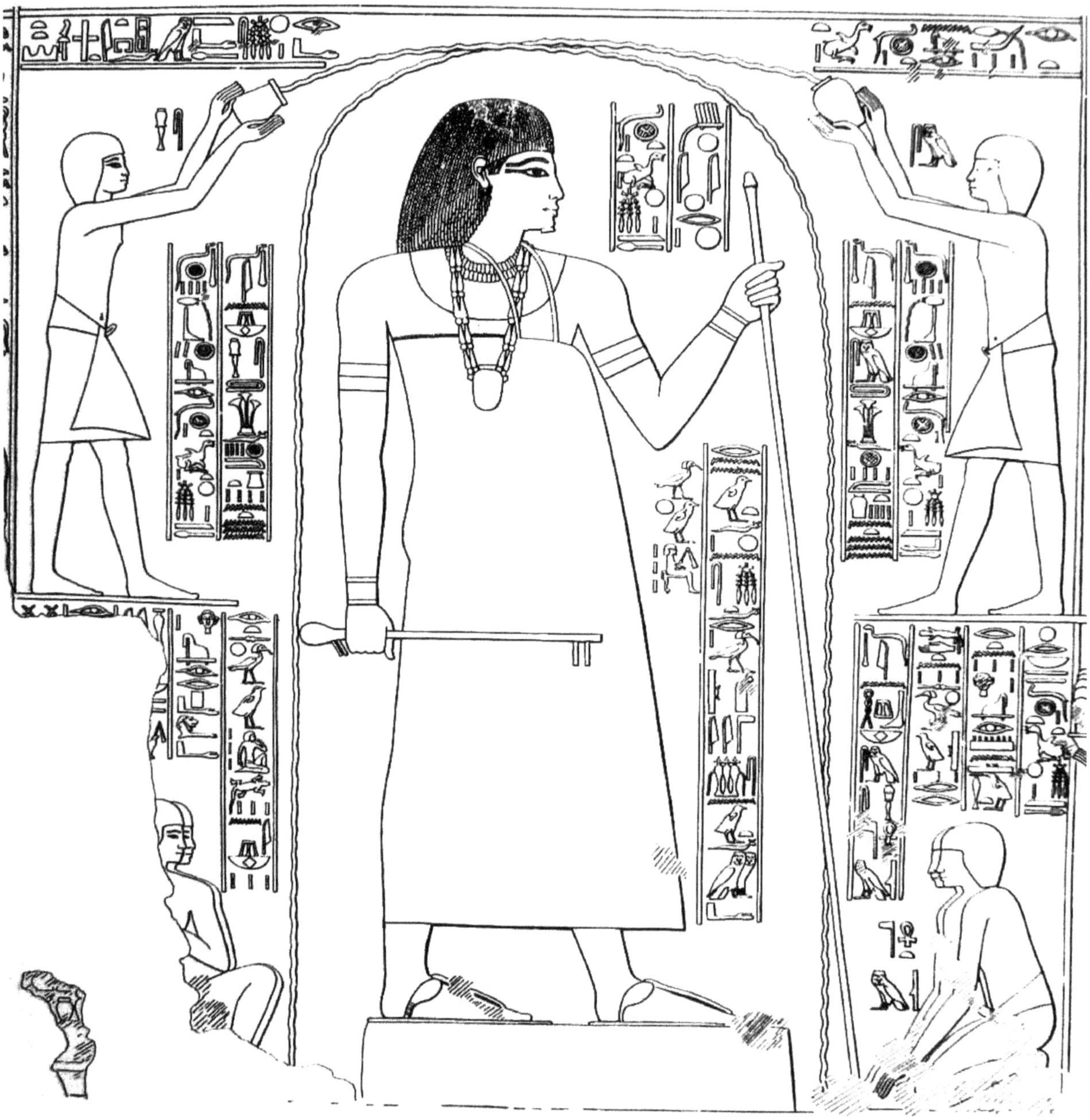

75. Sheikh Abd el-Gurnah, tomb of Ramose (TT 55)

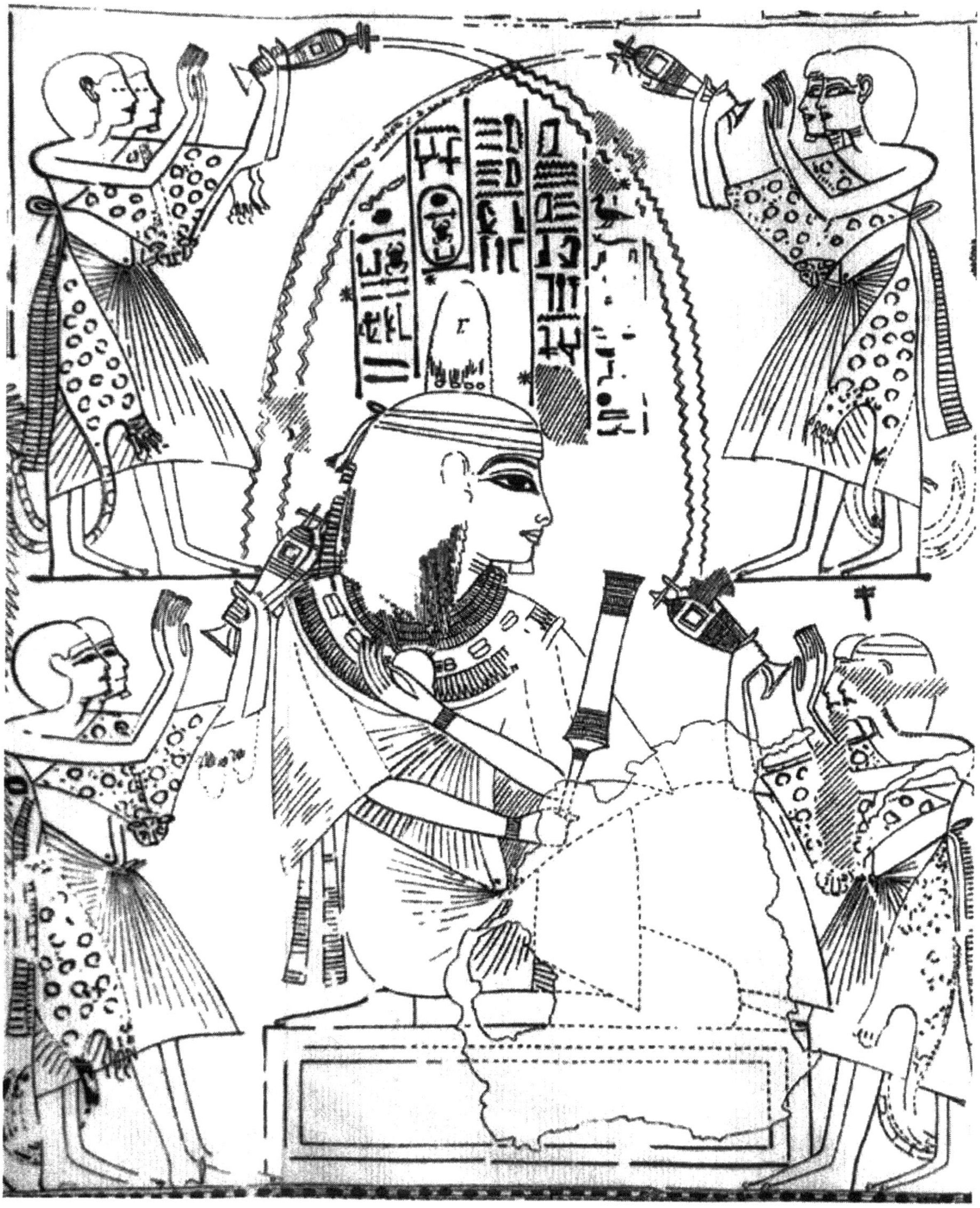

76. Sheikh Abd el-Gurnah, tomb of Userhat (TT 51). Drawing in N. DAVIES, *Two Ramesside Tombs*, 1927, pl. XI

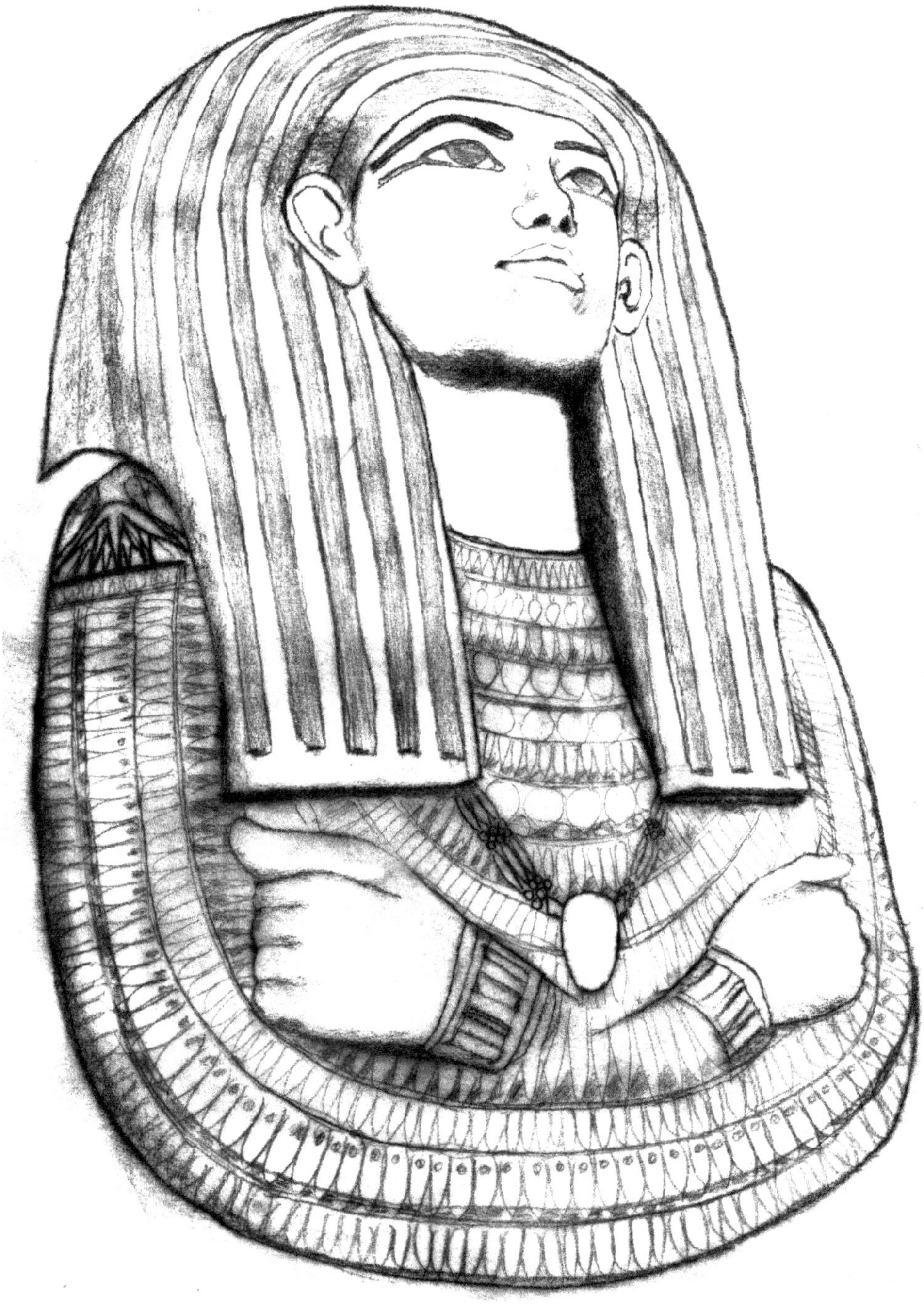

77. Coffin of Maherpa (JE 31378/CG 4219, Cairo Egyptian Museum)

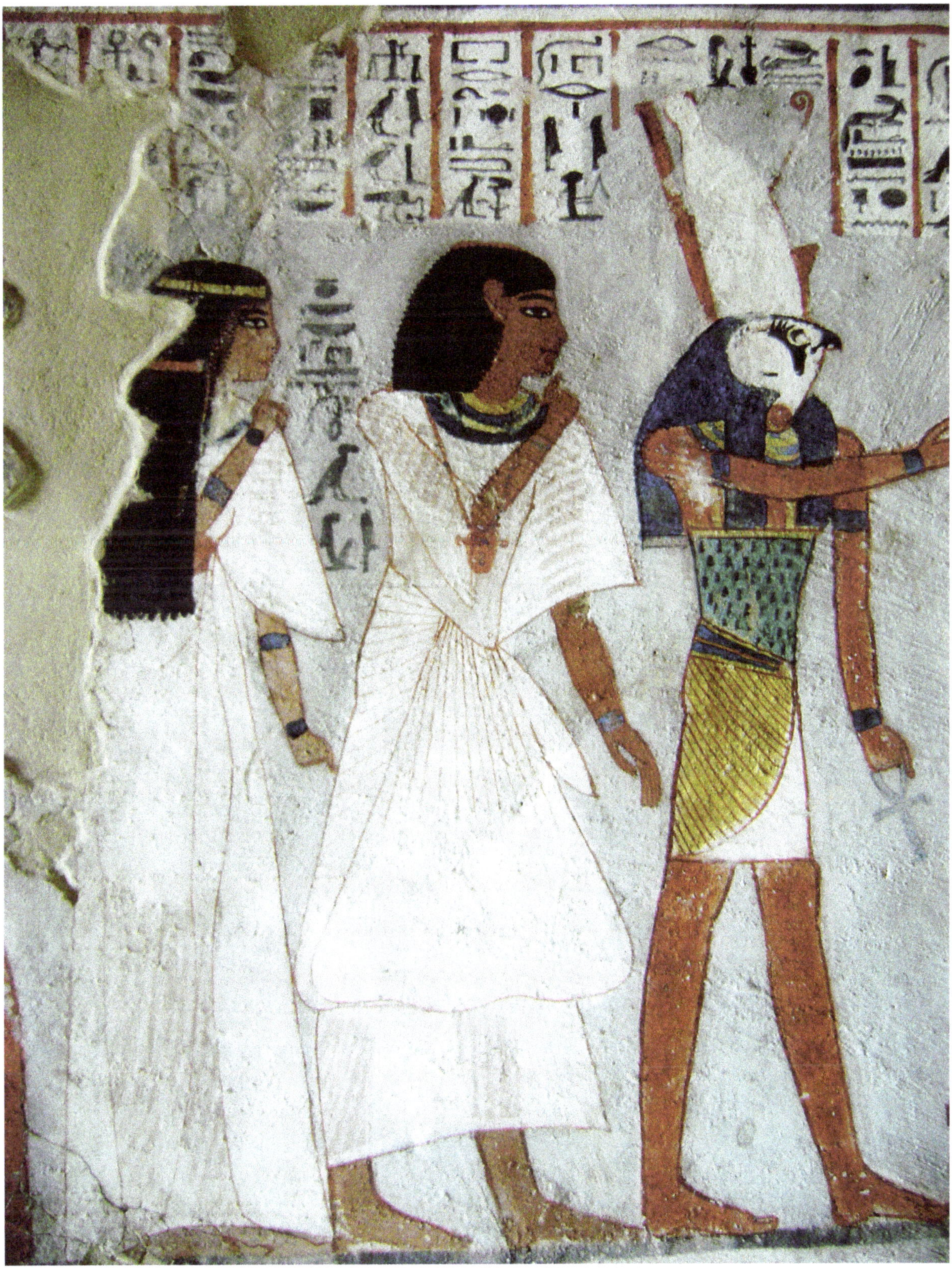

78. Dra Abu el-Naga, tomb of Rai (TT 255)

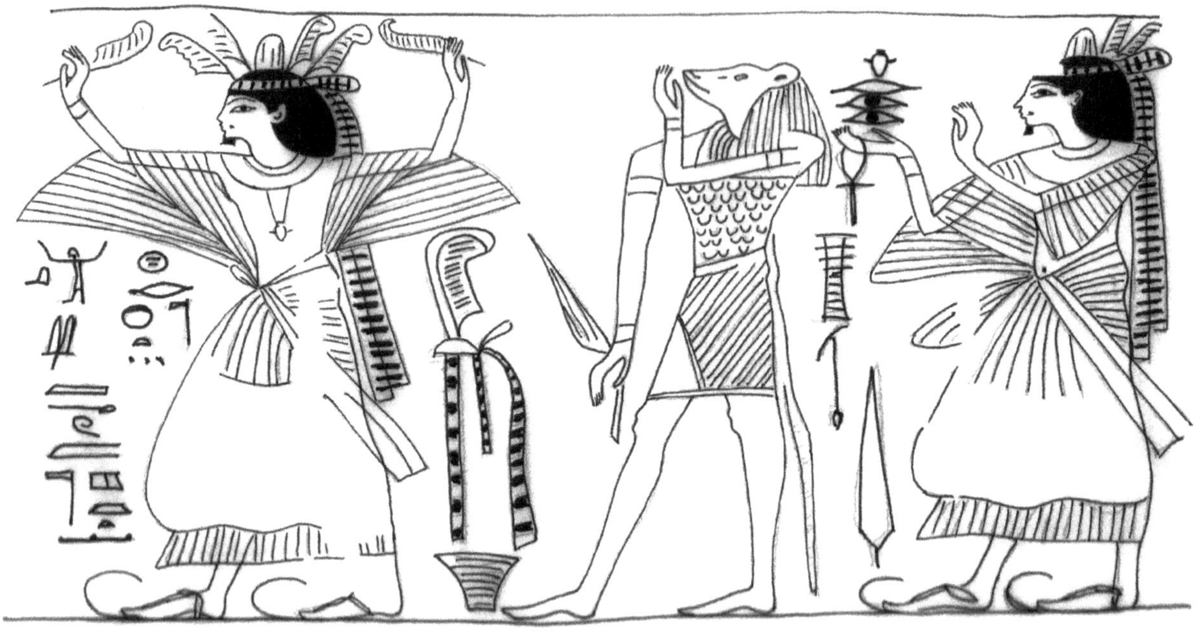

79. Funerary papyrus of Nesipakachuti (E 17401, Louvre Museum), vignette of the weighing of the heart (detail)

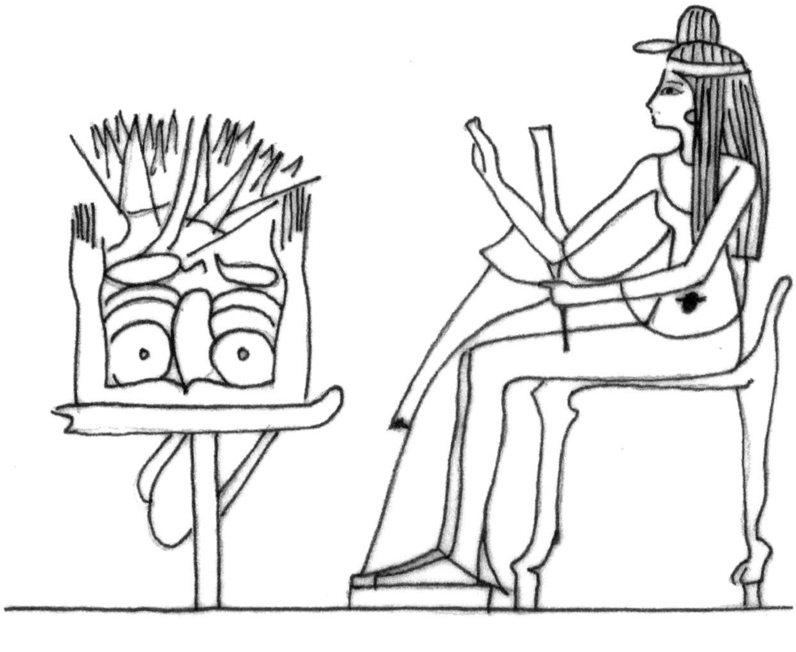

80. *Book of the Dead* of the lady Nesitanebicheru (British Museum), from Theban necropolis, Third Intermediate Period. Drawing after J. TAYLOR, *Death and the Afterlife in ancient Egypt*, 2001, p. 20.

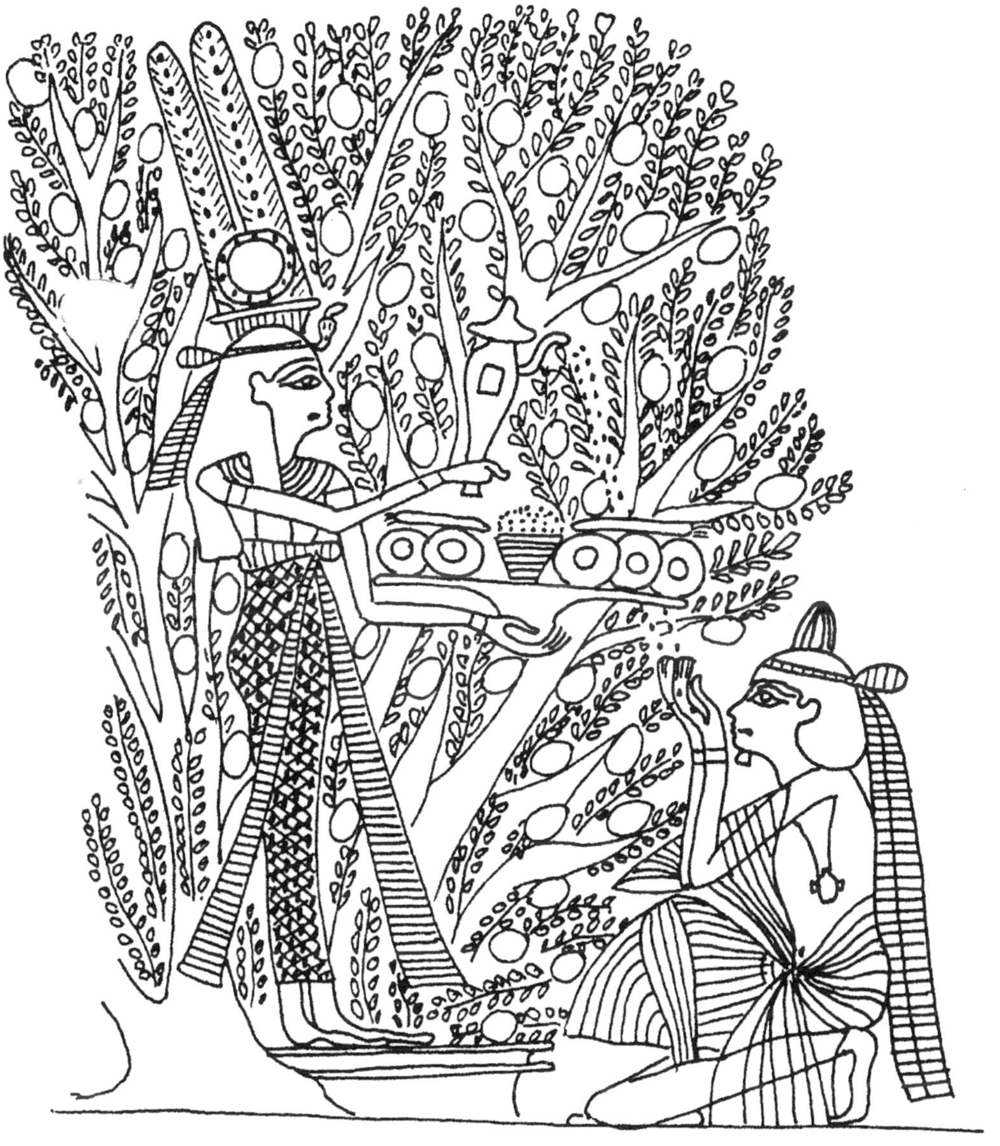

81. Coffin of a priest of Amun, from Theban necropolis, Third Intermediate Period. Drawing in A. NIWINSKI, *The Second Find of Deir el-Bahari,* II, 1999, p. 56

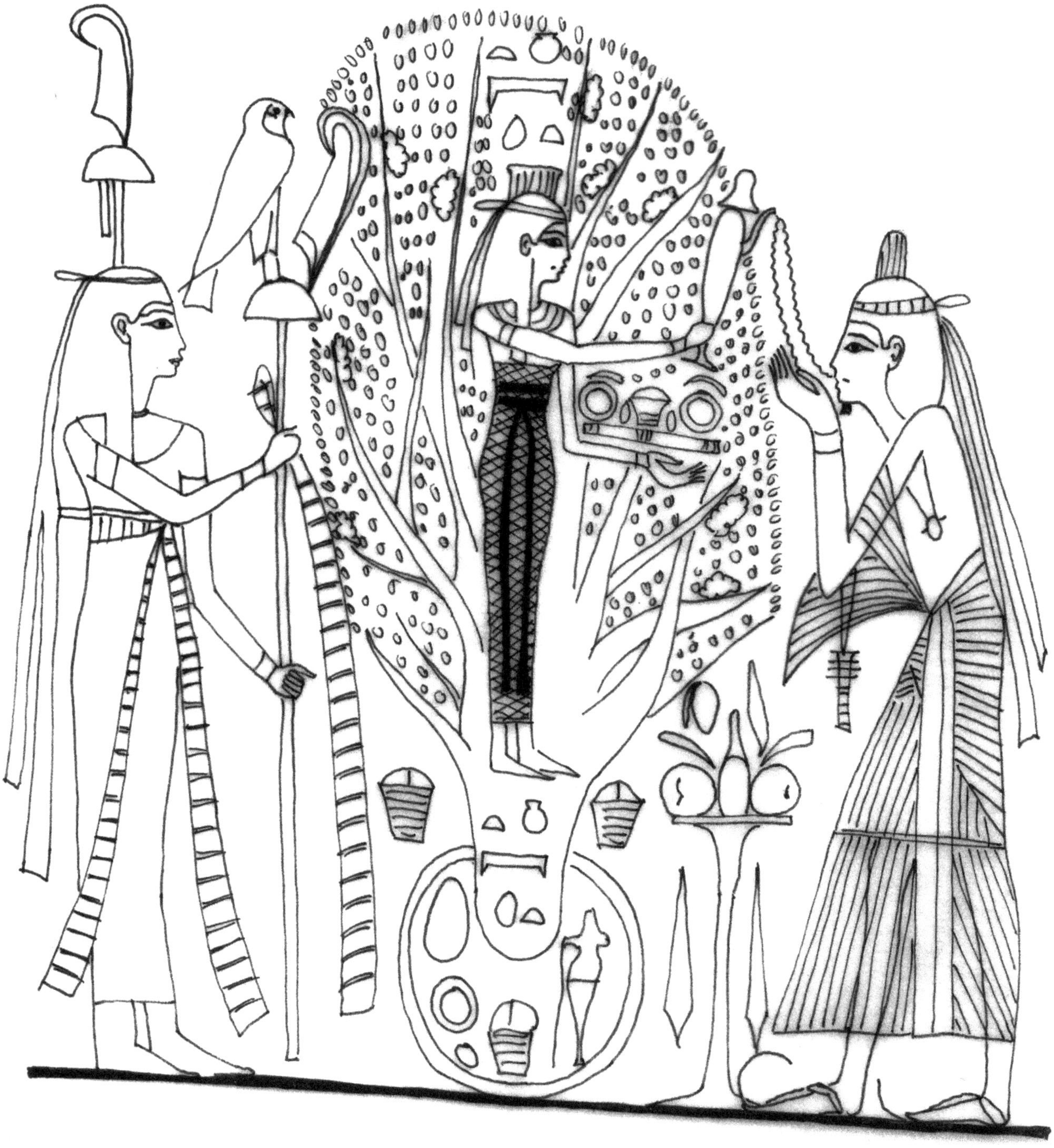

82. Outer coffin of Pakharu (CG 6122/6121, National Museum of Alexandria)

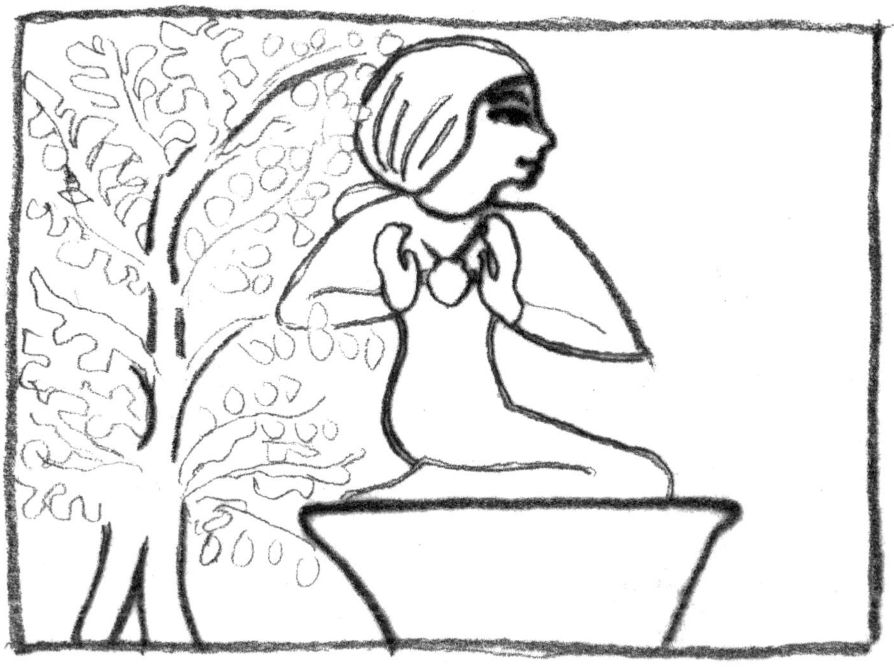

83. Pectoral of the lady Mehitkhati (British Museum), from Theban necropolis, Ramessid Period

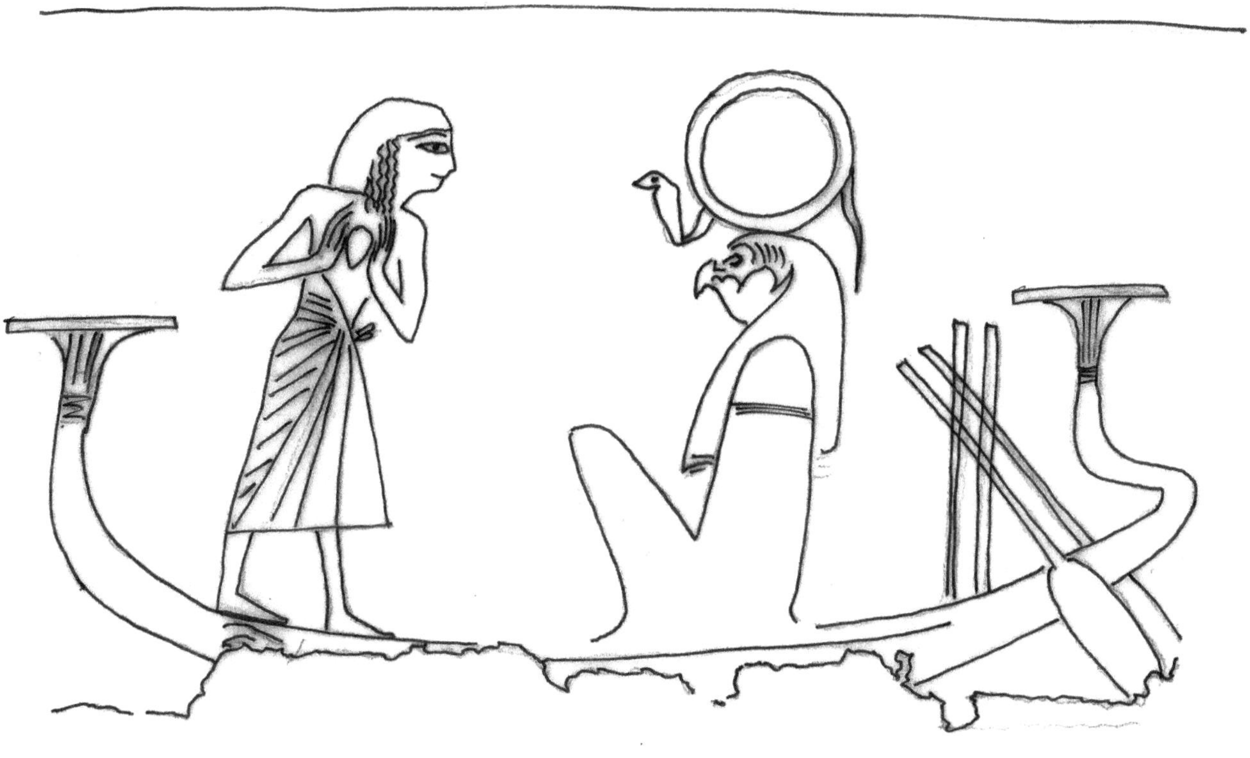

84. Vignette from the *Book of the Dead* of Neferenpet, Ramessid Period

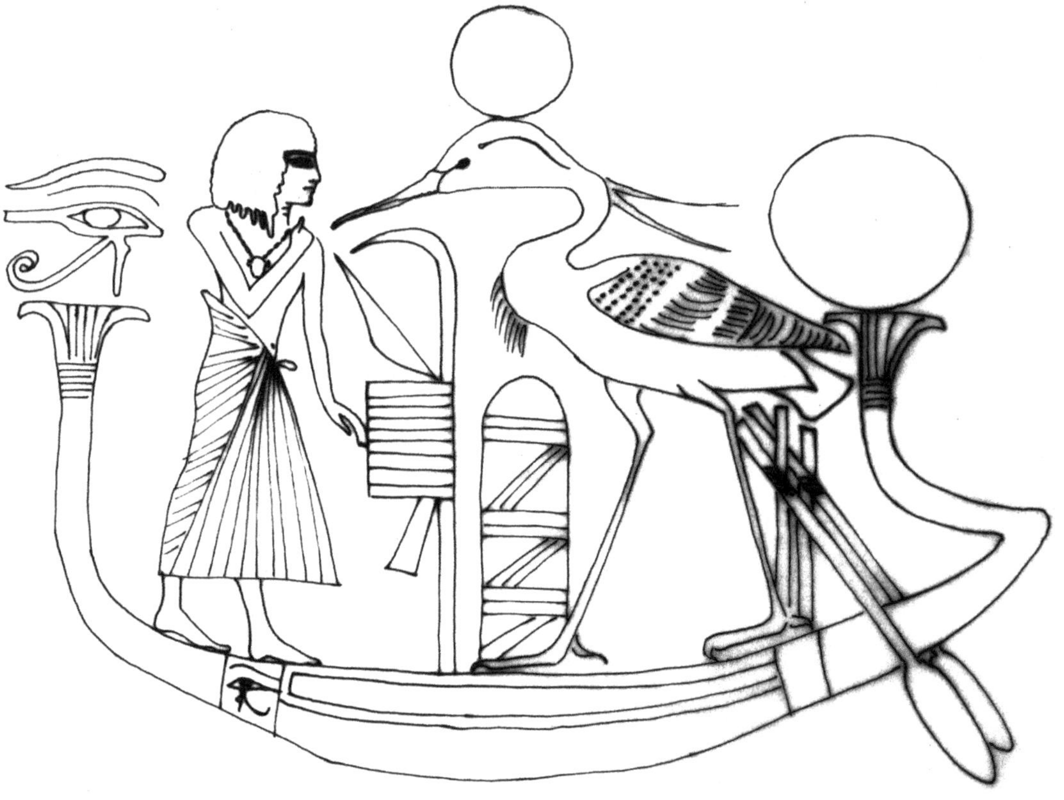

85. Deir el-Medina, tomb of Irinefer (TT 290)

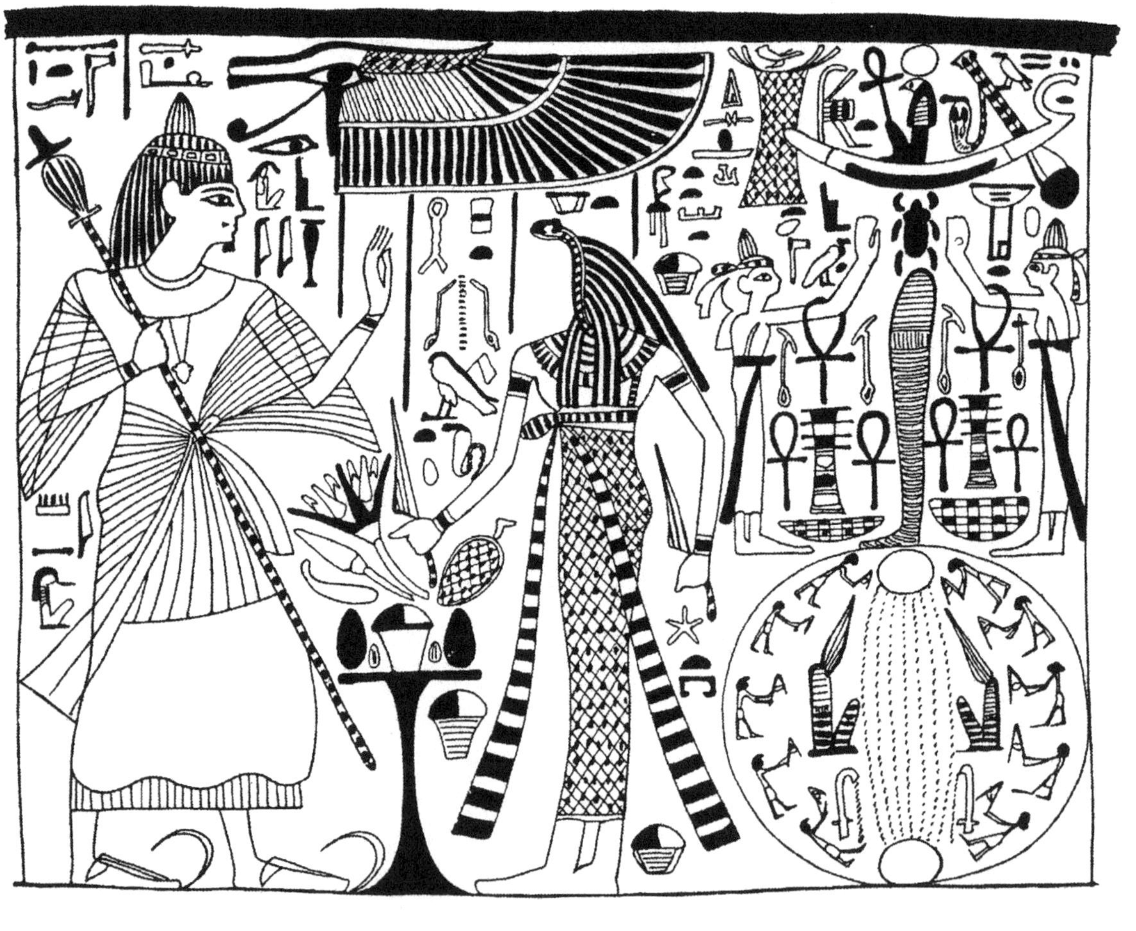

86. Coffin of a priest of Amun, from Theban necropolis, Third Intermediate Period. A. NIWINSKI, *The Second Find of Deir el-Bahari,* II, 1999, p. 6

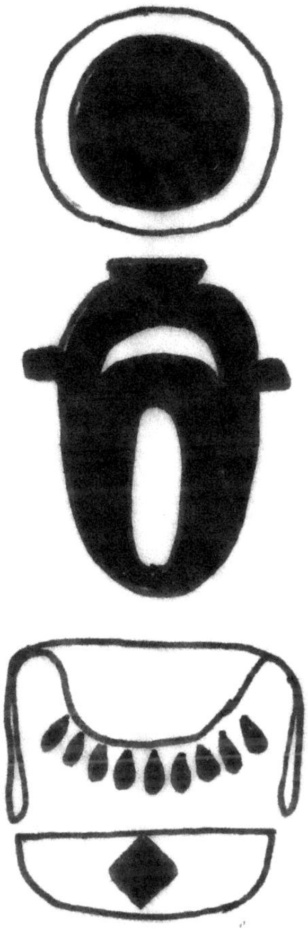

87. Coffin (BM 24793, British Museum), detail of the lid

88. Valley of the Kings, Tomb of Ramses VI (KV 9), Book of the Night (eigth hour). Drawing in A. PIANKOFF, *The Tomb of Ramses VI*, fig. 133

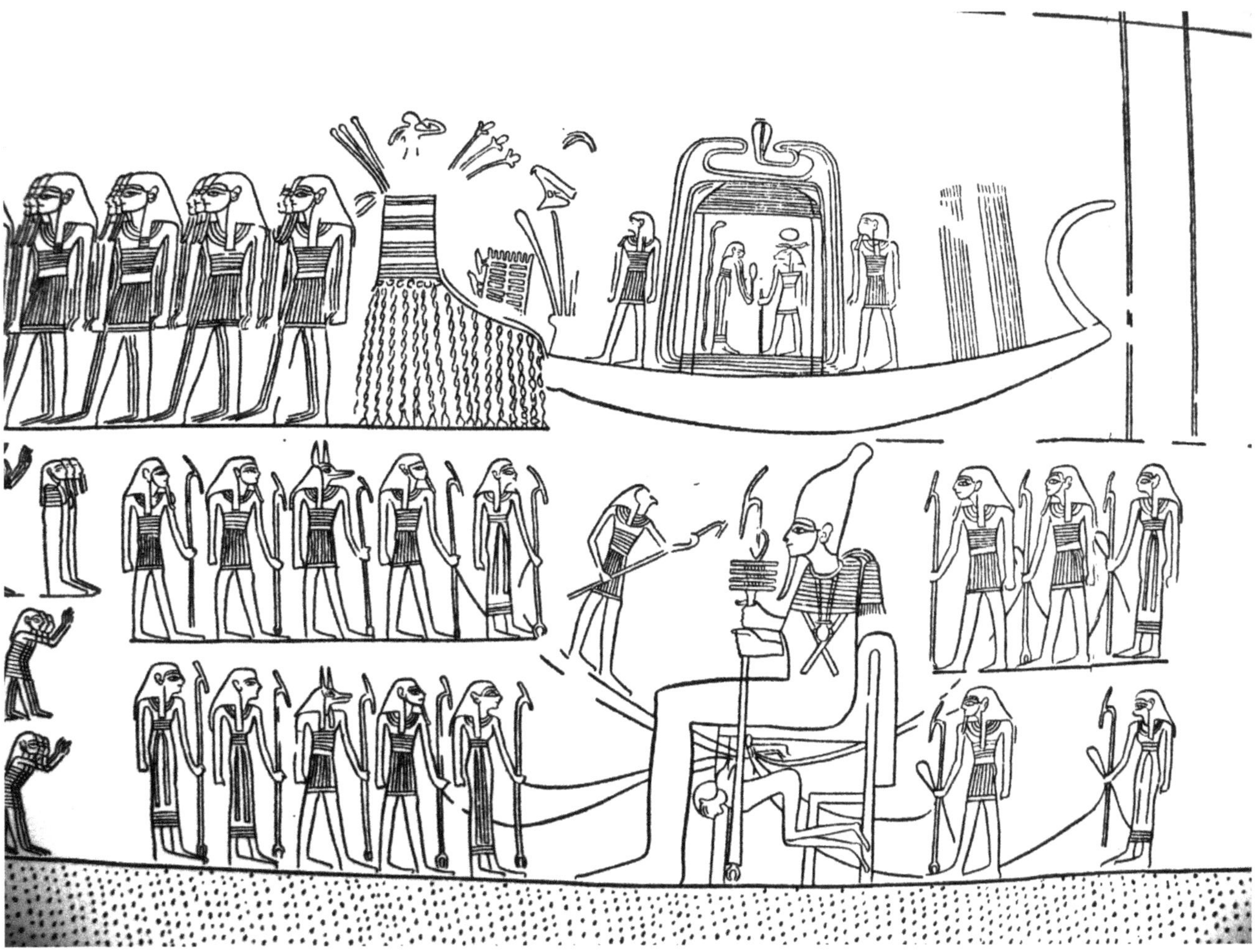

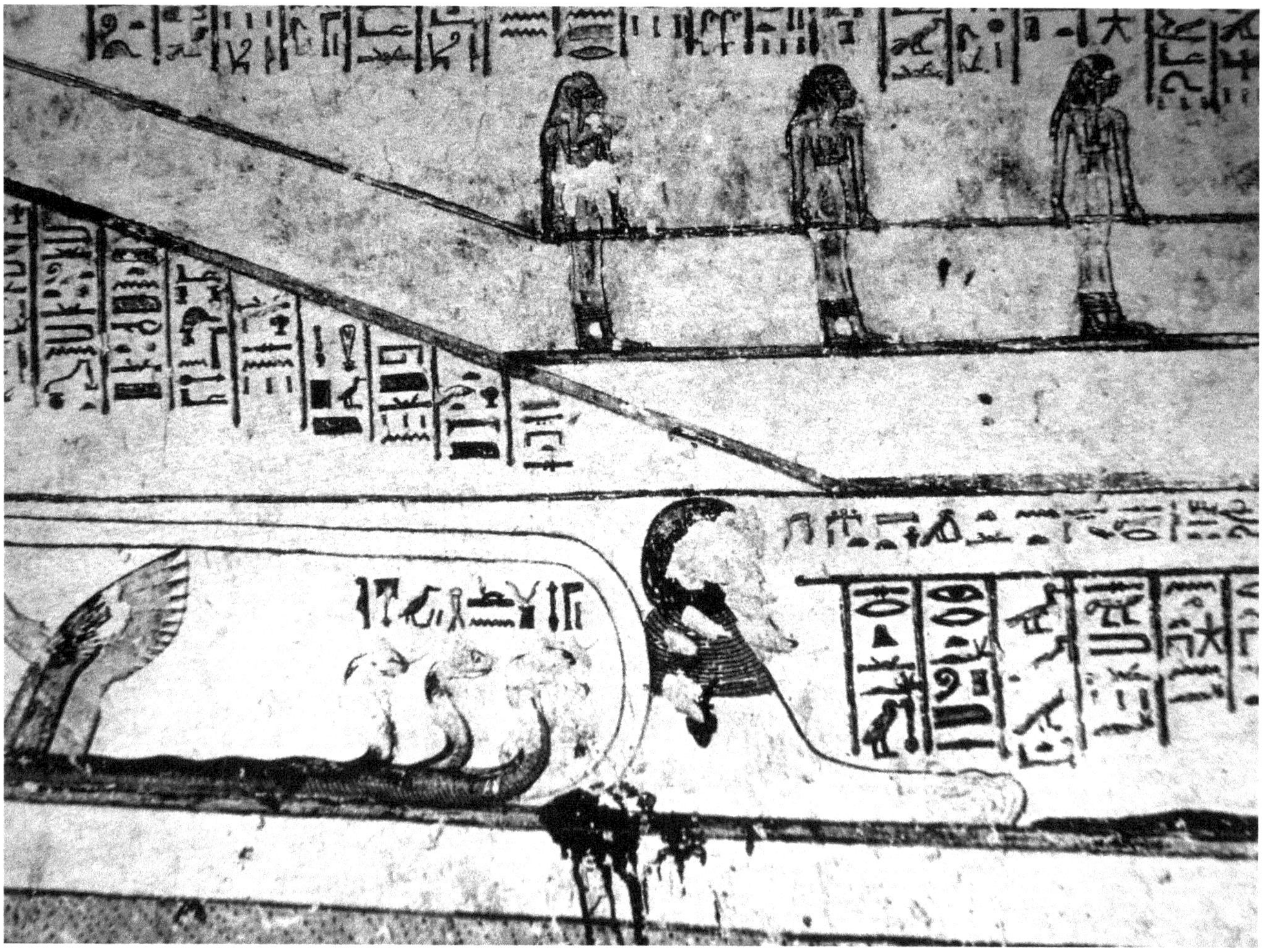

89. Valley of the Kings, Tomb of Ramses VI (KV 9), *Book of the Amduat* (fifth hour). Drawing in A. PIANKOFF, *The Tomb of Ramses VI*, Pl. 86

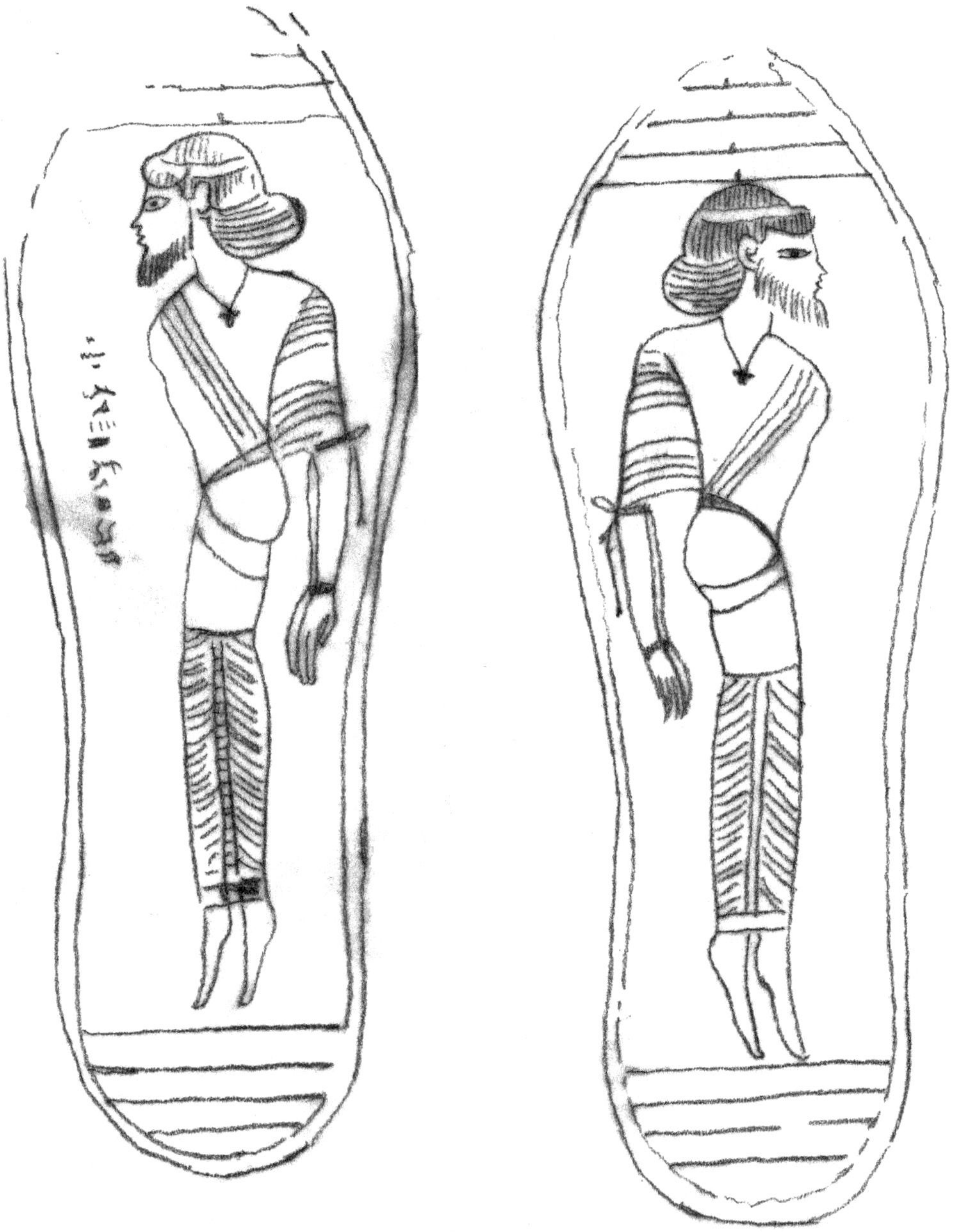

90. Coffin (Florence Egyptian Museum), outer decoration of the case (feet)

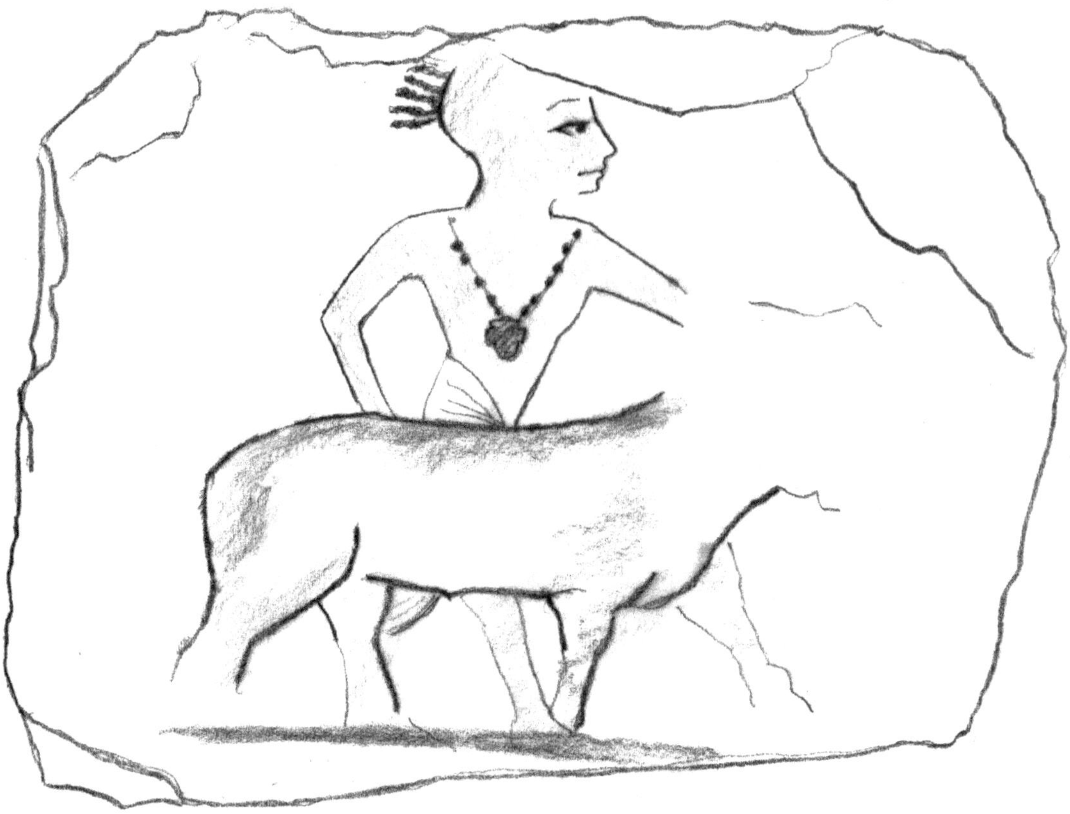

91. *Ostracon* (N 1562, Louvre Museum)

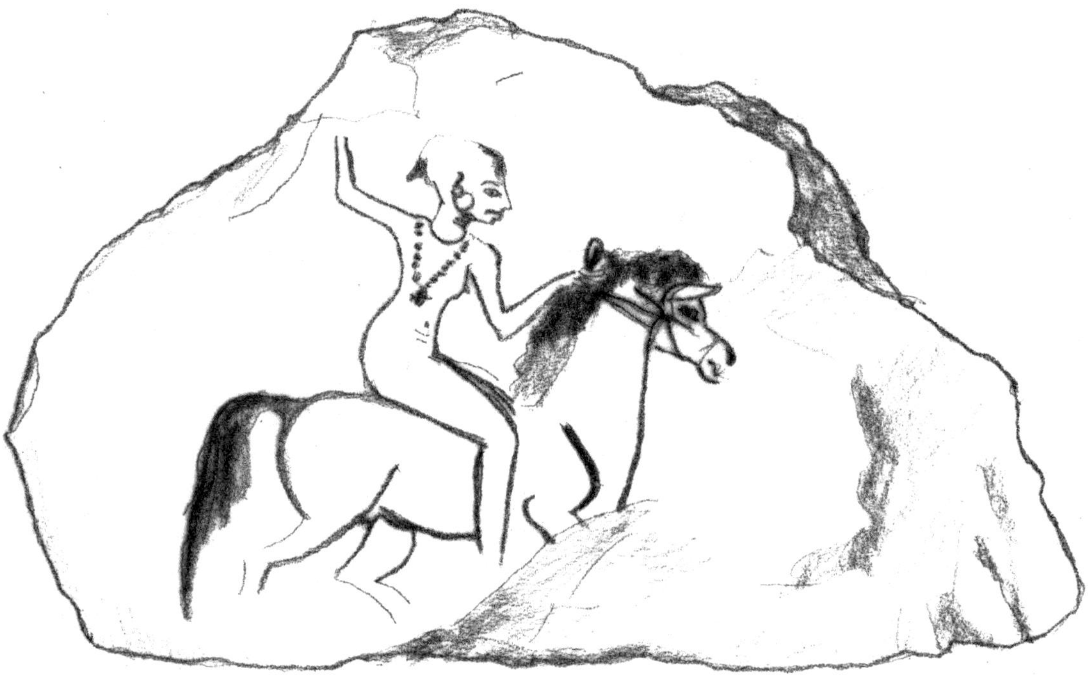

92. *Ostracon* (N 728, Berlin Egyptian Museum)

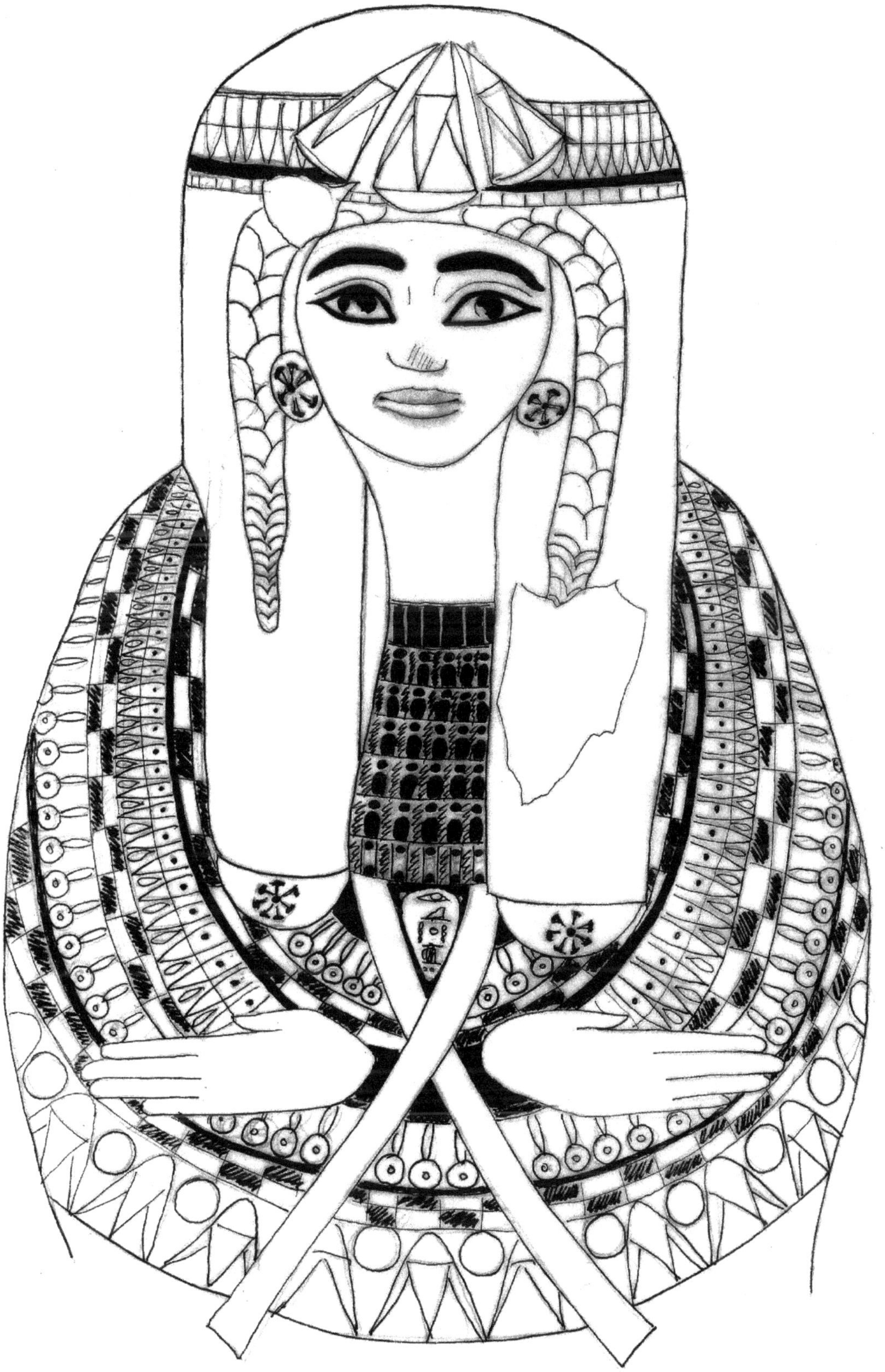

93. Coffin of an anonimous woman (SGL-AC-514, Sociedade de Geografia de Lisboa)

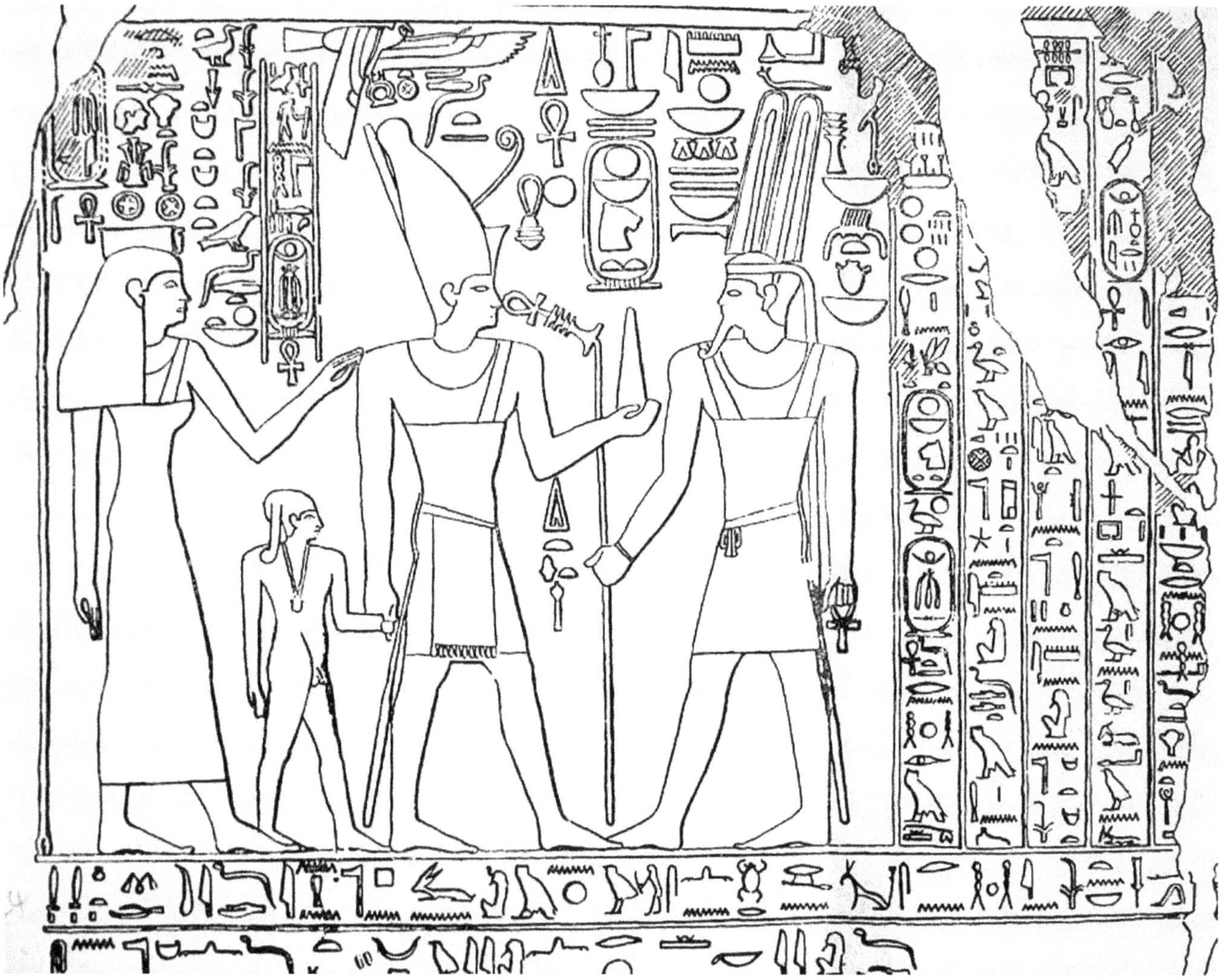

94. Donation stela. Drawing in I. HARARI, "Nature de la Stéle de Donation de Fonction du roi Ahmôsis a la reine Ahmès-Nefertari", *ASAE* 56 (1956), Pl. II

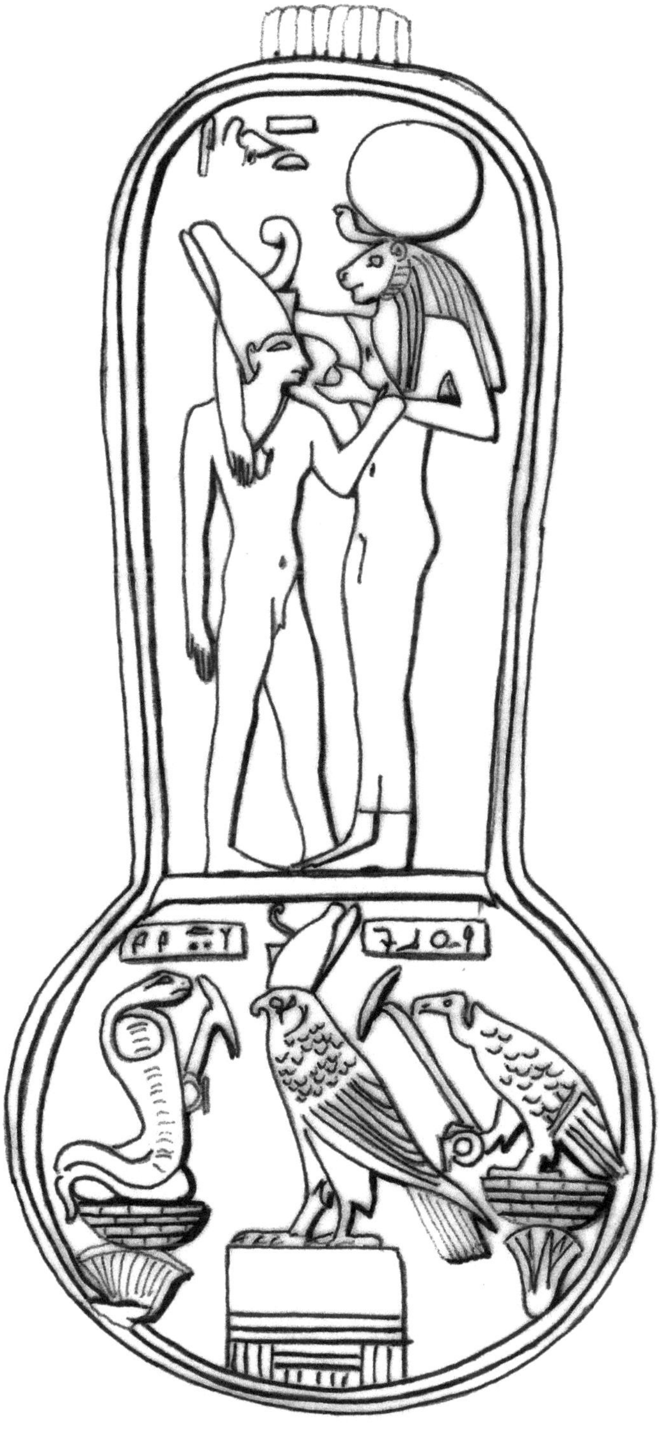

95. Counterpoise of *menat* necklace (41.160.104, Metropolitan Museum of Art), Third Intermediate Period

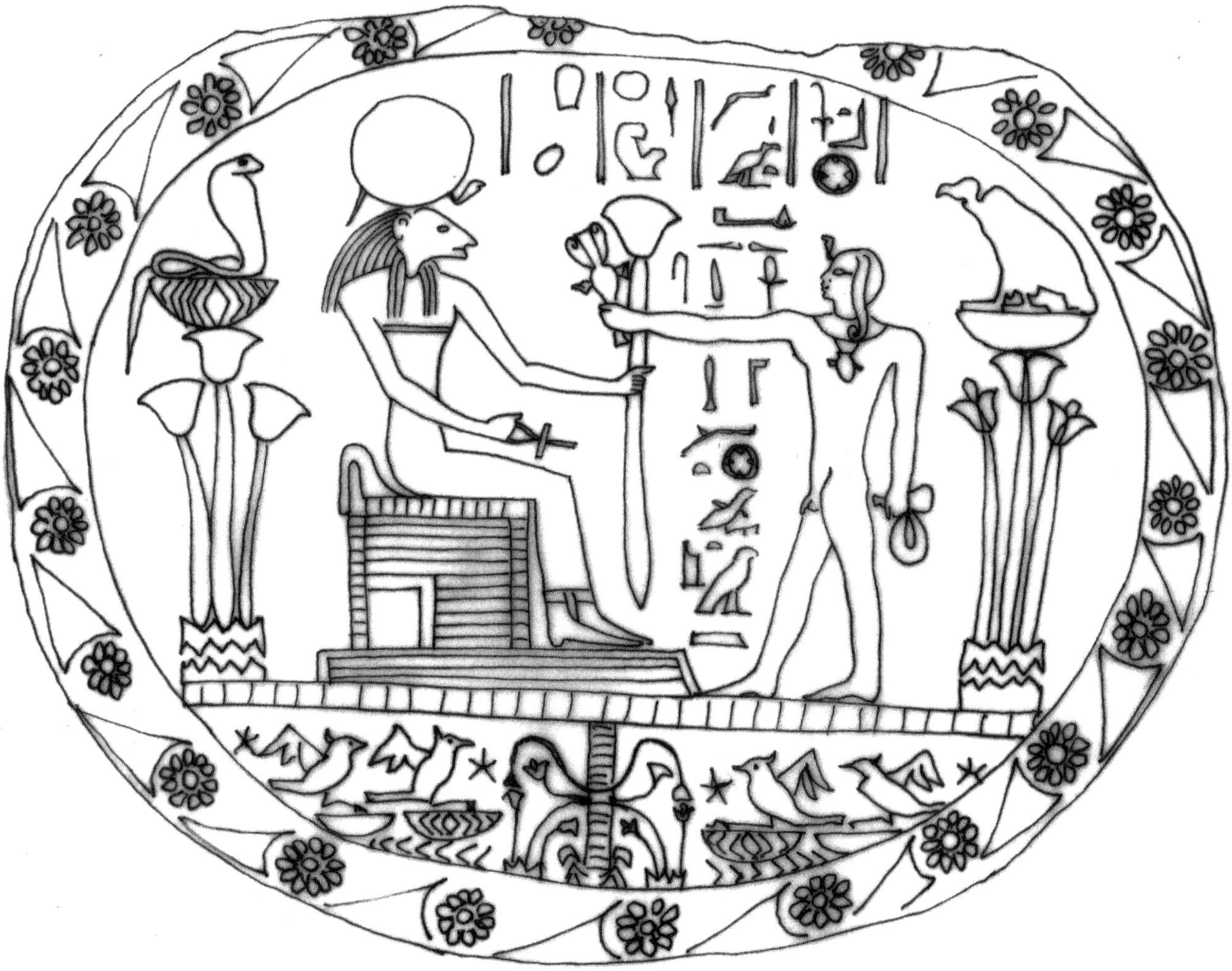

96. Fragment of a *menat* necklace (N 4434, Berlin Egyptian Museum), Third Intermediate Period

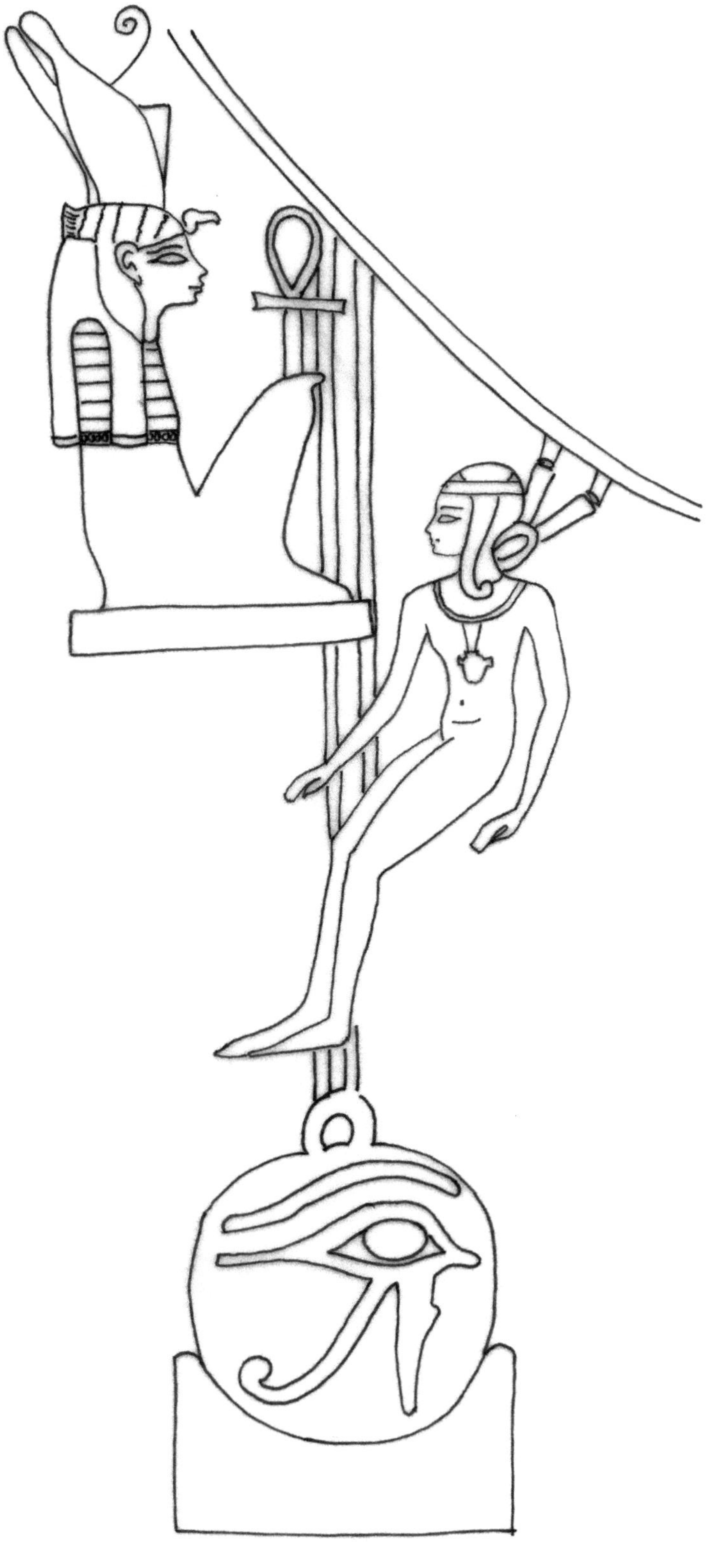

97. Cartonnage cover of the lady Tenkeret (JE 35055, Cairo Egyptian Museum), Third Intermediate Period, detail.

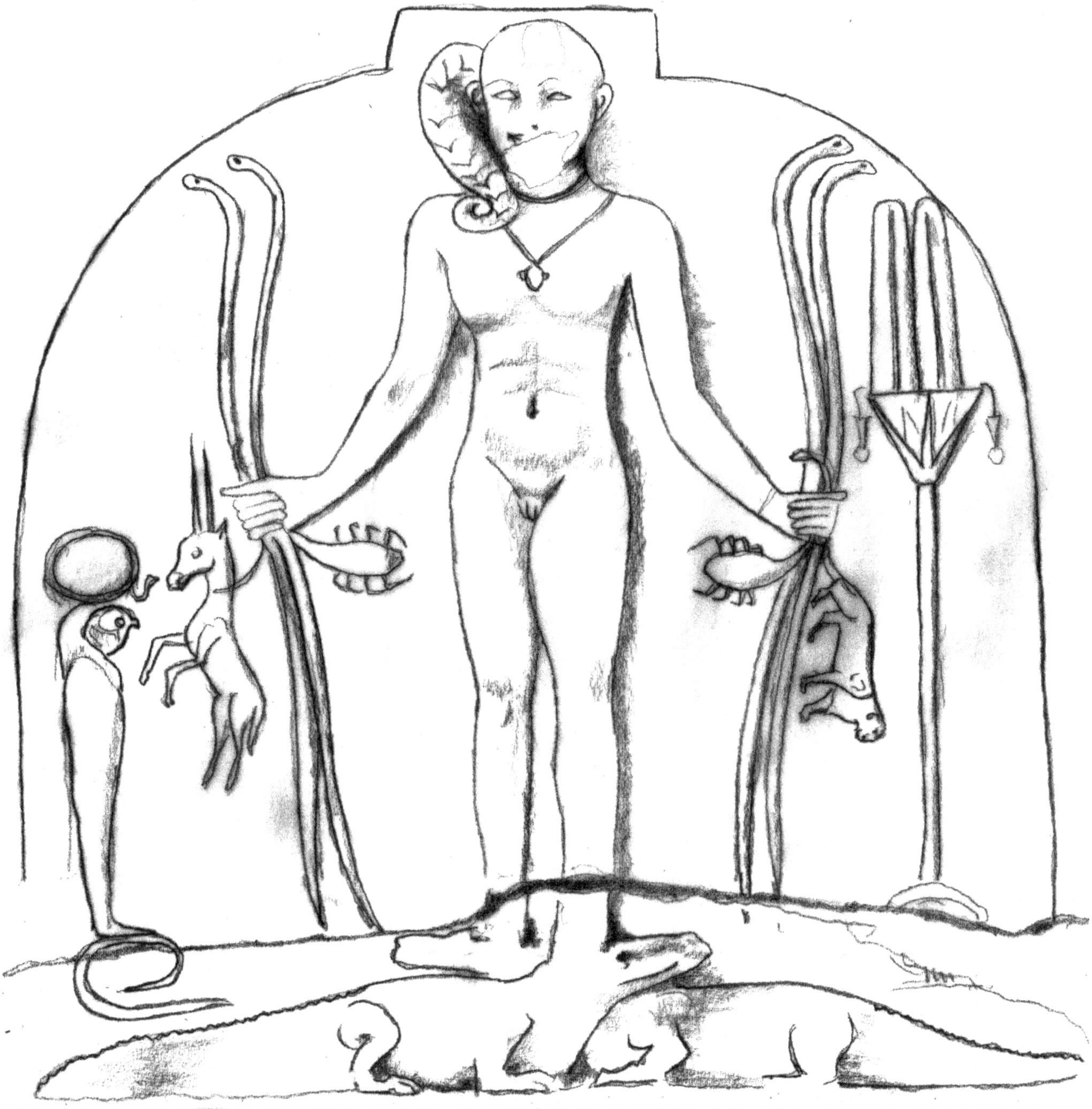

98. *Cippus* of Horpakhered (CG 9402, Cairo Egyptian Museum)

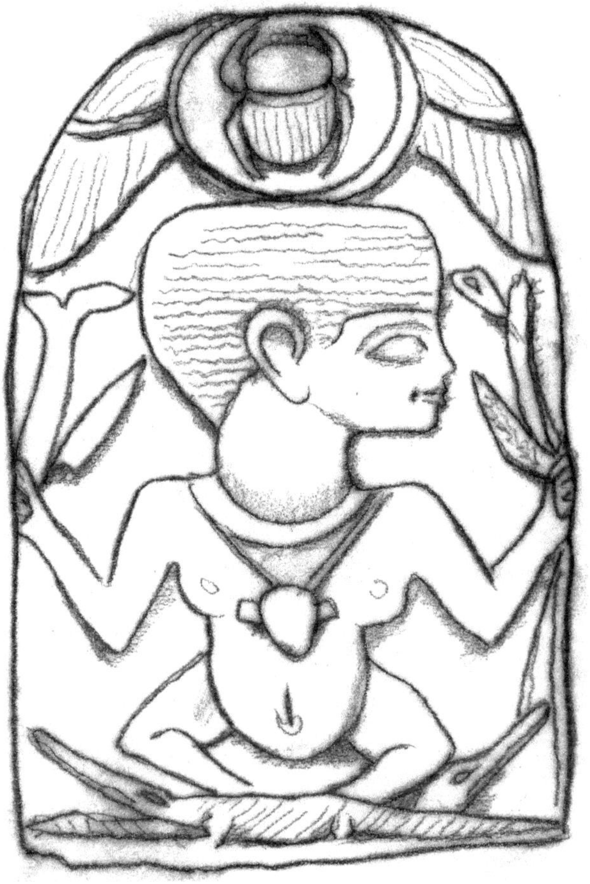

99. *Cippus*, (S 23-M-591, Museum of Fine Arts) from Meroe, Third Intermediate Period

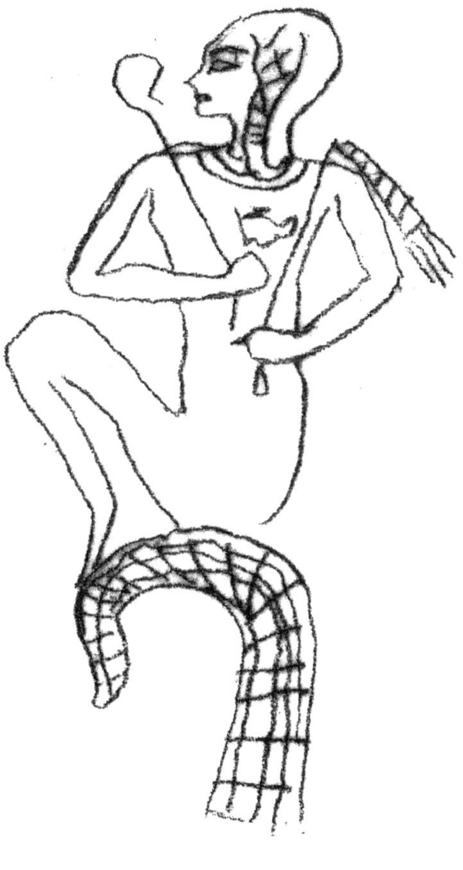

100. Milbank Papirus (OIM 10486, Oriental Institute), vignette of the weighing of the heart (detail)

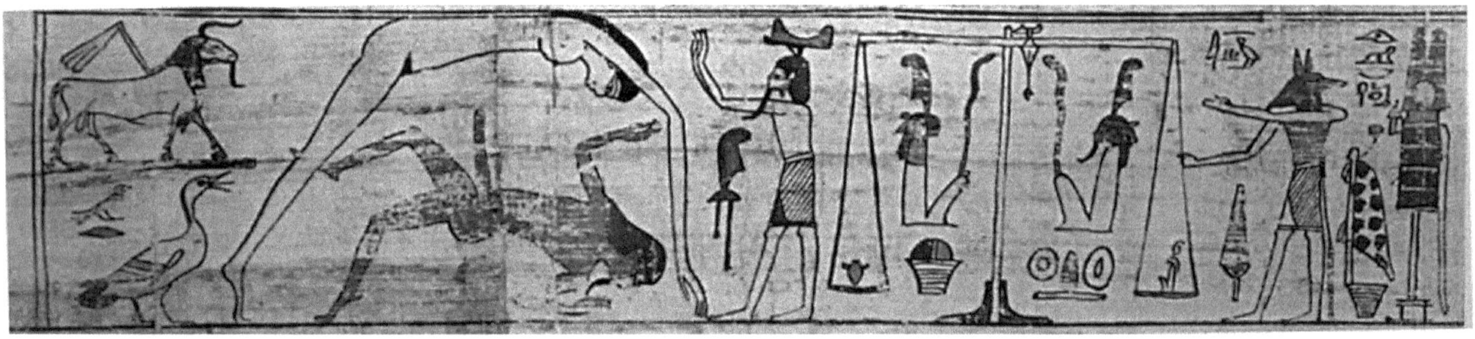

101. Funerary papyrus, from Theban necropolis, Third Intermediate Period. Photo after A. NIWINSKI, *Studies on Illustrated Theban Funerary Papyri*, pl. 29d

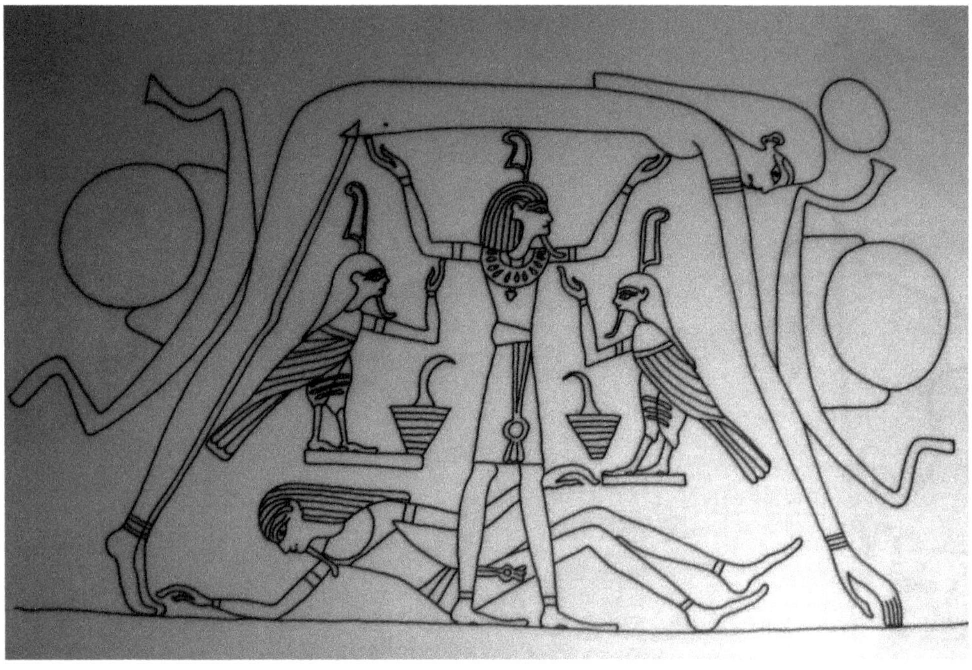

102. Leiden Papyrus AMS 34 (T.7). Drawing by Andrzej Niwinski

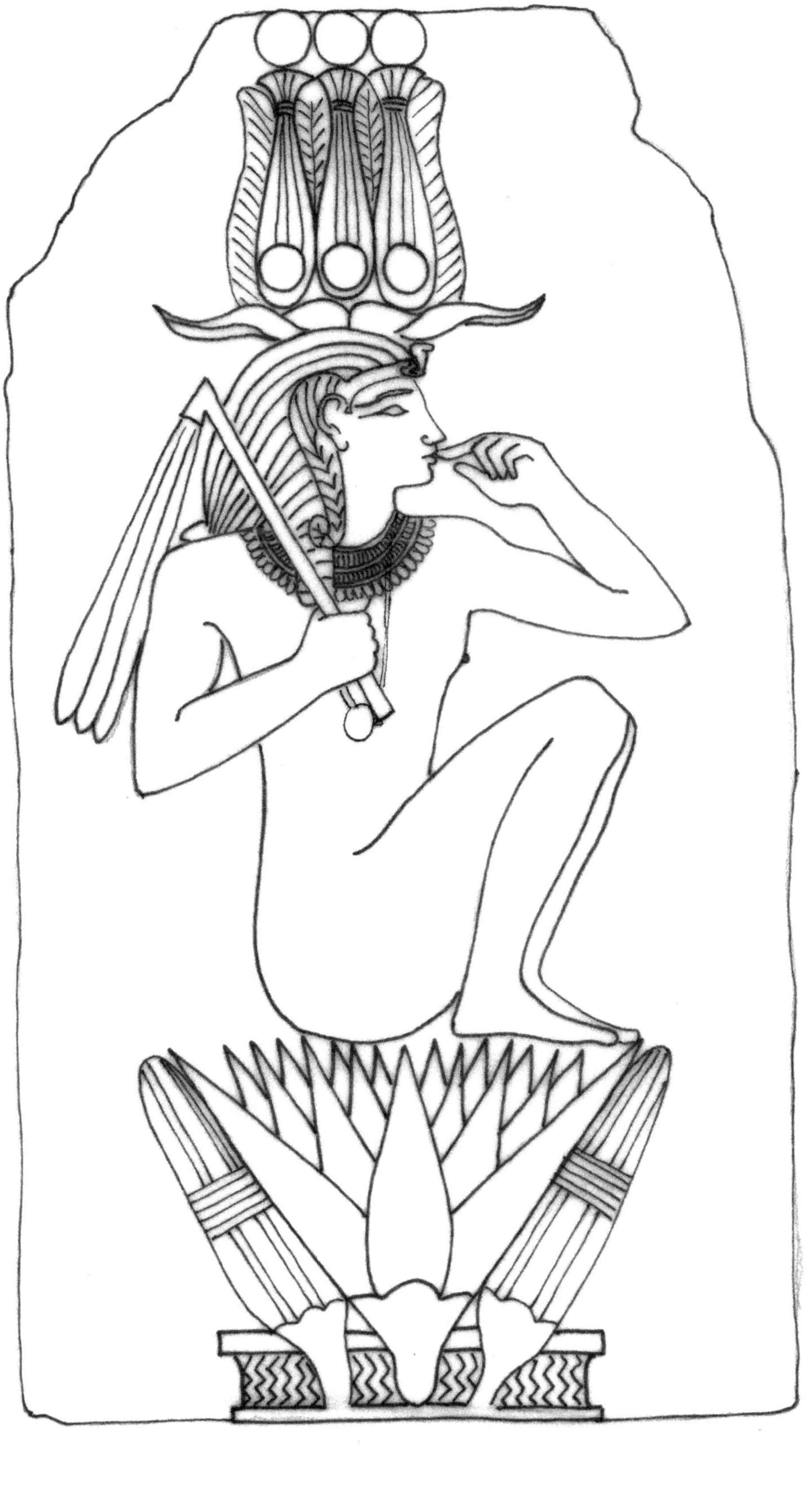

103. Plaque of Iuput II (1956.1485 National Museums of Scotland),
Third Intermediate Period

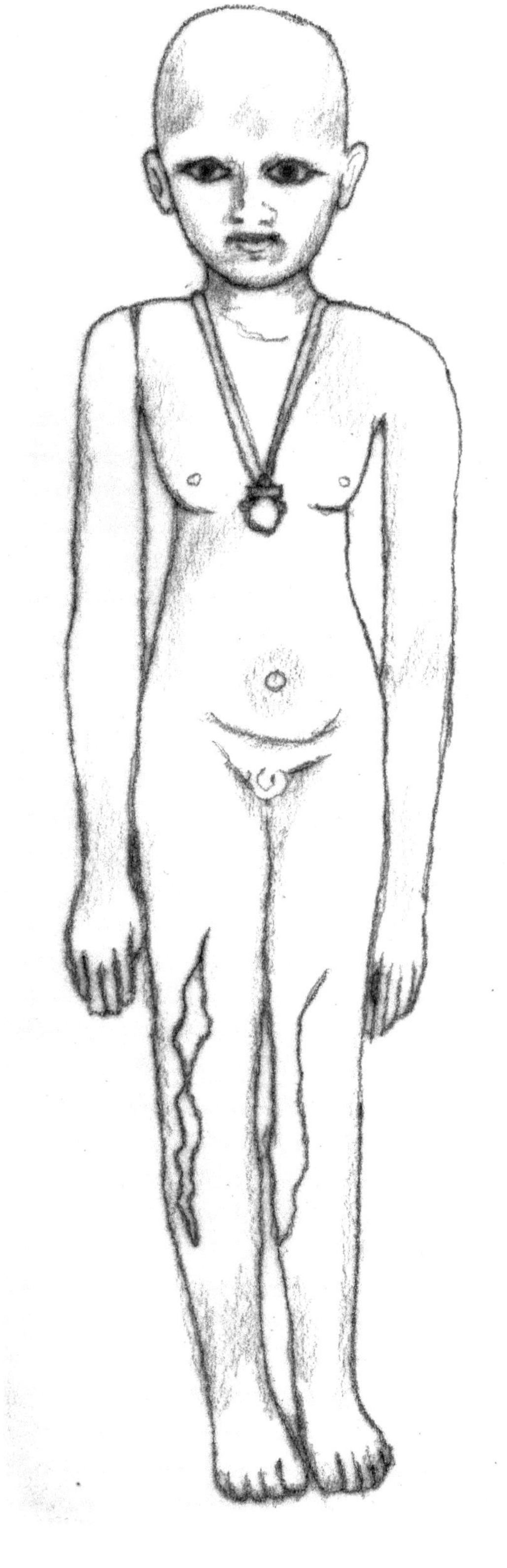

104. Statue of a divine child (SR 46380, Cairo Egyptian Museum), Greco-Roman Period

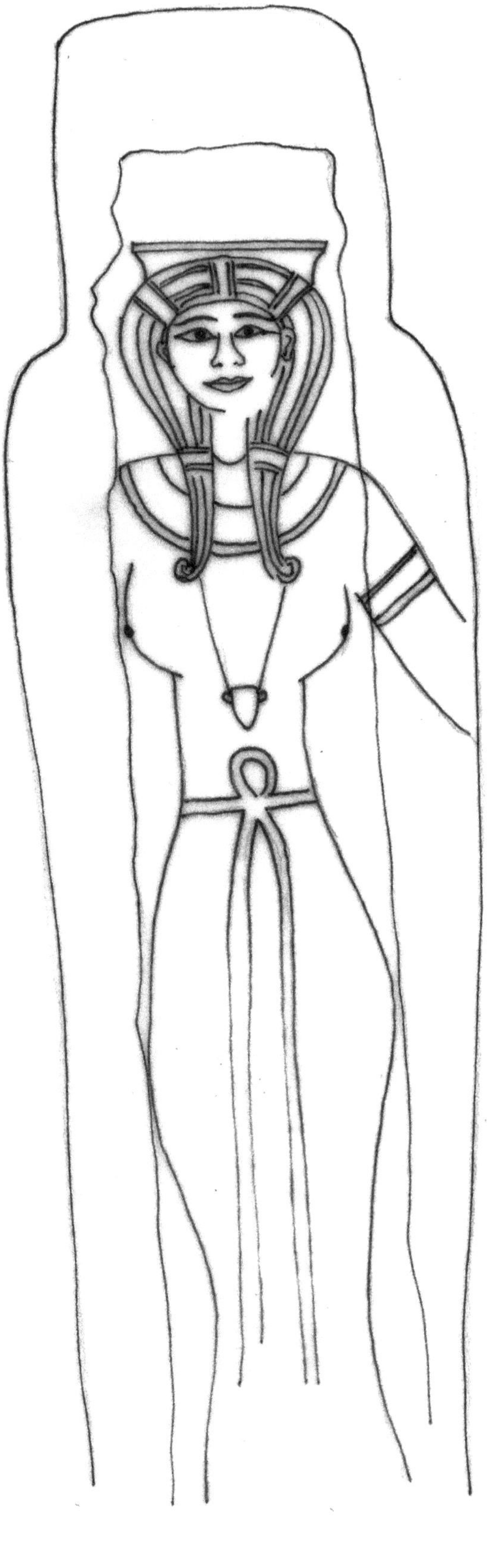

105. Coffin (E 332, Museu Nacional de Arqueologia de Lisboa), interior decoration of the bottom of the case

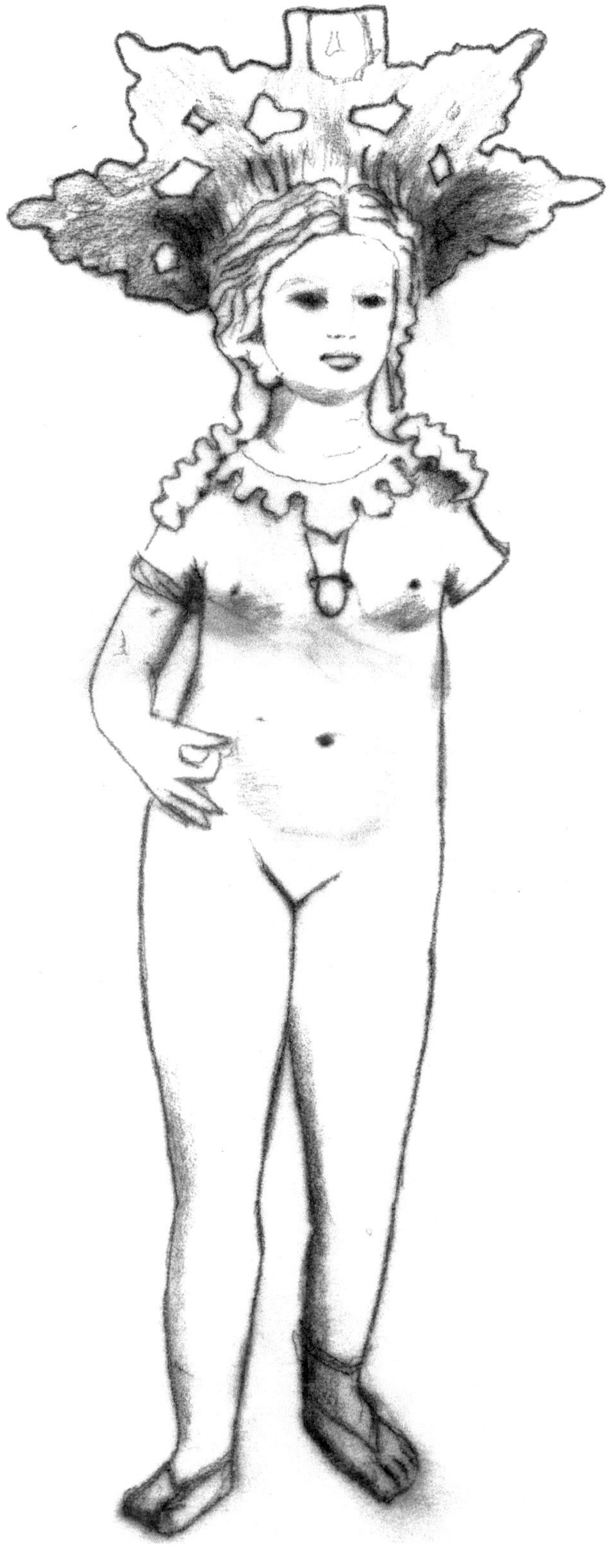

106. Sculpture of Isis-Aphrodite (X.0082, Brooklyn Museum), Greco-Roman Period

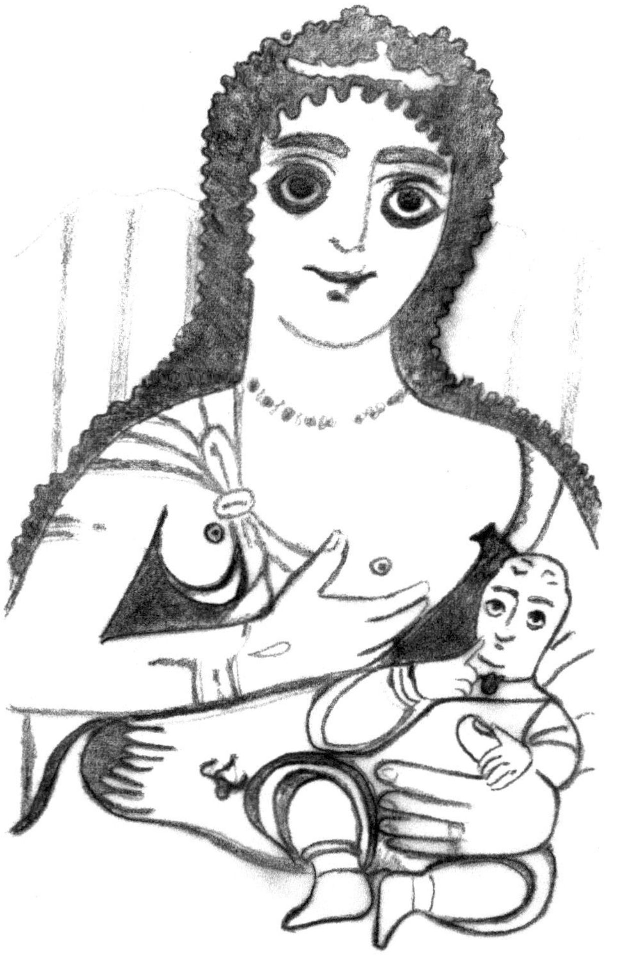

107. Isis and Harpokrates, wall painting from Karanis, Greco-Roman Period

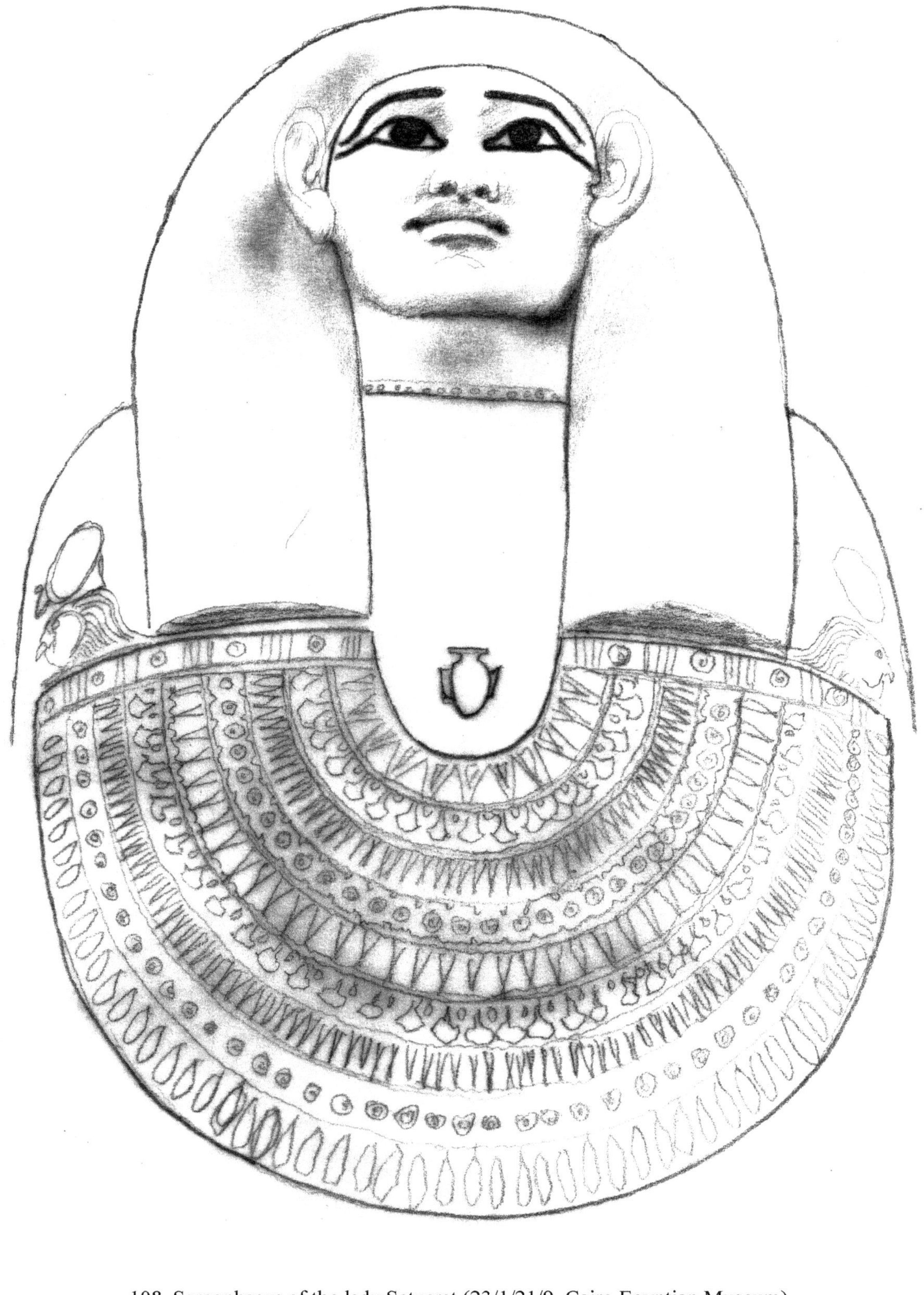

108. Sarcophagus of the lady Setueret (23/1/21/9, Cairo Egyptian Museum)

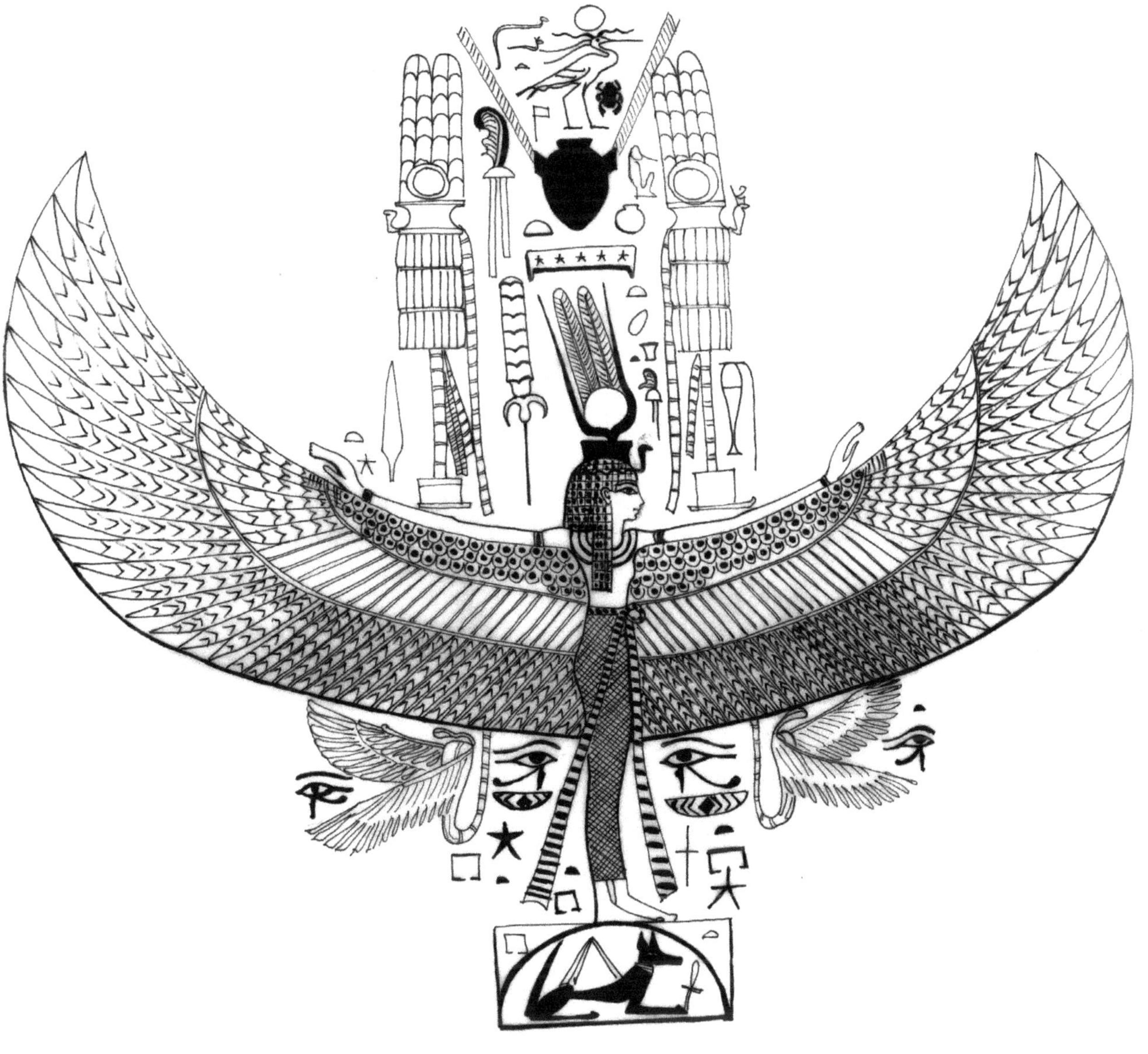

109. Coffin (CG 6191, Cairo Egyptian Museum), detail of the lid

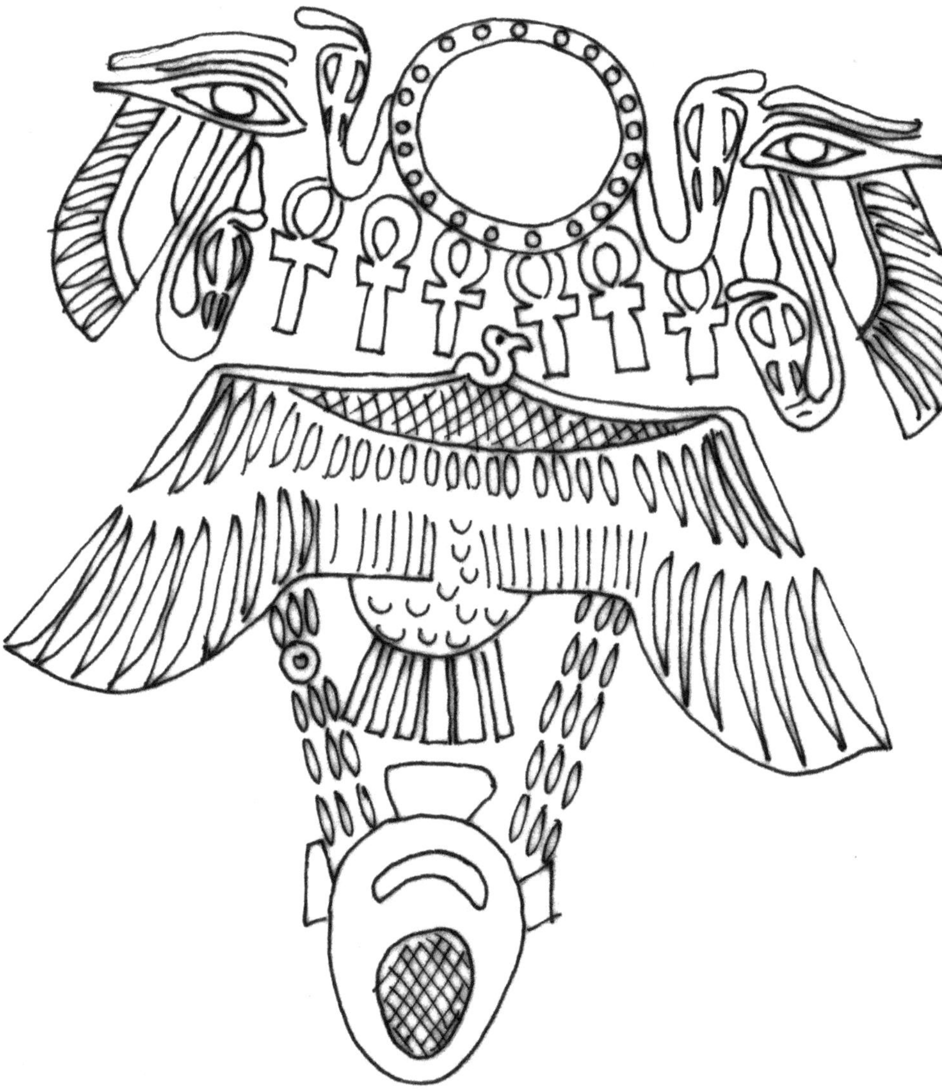

110. Coffin (Manchester), detail of the lid. Drawing by Andrzej Niwinski

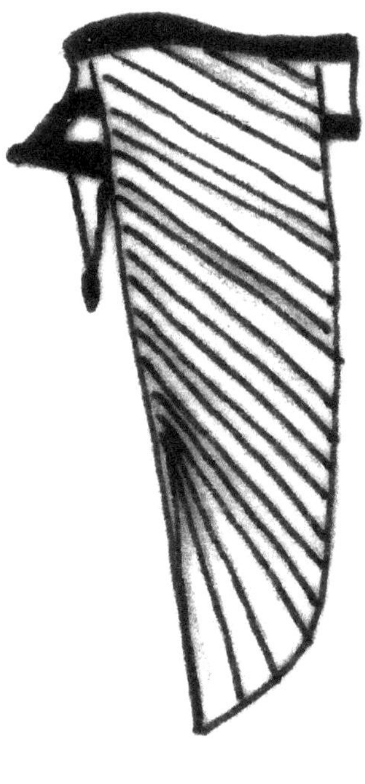

111. Coffin (N° inv. 228, Victoriamusset), detail of the outer decoration of the case

BIBLIOGRAPHY

Abreviations

ASAE	*Annales du Service des Antiquités de l'Égypte*, Cairo
ARTIS	*Revista do Instituto de História de Arte da Faculdade de Letras de Lisboa*, Lisboa
BMH	*Bulletin du Musée Hongrois des Beaux Arts*, Budapeste
BSEG	*Bulletin de la Societé d'Égyptologie de Genéve*, Genève
BACE	Bulletin of the Australian Centre for Egyptology, *Sydney*
BIFAO	*Bulletin de l'Institut Français d'Archéologie Oriental*, Cairo
CdÉ	*Chronique d'Égypte*, Bruxelles.
GM	*Göttinger Miszellen,* Götingen
CIV	Carter inventory number from the Tutankhamun's tomb
JARCE	*Journal of the American Research Center in Egypt*, New York
JEA	*Journal of Egyptian Archaeology*, London
JEOL	*Jaarbericht van het Vooraziatisch-Egyptish Genootschap* ,Ex Oriente Lux', Leiden
MMAF	*Bulletin of the Metropolitan Museum of Art*, New York
OMRO	*Oudheidkundige Mededelingen uit het Rijksmuseum van Oudheden te Leiden*, Leiden
RA	*Révue Archéologique*, Paris.
RdC	*Revue du Caire*, Cairo
Rd'É	*Révue d'Égyptologie*, Paris
RT	*Recueil de Travaux Relatifs à la Philologie et à l'Archéologie Égyptiennes et Assyriennes*, Paris.
ZÄS	*Zeitschrift für ägyptische Sprache und Altertumskunde*, Berlin, Lepzig

1. Grammars and Dictionaries

Luís Manuel de ARAÚJO (dir.), *Dicionário do Antigo Egipto*, Editorial Caminho, Lisboa, 2001

Alan GARDINER, *Egyptian Grammar. Being an Introduction to the Study of Hieroglyphs*, Griffith Institute, Ashmolean Museum, Oxford, 1994

Wolfgang HELCK, Eberhard OTTO, Wolfhart WESTENDORF (ed.), *Lexikon der Ägyptologie*, 7 volumes, Otto Harrassowitz, Wiesbaden, 1975-1986

Raymond FAULKNER, *A Concise Dictionary of Middle Egyptian*, Griffith Institute, Oxford, 1999

Christian LEITZ, *Lexikon der Ägyptichen Götter und Götterbezeichungen*, vol. I, Uitgeverij Peeters en Departement Ossterse Studies, Louvain, Paris, Dudley, 2002

Bernardette MENU, *Petite Grammaire de l'Égyptien Héroglyphique à l'usage des débutants*, Librairie Orientaliste Paul Geuthner, Lausanne, 1997

Donald REDFORD (dir.), *Oxford Ecyclopedia of Ancient Egypt*, Oxford University Press, Oxford, 2001

2. Catalogues and Exhibitions

Ägyptisches Museum Berlin, Östlicher Stürlerbau am Schloss Charlottenburg, Berlin, 1967

Album du Département Égyptien, Musées Royaux d'Art et d'Histoire, Fondation Egyptologique Reine Elisabeth, Buxelles, 1934

Aménophis III, le Pharaon-Soleil, Réunion des Musées Nationaux, Paris, 1993

Brigitte AFFHOLDER-GÉRARD, Marie-Jeanne CORNIC, *Angers, Musée Pincé: Collections Égyptiennes*, Réunion des Musées Nationaux, Paris, 1990

Guillemette ANDREU, Marie-Hélène RUTSCHOWS-CAYA, Christiane ZIEGLER, *Ancient Egypt at the Louvre*, Hachette, Paris, 1997

Luís Manuel de ARAÚJO, *Antiguidades Egípcias*, I, Museu Nacional de Arqueologia, Lisboa, 1993

Luís Manuel de ARAÚJO, *Arte Egípcia: Colecção Calouste Gulbenkian*, Museu Calouste Gulbenkian, Lisboa, 2006

Luís Manuel de ARAÚJO, Paula BASSO, *A Farmácia no Mundo Pré-Clássico e nas Culturas Tradicionais*, Museu da Farmácia, Lisboa, 2008

L'Art Égyptien au Temps des Pyramides, Réunion des Musées Nationaux, Paris, 1999

Ausgewhälte Werke der Ägyptischen Sammlung, Hannover, 1958

Lawrence BERMAN, Kenneth BOHAC, *Catalogue of Egyptian Art*, Cleveland Museum of Art, Cleveland, 1999

Samuel BIRCH, *Catalogue of the collection of Egyptian Antiquities at Alnwick Castle*, R. Clay, Sons and Taylor Printers, London, 1880

Gun BJÖRKMAN, *A Selection of the Objects in the Smith Collection of Egyptian Antiquities at the Linköping Museum*, Almqvist & Wiksell, Stockholm, 1971

William BRASHEAR & others, *Belser Kunstblibliothek: Die Meisterwerke aus dem Ägyptischen Museum Berlin*, Belser Verlag, Stuttgart, Zurich, 1980

Emma BRUNNER-TRAUT, Hellmut BRUNNER, *Die Ägyptishe Sammlung der Universität Tübingen*, Verlag Philipp von Zabern, Mainz am Rhein, 1981

John COONEY, *Catalogue of Egyptian antiquities in the British Museum*, IV: *Glass*, British Museum Publisher, London, 1970

Jean-Pierre CORTEGGIANI, *L'Égypte des Pharaons au Musée du Caire*, Hachette, Paris, 1986

Silvio CURTO, *L'antico Egitto nel Museo Egizio di Torino*, Tipografia Torinese Editrice, Turim, 1984

Silvio CURTO, Anna Maria DONADONI ROVERI, Alessandro ROCCATI, *The Museums of Turin: The Egyptian Museum*, Daniela Piazza Editore, Turim, 1989

Sue D'AURIA, Peter LACOVARA, Catharine ROEHRING, *Mummies & Magic: The Funerary Arts of Ancient Egypt*, Museum of Fine Arts, Boston, 1988

Michel DEWACHTER, *Musée Champollion: La Collection Égyptienne*, Figeac, 1986

Arne EGGEBRECHT, *Ägyptens Aufstieg zur Weltmacht*, Verlag Philipp von Zabern, Mainz am Rhein, 1987

Arne EGGEBRECHT, *Ägypten geheimnis der grabkammern: Suche nach unster-blichkeit*, Verlag Philipp von Zabern, Mainz, 1993

Jean-Yves EMPEREUR, *Petit Guide du Musée Greco-Romain d'Alexandrie*, Harpo-crates Publishing, Alexandria, 2000

Richard FAZZINI, James ROMANO, Madeleine CODY, *Art for Eternity: Masterworks from Ancient Egypt*, Brooklyn Museum of Art, Scala Publishers, Brooklyn, 1999

Florence Dunn FRIEDMAN, *Gifts of the Nile:Ancient Egyptian Faience*, Thames & Hudson and Rhode Island School of Design Museum of Art, Rhode Island, 1998

Brigitte GRATIEN, Françoise LE SAOUT, *Nubie: Les cultures antiques di Soudan à travers les explorations et les fouilles françaises et franco-soudanaises*, Université Charles de Gaulle, Lille, 1994

Henry HALL, *Catalogue of Egyptian Scarabs in the British Museum*, vol. I: Royal Scarabs, Trustees of the British Museum, London, 1913

Fekri HASSAN, *Greco-Roman Museum*, National Center for Documentation of Cultural and Natural Heritage & Supreme Council of Antiquities, Cairo, 2002

William HAYES, *The Scepter of Egypt: A Background for the Study of the Egyptian Antiquities in the Metropolitan Museum of Art*, 2 vols., Metropolitan Museum of Art, New York, 1990

Svetlana HODJADH, Oleg BERLEV, *The Egyptian Reliefs and Stelae in the Pushkin Museum of Fine Arts in Moscow*, Aurora Art Publishers, Leningrad, 1982

Erik HORNUNG, Betsy BRYAN, *The Quest of Immortality: Treasures of Ancient Egypt*, National Gallery of Art, Washington, 2002
Mogens JORGENSEN, *Catalogue Egypt II (1550-1080 B.C.)*, Ny Carlsberg Glyptotek, Copenhagen, 1998
Mogens JORGENSEN, *Catalogue Egypt III: Coffins, Mummy adornments and Mummies from the Third Intermediate, Late Ptolemaic and Roman Periods (1080 BC-AD 400)*, Ny Carlsberg Glyptotek, Copenhaga, 2001
Timothy KENDALL, *Kerma and the Kingdom of Kush (2500-1500 B. C.): The Archaeological Discovery of an Ancient Nubian Empire*, National Museum of African Art, Washington, 1997
Gabrielle KUENY, Jean YOYOTTE, *Grenoble, Musée des Beaux-Arts. Collection Égyptienne*, Reunion des Muséss Nationaux, Paris, 1979
Peter LACOVARA, Betsy TROPE, *The Realm of Osiris: Mummies, Coffins and Ancient Egyptian Funerary Arts in the Michael C. Carlos Museum,* Emory University, Atlanta, 2001
Georges LEGRAIN, *Collection Hoffmann: Catalogue des Antiquités Égyptiennes*, Paris, 1894
Leben und Tod im Älten Agypten: Meisterwerke aus dem Reichmuseum fur Altertümer in Leiden, Gustav Lubcke Museum, Hamm, 1999
Les artistes de Pharaon: Deir el-Médineh et la Valée des Rois, Éditions de la Réunion des Musées Nationaux, Paris, 2002
Noël MAHÉO, Olivier PERDU, Elsa RICKAL (coord.), *La collection Égyptienne du Musée de Picardie*, Réunion des Musées Nationaus, Paris, 1994
Gamal MOKHTAR & others, *Egipto, Creador de la Civilizacion*, Oficina Cultural de la Embajada de Egipto, Madrid, 1992
Philippe de MONTEBELLO, *Egyptian Art*, Metropolitan Museum of Art, New York, 1994
István NAGY, *Guide to the Egyptian Collection,* Museum of Fine Arts of Budapest, Budapest, 1999
Nubian Museum, Ministery of Culture, Cairo, 1998
Hanna PHILIPP, *Terrakotten aus Ägypten im Ägyptischen Museum Berlin*, Gebr. Mann Verlag, Berlin, 1972
Stephen QUIRKE, A.J. SPENCE, *The British Museum book of Ancient Egypt*, The British Museum Press, London, 1992
Suzanne RATIÉ, *Annecy, Musée-châtêau; Chambéry, Musées d'Art et d'Histoire; Aix-les-Bains, Musée Archéologique: Collections Égyptiennes*, Réunion des Musées Nationaux, Amiens, 1999
Anna Maria DONADONI ROVERI, *Museo Egizio*, Barisone Editore, Turin, s/d
Mohamed SALEH, Hourig SOUROUZIAN, *The Egyptian Museum: The Official Catalogue*, Verlag Philipp von Zabern, Mainz, 1987
Helmut SATZINGER, *Das Kunsthistorische Museum in Wien: Die Ägyptisch-Orientalische Sammlung*, Verlag Philipp von Zabern, Mainz am Rhein, 1994
Cinthia May SHEIKHOSLESLAMI, *The Egyptian Museum at the Millenium: a Special Exhibition in honor of the VIIIth International Congress of Egyptologists*, Cairo, 2000
Hans SCHNEIDER, Maarten RAVEN, *De Egyptische Oudheid: Een inleiding aan de hand van de Egyptische verzameling in het Rijksmuseum van Oudheden te Leiden*, Leiden, 1981
Wilfried SEIPEL, *Ägypten: Götter, Gräber und die Kunst – 4000 Jahre Jeinseitsglaube*. Vol. I, Schlossmuseum, Linz, 1989
Wilfried SEIPEL, Elfriede HASLAUER, *Ägypten im Kunsthistorischen Museum Wien*, Medien, Vienna, 2001
Lunsingh SCHEURLEER, *Egypte, Geschenk van de Nijl*, Allard Pierson Museum, Amsterdam, 1992
Birgit SCHLICK-NOLTE, Vera HÜLSHOFF, *Liebieghaus-Museum Alter Plastik. Aegyptische Bildwerke,* vol. I: *Skarabäen, Amulette und Schmuck*, Museum Alter Plastik, Melsungen, 1990
Gerry SCOTT, *Ancient Egypt Art at Yale*, Yale University Art Gallery, Yale, New Haven, 1986
Stephen SPURR, Nicholas REEVES, Stephen QUIRKE, *Egyptian Art at Eton College: Selections from the Myers Museum*, The Metropolitan Museum of Art & Eton College, New York, 1999
Francesco TIRADRITTI (ed.), *Tesouros do Egito do Museu Egípcio do Cairo*, Manole, São Paulo, 1998
Bernhard VOGEL (dir.), *Meisterwerke Altägyptischer Keramik: 5000 Jahre Kunst und Kunstlandwerk aus Ton und Fayence*, Höhr-Grenzhausen, Rastal-Haus, 1978
Karl-Heinz PRIESE (ed.), *Ägyptisches Museum*, Verlag Philipp von Zabern, Mainz, 1991
Susan WALKER, Peter HIGGS, *Cleopatra of Egypt: from history to myth*, The British Museum Press, London, 2001
Steffen WENIG, *Africa in Antiquity: The Arts of Ancient Nubia and the Sudan*, 2 volumes, Brooklyn Museum, Brooklyn, 1978
Dietrich WILDUNG, *Egyptian Art in Berlin: Masterpieces in the Bodemuseum and in Charlottenburg*, Ägyptisches Museum und Papyrussammlung, Staatliche Museen zu Berlin, Verlag Phillip von Zabern, Mainz am Rhein, 1998

Catalogue of the Cairo Egyptian Museum

CG 1-1294
Von Ludwig BORCHARDT, *Catalogue Général des Antiquités Égyptiennes du Musée du Caire,* N° 1-1294: *Statuen und statuetten von königen und privatleuten in Museum von Kairo,* Berlin, 1925
CG 5218-6000, 12001-13595
George REISNER, *Catalogue Général des Antiquités Égyptiennes du Musée du Caire*, n° 5218-6000, 12001-13595: *Amulets* I-II, IFAO, Cairo, 1907-1958
CG 6001-6029
Émile CHASSINAT, *Catalogue Général des Antiquités Égyptiennes du Musée du Caire*, n° 6001-6029: *La*

seconde trouvaille de Deir el-Bahri (sarcophages), Leipzig, 1909

CG 6069-6082

Andrzej NIWINSKI, *Catalogue Général des Antiquités Égyptiennes du Musée du Caire*, n° 6069-6082: *The second find of Deir el-Bahri (Coffins)*, Supreme Council of Antiquities of Egypt, Institut of Archaeology of the Warsaw University & Polish Centre of Mediterrean Archaeology in Cairo, Cairo, 1999

CG 9401-9449

Émile CHASSINAT, *Catalogue Général des Antiquités Égyptiennes du Musée du Caire*, n° 9401-9449: *Textes et dessins magiques*, Cairo, 1903

CG 31271-31670

Arthur WEIGALL, *Catalogue Général des Antiquités Égyptiennes du Musée du Caire*, n° 31271-31670: *Weights and balances*, Cairo, 1908

CG 38001-39849

Georges DARESSY, *Catalogue Général des Antiquités Égyptiennes du Musée du Caire*, n° 38001-39849: *Statues de divinités*, I-II, Cairo, 1905-1906

CG 41001-41041

Alexandre MORET, *Catalogue Général des Antiquités Égyptiennes du Musée du Caire*, n° 41001-41041: *Sarcophages de l'Époque Bubastite à l'Époque Saïte*, I-II, Cairo, 1913

CG 41042-41072

Henry GAUTHIER, *Catalogue Général des Antiquités Égyptiennes du Musée du Caire*, n° 41042-41072: *Cercueils anthropoïdes des prêtres de Montu*, I-II, Cairo, 1913

CG 42192-42250

Georges LEGRAIN, *Catalogue Général des Antiquités Égyptiennes du Musée du Caire*, n° 42192-42250: *Statues et statuettes de rois et de particuliers*, I-III, Cairo, 1914

CG 46530-48575

Percy NEWBERRY, *Catalogue Général des Antiquités Égyptiennes du Musée du Caire*, n° 46530-48575: *Funerary statuettes and model sarcophagi*, I-III, Cairo, 1930-1957

CG 51001-51191

James QUIBELL, *Catalogue Général des Antiquités Égyptiennes du Musée du Caire*, n° 51001-51191: *The tomb of Yuaa and Thuiu*, Cairo, 1908

CG 52001-53855

Émile VERNIER, *Catalogue Général des Antiquités Égyptiennes du Musée du Caire*, n° 52001-53855: *Bijoux et orfèvreries*, Tomes I-II, Cairo, 1927

CG 61001-61044

Georges DARESSY, *Catalogue Général des Antiquités Égyptiennes du Musée du Caire*, n° 61001-61044: *Cercueils des cachettes royales*, Cairo, 1909

CG 61051-61100

Grafton Eliot SMITH, *Catalogue Général des Antiquités Égyptiennes du Musée du Caire*, n° 61051-61100: *The royal mummies*, Cairo, 1912

3. Archaeology

Description de l'Égypte publiée par les ordres de Napoléon Bonaparte, Taschen, Köln, 2002

Jan ASSMANN, *Das Grab des Amenemope (TT41)*, Verlag Philipp von Zabern, Mainz am Rhein, 1991

Edward AYRTON, Charles CURRELY, Arthur WEIGALL, *Abydos*, Part III, 1904, The Egypt Exploration Fund, London, 1904

Alessandro BARSANTI, 'Fouilles autour de la Pyramide d'Ounas: Les tombeaux de Psammétique et de Setariban', *ASAE* 1 (1900), pp. 161-166

Alessandro BARSANTI, 'Fouilles autour de la Pyramide d'Ounas: Tombeau de Petneit', *ASAE* 2 (1901), pp. 97-104

Alessandro BARSANTI, 'Sur la découverte du puits d'Ouazhoru à Sakkarah', *ASAE* 3 (1903), pp. 209-212

Freiherr von BISSING, 'Tombeau d'Époque Romaine à Akhmîn', *ASAE* 51 (1951), pp. 553-576

Urbain BOURIANT, 'Tombeau de Harmhabi', *MMAF* 5 (1891), pp. 413-433

Bernard BRUYÈRE, *Rapport sur les Fouilles de Deir el-Mèdineh (1928)*, IFAO, Cairo, 1929

Bernard BRUYÈRE, *Rapport sur les Fouilles de Deir el Mèdineh (1930)*, IFAO, Cairo, 1933

Guy BRUNTON, *Mostagedda and the Tasian culture*, British Museum Expedition to Middle Egypt (1928-1927), London, 1937

Howard CARTER, *The tomb of Tutankhamen. Discovered by the late earl of Carnavon and Howard Carter*, vol. II, Cassell and Company, Ltd., London-Toronto, 1923

Lady William CECIL, 'Report on the work done at Aswân', *ASAE* 4 (1904), pp. 59-65

Mohamed CHABAN, 'Fouilles dans la nécropole de Saqqarah', *ASAE* 19 (1919), pp. 208-215

Émile CHASSINAT, *Le Temple de Dendara*, vol. II-V, IFAO, Cairo, 1934-1947

Georges DARESSY, 'Les sépultures des prètres d'Ammon à Deir el-Bahari', *ASAE* 1 (1900), pp. 141-148

Georges DARESSY, 'Tombe de Hor-kheb à Saqqarah', *ASAE* 4 (1904), pp. 76-82

Georges DARESSY, 'Les cercueils des prètres d'Ammon (Deuxième trouvaille de Deir el-Bahari)', *ASAE* 8 (1907), pp. 3-38

François DAUMAS, *Les Mammisis de Dendara*, IFAO, Cairo, 1959

François DAUMAS, Bernard LENTHÉRIC, *Le Temple de Dendara*, vol. IX, IFAO, Cairo, 1987

Norman de Garis DAVIES, *The Tomb of Two Sculptors at Thebes*, The Metropolitan Museum of Art, New York, 1925

Norman de Garis DAVIES, *Two Ramesside Tombs at Thebes*, The Metropolitan Museum of Art, New York, 1927

Norman de Garis DAVIES, *The Tomb of the Vizier Ramose. Mond Excavations at Thebes*. II. Egypt Exploration Society, London, 1941

Norman de Garis DAVIES, *Seven Private Tombs. Mond Excavations at Thebes*. II. Egypt Exploration Society, London, 1948

Theodore DAVIS, *The tomb of Siptah, the Monkey tomb and Gold tomb*, Egypt Exploration Society, London, 1908

Étienne DRIOTON, Jean-Philippe LAUER, 'Les tombes jumelées de Neferibrê-sa-Neith et de Ouahibrê-Men', *ASAE* 51 (1951) pp. 469-490

Mohammed EFFENDI, 'Fouilles dans la nécropole de Saqqarah', *ASAE* 19 (1920), pp. 208-215

Reginald ENGELBACH, *Harageh*, British School of Archaeology in Egypt, London, 1923

Ahmed FAKHRY, 'Bahria and Farafra Oases: Third preliminary report on the new discoveries', *ASAE* 40 (1940), pp. 856-861

Ahmed FAKHRY, *The Egyptian Deserts: Bahria Oasis*, vol. 1, Government Press, Cairo, 1942

Erika FEUCHT, *Das Grab des Nefersecheru (TT 296)*, Verlag Philipp von Zabern, Mainz am Rhein, 1985

Henri FRANKFORT, *The Cenotaph of Seti I at Abydos*, 2 volumes, Egypt Exploration Society, London, 1933

Henri FRANKFORT, *Kingship of the Gods. A study of Ancient Near Eastern Religion as the integration of Society and Nature*, University of Chicago, Chicago, London, 1978

Henri GAUTHIER, 'Une tombe d'époque saite à Heliopolis', *ASAE* 27 (1927), pp. 1-18

Zakaria GONEIM, *Horus Sekhem-khet, the unfinished step pyramid at Saqqara*, IFAO, Cairo, 1957

Labib HABACHI, 'Athribis in the XXVI Dynasty', *BIFAO* 82 (1982), pp. 36-235

Jochen HALLOF, Hans van den BERG & others, *Le Temple de Dendara: La Porte d'Isis*, IFAO, Cairo, 1999

Ahmed HAMADA, 'Une troisiéme tombe à El-Fostat', *ASAE* 38 (1938), pp. 479-492

John Richard HARRIS, *Lexicographical Studies in Ancient Egyptian Minerals*, Akademie Verlag, Berlin, 1961

Selim HASSAN, *Excavations at Gîza*, vol. IV (1932-1933), Service des Antiquités de l'Égypte, Cairo, 1943

Selim HASSAN, *Excavations at Gîza*, vol. V (1933-1934), Service des Antiquités de l'Égypte, Cairo, 1944

Eva HOFMANN, *Das Grab des Neferrenpet Gen. Kenro (TT 178)*, Verlag Philipp von Zabern, Mainz am Rhein, 1995

Richard LEPSIUS, *Denkmäler aus Aegypten und Aethiopien*, 12 vol., Berlin, 1849-1859

Ahmed KAMAL, 'Rapport sur les fouilles de Said Bey Khachaba au Deir el-Gabroui', *ASAE* 13 (1933), pp. 161-178

Gustave LEFEBVRE, *Le tombeau de Petosiris*, 2 volumes, IFAO, Cairo, 1924

Charles MAYSTRE, *Tombes de Deir el-Médineh: La tombe de Nebenmât (nº 219)*, MIFAO, vol. 71, IFAO, Cairo, 1936

Anne MINAUL-GOUT, *Balat II: Le mastaba d'Ima-Pepi*, Institut Français d'Archaeo-logie Orientale du Caire, Cairo, 1992

Pierre MONTET, *Les constructions et le tombeau d'Osorkon II à Tanis*, Paris, 1947

Pierre MONTET, *Les constructions et le tombeau de Psousennès I à Tanis*, Paris, 1951

Pierre MONTET, *Les constructions et le tombeau de Chéchanq III à Tanis*, Paris, 1960

Alexandre MORET, 'De l'expression *iᶜ ib*', *RT* 14 (1893), pp. 120-123

Alexandre MORET, 'Le jugement du roi mort dans les Texts des Pyramides de Saqqarah', *Annuaire*, École Pratique des Hautes Études, Paris, 1922

Alexandre MORET, 'La doctrine de Maât', *RdÉ* 4 (1940), pp. 1-14

Jacques de MORGAN, *Fouilles à Dachour en 1894-1895*, Adolphe Holzhausen, Vienna, 1903

Édouard NAVILLE, *The Temple of Deir el-Bahari*, Part III, Egypt Exploration Fund, London, 1898

Maged NEGM, *The Tomb of Simut called Kyky – Theban Tomb 409 at Qurnah*, Aris & Philips Ltd., Warminster, 1997

Paul NICHOLSON, Ian SHAW (eds), *Ancient Egyptian Materials and Techonology*, University Cambridge Press, Cambridge, 2001

William Flinders PETRIE, *Dendereh*, Egypt Exploration Fund, London, 1900

William Flinders PETRIE, *Abydos*, vol. I, Egypt Exploration Fund, London, 1902

William Fliders PETRIE, *Historical Studies*, British School of Archaeology in Egypt, London, 1911

William Fliders PETRIE & others, *Lahun*, vol. II, British School of Archaeology in Egypt, London, 1923

William Fliders PETRIE, *Objects of daily use*, British School of Archaeology in Egypt, London, 1927

Serge SAUNERON, *Esna*. vol. V*: Les Fêtes religieuses d'Esna aux derniers siécles du paganisme*, IFAO, Cairo, 1662

Serge SAUNERON, *Esna*. vol. II, IFAO, Cairo, 1963

Serge SAUNERON, *Esna*. vol. III, IFAO, Cairo, 1968

Georg STEINDORFF, *Aniba*, 2 volumes, Service des Antiquités d'Égypte, Mission Archéologique de Nubie (1929-1934), Glückstadt, Hamburgo, New York, 1937

Mario TOSI, Mohamed NASR, *The Tomb of Pashed and the Valley of the Artisans*, Casa Editrice Bonechi, Florença, 2001

Michel VALLOGGIA, 'Rapport préliminaire sur la troisiéme campagne de fouilles du mastaba V à Balat (Oasis de Dakhleh)', *BIFAO* 80 (1980), pp. 97-128

Michel VALLOGGIA, *Balat I: Le mastaba de Medou-nefer*, IFAO, Cairo, 1986

Jacobus van DIJK, 'Entering the House of Hearts: An addition to Chapter 151 in the Book of the Dead of Qenna', *OMRO* 75 (1995), pp. 7-11

Jacques VANDIER, *Tombes de Deir el-Médineh: La tombe de Nefer-Abou*, MIFAO, vol. 69, IFAO, Cairo, 1935

Philippe VIREY, 'La tombe des vignes à Thèbes', *RT* 20 (1898), pp. 210-223

Philippe VIREY, 'La tombe des vignes à Thèbes (suite)', *RT* 22 (1900), pp. 83-97

4. Texts

Luís Manuel de ARAÚJO, *Mitos e Lendas do Antigo Egipto*, Livros & Livros, Lisboa, 2005

Paul BARGUET, *Le Livre des Morts des Anciens Égyptiens*, Litteratures Anciennes du Proche-Orient, Les Éditions du Cerf, Paris, 1967

Paul BARGUET, *Les Textes des Sarcophages Égyptiens du Moyen Empire*, Les Éditions du Cerf, Paris, 1986

André BARUCQ, François DAUMAS, *Hymnes et Priéres de l'Égypte Ancienne,* Les Éditions du Cerf, Paris, 1980

Joris BORGHOUTS, Dirk van der PLAS, *The Egyptian Coffin Texts*, vol. VIII: *Coffin Texts Word Index*, Publications Interuniversitaires de Recherches Égyptologiques Informatisées, Utrecht, Paris, 1998

James BREASTED, 'The Philosophy of a Memphite Priest', *ZÄS* 39 (1901), pp. 39-54

Theodore DAVIS, *The Funeral Papyrus of Iouiya. With an Introduction by Édouard Naville*, Archibald Constable and Co., Ltd., London, 1908

Adrian DE BUCK, *The Egyptian Coffin Texts. Texts of Spells*, 7 volums, The University Chicago Press, Oriental Institute Publications, Chicago, 1935-1961

Adolf ERMAN, *Ancient Egyptian Poetry and Prose*, Dover Publications, New York, 1995

James WASSERMANN (ed.), *The Egyptian Book of the Dead (The book of going forth by day)*, The American University of Cairo Press, Cairo, 1998

Raymond FAULKNER, *The Ancient Egyptian Pyramid Texts*, Oxford University Press, Oxford, 1969

Raymond FAULKNER, Eva DASSOW (ed.), *The Egyptian Book of the Dead: The Book of Going Forth by Day,* The American University in Cairo Press, Cairo, 1998

Alan GARDINER, *Notes on the story of Sinuhe*, Librairie Honoré Champion, Paris, 1916

Alan GARDINER, 'A stele in the Macgregor Collection', *JEA* 4 (1918), pp. 188-189

Alan GARDINER, *Late Egyptian Stories*, Bibliotheca Aegyptiaca, I, Fondation Égyptologique Reine Élizabeth, Bruxelles, 1932

Alan GARDINER, 'Davie's Copy of the Great Speos Artemidos Inscription', *JEA* 32 (1946), pp. 43-46

Henri GAUTHIER, *La Grande Inscription Dédicatoire d'Abydos*, Col. Bibliothèque d'Étude, IV, IFAO, Cairo, 1912

Jean-Claude GOYON, *Rituels Funéraires de l'ancienne Égypte*, Édition du Cerf, Paris, 1972

Pierre GRANDET, *Le Papyrus Harris I (BM 9999)*, vol. I, Col. Bibliothèque d'Étude, IFAO, Cairo, 1994

Pierre GRANDET, *Hymnes de la religion d'Aton*, Éditions du Seuil, Paris, 1995.

François-René HERBIN, *Le Livre de Parcourrir l'Éternité*, Peeters: Orientalia Lovaniensia Analecta, Louvaina, 1994

Moharam KAMAL, 'The stela of *s ḥtp ib rꜥ* in the Egyptian Museum', *ASAE* 38 (1938), pp. 265-288

Gustave LEFEBVRE, *Romans et Contes Égyptiens de l'Époque Pharaonique,* Librairie d'Amérique et d'Orient Adrien Maisonneuve, Paris, 1988

Richard LEPSIUS, *Das Totenbuch der Ägypter nach dem Einem Vorworte zum Ersten Male Herausgegeben*, Leipzig, 1842

François LEXA, *Papyrus Insinger: Les Enseignements Moraux d'un Scribe Égyptien du Premier Siécle Aprés J. C.*, 2 vol., Librairie Orientaliste Paul Geuthner, Paris, 1926

Miriam LICHTHEIM, *Ancient Egyptian Literature*, vol. I: The Old and the Middle Kingdom, University of California Press, Berkeley, Los Angeles, London, 1973

Miriam LICHTHEIM, *Ancient Egyptian Literature*, vol. II: The New Kingdom, University of California Press, Berkeley, Los Angeles, London, 1976

Miriam LICHTHEIM, *Ancient Egyptian Literature*, vol. III: The Late Period, University of California Press, Berkeley, Los Angeles, London, 1980

Victor LORET, *L'Inscription d'Ahmés fils d'Abana*, col. Bibliothèque d'Étude, III, IFAO, Cairo, 1910

Gaston MASPERO, *Mémoires de Sinouhit*, col. Bibliothèque d'Étude, I, IFAO, Cairo, 1908

Gaston MASPERO, *Hymne au Nil*, col. Bibliothèque d'Étude, V, IFAO, Cairo, 1912

Gaston MASPERO, *Les Enseignements d'Amenemhaît I à son fils Sanouasrît I*, Col. Bibliothèque d'Étude, VI, IFAO, Cairo, 1914

Bernard MATHIEU, *La Poesie Amoureuse de l'Égypte Ancienne: Recherches sur un genre littéraire au Nouvel Empire*, Bibliothéque d'Étude, 115, Institut Français d'Archéologie Oriental, Cairo, 1996

Richard PARKINSON, *The Tale of the Eloquent Peasant*, Griffith Institute & Ashmolean Museum, Oxford, 1991

Alexandre PIANKOFF, 'Les Compositions Théologiques du Nouvel Empire Égyptien', *BIFAO* 41 (1942), pp. 121-128

Alexandre PIANKOFF, 'Les Grandes Compositions Religieuses du Nouvel Empire et la Réforme d'Amarna', *BIFAO* 41 (1942), pp. 285-300

Alexandre PIANKOFF, 'Le Livre des Quererets', *BIFAO* 41 (1942), pp. 1-1

Alexandre PIANKOFF, 'Le tableau d'Osiris et les divisions V, VI et VII du Livre des Portes (suite)', *ASAE* 55 (1958), pp. 157-165

Alexandre PIANKOFF, *Le Livre des Portes*, vol. II, IFAO, Cairo, 1961

Alexandre PIANKOFF, *The Pyramid of Unas*, Bollingen Series, XL: Egyptian Religious Texts and Representations, vol. 5, Princeton University Press, Princeton, 1968

Alexandre PIANKOFF, Natacha RAMBOVA, *The Shrines of Tut-ankh-amon*, Bollingen Series, XL: 2, Pantheon Books, New York, 1955

Alexandre PIANKOFF, Natacha RAMBOVA, *Mythological Papyri*, Bollingen Series, XL: Egyptian Religious Texts and Representations, vol. 3, Pantheon Books, New York, 1957

James PRITCHARD, *The Ancient Near East*, vol. I: An anthology of texts and pictures, Princeton University Press, Princeton, 1958

Suzanne RATIÉ, *Le papyrus de Neferoubenef (Louvre III 93)*, IFAO, Cairo, 1968

Odette RENAUD, *Le Dialogue du Désespéré avec son Âme: une interpretation littéraire*, Cahiers de la Société d'Égyptologie, vol. 1, Genebra, 1991

Kurt SETHE, *Urkunden der 18. Dynastie: Historisch Biographische Urkunden*, vol. I, J. C. Hinrich Sche Buchhandlung, Leipzig, 1906

Kurt SETHE, *Urkunden der 18. Dynastie: Historisch Biographische Urkunden*, vol. II, J. C. Hinrich Sche Buchhandlung, Leipzig, 1907

Kurt SETHE, *Urkunden der 18. Dynastie: Historisch Biographische Urkunden*, vol. III, J. C. Hinrich Sche Buchhandlung, Leipzig, 1909

Kurt SETHE, *Dramatische Texte zu Altaegyptischen Mysterienspielen*, J. C. Hinrich Sche Buchhandlung, Leipzig, 1928

Heinrich SCHÄFER, *Principles of Egyptian Art*, Griffith Institute, Oxford, 1986

Siegfried SCHOTT, *Urkunden Mythologischen Inhalts*, J. C. Hinrich Sche Buchhandlung, Leipzig, 1920

Siegfried SHOTT, *Les Chants d'Amour de l'Égypte Ancienne*, Librairie Maisonneuve, Paris, 1956

Rogério SOUSA, *Os Doces Versos: Poemas de Amor no Antigo Egipto*, Fafe, 2001

Paul TRESSON, *L'Inscription d'Ouni*, Col. Bibliothèque d'Étude, VIII, IFAO, Cairo, 1919

Paul TRESSON, *La Stéle de Koubân*, Col. Bibliothèque d'Étude, IX, IFAO, Cairo, 1922

Alexandre VARILLE, 'L'Hymne au Soleil des Architectes d'Aménophis III Souti et Hor', *BIFAO* 41 (1942), pp. 25-30

Pascal VERNUS, *Chants d'Amour de l'Égypte Antique*, Imprimerie Nationale Éditions, Paris, 1992

Pascal VERNUS, *Sagesses de l'Égypte pharaonique*, Impremerie Nationale Éditions, Paris, 2001

John WILSON, 'The Memphite Theology of Creation', in James Pritchard, *The Ancient Near East: An Anthology of Texts and Pictures*, I, Princeton University Press, New Jersey, 1973, pp. 1-2

5. Specific Bibliography

Carol ANDREWS, *Amulets of Ancient Egypt*, University of Texas Press, 1998

Carol ANDREWS, 'Amulets', in Donald Redford (ed), *The Oxford Encyclopedia of Ancient Egypt*, vol. I, Oxford University Press, Oxford, 2001, pp. 75-82

Rudolf ANTHES, ‚Das steinharte Herz', in *Jahrbuch für Antike und Christentum*, 4, Ashendorffsche Verlagsbuchhandlung, Münster, Westfalen, 1961, pp. 77-107

Luís Manuel de ARAÚJO, 'Um escaravelho do coração numa colecção privada portuguesa', *Museu* 9 (2000), pp. 7-27

Jan ASSMANN, *Ägypten Theologie und Frömmigkeit einer fhühen Hochkultur*, Kohlhmmer, Köhln, Stuttgart, Berlin, 1991

Jan ASSMANN, ‚Zur Geschichte des Herzens im alten Ägypten', in *idem* (ed.) *Die Erfindung des inneren Menschen: Studien zur reliogiösen Anthropologie.* (Studien zum Verstehen fremder Religionen, 6, Gütersloch, 1993, pp. 81-113

Sydney AUFRÉRE, 'Cœur, l'annulaire gauche, Sekhmet et les maladies cardiaques', *RdÉ* 36 (1985), pp. 21-34

Thiery BARDINET, *Les papyrus médicaux de l'Égypte pharaonique,* Fayard, Paris, 1995

Daphna BEN-TOR, *The Scarab: A reflection of Ancient Egypt*, The Israel Museum, Jerusalem, 1989

Susanne BICKEL, 'Heliopolis et le tribunal des dieux', *Études sur l'Ancien Empire et la nécropole de Saqqâra dédiées à Jean-Philippe Lauer*, Université de Paul Valéry, Montpellier, 1997, pp. 113-122

Samuel BIRCH, 'On formulas relating to the heart', *ZÄS* 4 (1866), pp. 89-92

Samuel BIRCH, 'On formulas relating to the heart', *ZÄS* 5 (1867), pp 16-17

Samuel BIRCH, 'On formulas of three royal coffins', *ZÄS* 7 (1869), pp. 49-53

Samuel BIRCH, 'On formulas relating to the heart', *ZÄS* 8 (1870), pp 30-34

Van der BROEK, *The myth of the Phoenix according to Classical and early Christian Traditions*, E. J. Brill, Leiden, 1972

Helmut BRUNNER, ‚Herz', in Wolfgang Helck, Wolfhart Westendorf (ed.), *Lexikon der Ägyptologie,* II, Otto Harrassowitz, Wiesbaden, 1977, col 1158-1168

Helmut BRUNNER, ‚Das Herz als Sitz des Lebensgeheimnisses', in *Das hörende Herz. Kleine Schriften zur religions und Geitesgeschichte Ägyptens,* Orbis Biblicus et Orientalis, 80, Göttingen, Fribourg, 1988, pp. 6-7

Helmut BRUNNER, ‚Das Herz im ägyptischen Glauben', in *Das hörende Herz. Kleine Schriften zur religions und Geitesgeschichte Ägyptens,* Orbis Biblicus et Orientalis, 80, Göttingen, Fribourg, 1988, pp. 8-41

Helmut BRUNNER, ‚Das hörende Herz', in *Das hörende Herz. Kleine Schriften zur religions und Geitesgeschichte Ägyptens,* Orbis Biblicus et Orientalis, 80, Göttingen, Fribourg, 1988, pp. 3-5

Adrian de BUCK, ‚Een groep dodenboekspreuken betreffende het hart', *JEOL* 9 (1944), pp. 9-24

Adrian de BUCK 'Un chapitre de Psychologie Egyptienne', *Cd'É* 41 (1946), pp. 17-24

Max BURCHARDT, ‚Das herz des Bata', *ZÄS* 50 (1912), pp. 118-119

Emil BUZOV, 'The role of the Heart in the purification', in A. Amenta (ed), *L' Acqua nell'antico Egitto: vita rigenerazione, incantesimo, medicamento – Proceedings of the First International Conference for Young Egyptologists*, vol. III, L'Erma di Bretschneider, Roma, 2005, pp. 273-281

Jean CAPART, 'Une liste d'amulettes', *ZÄS* 45 (1908-09), pp. 14-22

Albert de CALUWE, 'Les bandelettes de momie du Musée Vleeshuis d'Anvers', *JEA* 79 (1993), pp. 199-214

Jacques-Jean CLÈRE, 'Un passage de la stèle du général Antef (Glyptothèque Ny Carlsberg, Copenhague)', *BIFAO* 30 (1931), pp. 425-447

Michel DEWATCHER, 'Le scarabée funéraire de Néchao II et deux amulettes inédites du Musée Jacquemart-André', *Rd'É* 37 (1986), pp. 53-62

Étienne DRIOTON, 'Note sur un cryptogramme récemment découvert à Athribis', *ASAE* 38 (1938), pp. 109-116

Étienne DRIOTON, 'Le jugement des âmes dans l'ancienne Égypte', *RdC* (1949), pp. 1-20

Étienne DRIOTON, 'Scarabées à maximes', *Annals of the Faculty of Arts*, Vol. I, Fouad University Press, Cairo, 1951, pp. 55-71

Étienne DRIOTON, 'Maximes morales sur des scarabées égyptiens', *Hommages à Waldemar Deonna*, Latomus, vol. 28, Berchem, Bruxelles, 1957, pp. 197-202

Gertie ENGLUND, *Akh - une notion religeuse dans l'Égypte pharaonique*, Boreas 11, Uppsala Studies in Ancient Mediterranean and Near Eastern Civilizations, Acta Universitatis Upsaliensis, Uppsala, 1978

Gertie ENGLUND, 'Gods as a frame of reference. On thinking and concepts of thought in Ancient Egypt', in *The Religion of Ancient Egypt. Cognitive structures and popular expressions. Proceedings of Symposia in Uppsala and Bergen*, Uppsala, 1987, pp. 7-28

Gertie ENGLUND, 'The treatment of opposites in temple thinking and wisdom literature', Idem (ed) *The religion of ancient Egyptians: Cognitive structures and popular expressions. Proceedings of Symposia in Uppsala and Bergen 1987 and 1988*, Acta Universitatis Upsaliensis, Boreas, Uppsala Studies in Ancient Mediterranean and Near Eastern Civilizations, 20, Uppsala, 1987, pp. 77-88

Julia FALKOVITCH, 'L'usage des amulettes égyptiennes', *BSEG* 16 (1992), pp. 20-26

Hanane GABER, 'Les scarabées de coeur à tête humaine à la lumière d'une variante de la pesée du coeur' in Goyon, J.-C., Cardin, C., *Proceedings of the Ninth International Congress of Egyptologists*, Vol. I, Peeters Publishers & Department of Oriental Studies, Leuvein, Paris, Dudley, 2007, pp. 743-748

Hans GOEDICKE, 'The Riddle of Sinuhe's Flight', *RdÉ* 35 (1984), pp. 95-103

Beatrice GOFF, *Symbols of Ancient Egypt in the Late Period. Twenty-first Dynasty*. Col. Religion and Society, 13, Mouton Publishers, Paris, New York, 1979

Jean-Claude GOYON, 'Momification et recomposition du corps divin: Anubis et les canopes', J. Kamstra, H. Milde, K. Wagtendonk (ed.), *Funerary symbols and Religion. Essays dedicated to Professor M. Heerma van Voss on the occasion of his retirement from the Chair of the History of Ancient Religions at the University of Amsterdam*, J. H. Kok, Kampen, 1988, pp. 34-44

Liselotte GREVEN, *Der Ka in theologie und Königskult der Ägypter des Alten Reiches*, Verlag J. J. Augustin, Glückstad, Hambourg, New York, 1952

Alice GRENFELL, 'The *ka* on Scarabs', *RT* 37 (1915), pp. 77-93

Gwyn GRIFFITHS, 'Eight funerary paintings with judgement scenes in the Swansea Wellcome Museum', *JEA* 38 (1952), pp. 228-252

Nadine GUILHOU, 'Les parties du corps dans les textes de la pyramide d'Ounas: pensée religieuse et pratiques funéraires', in *Études sur l'Ancien Empire et la nécropole de Saqqâra dédiées à Jean-Philippe Lauer*, Université de Paul Valéry, Montpellier, 1997, pp. 221-231

Mohamed HAMZA, 'The correct readind of the place-name *ḥwt tꜣ ḥr ib*', *ASAE* 38 (1938), pp. 197-208

Ibrahim HARARI, 'Nature de la Stéle de Donation de Fonction du roi Ahmôsis a la reine Ahmès-Nefertari', *ASAE* 56 (1956), pp. 1-63

Susan HOLLIS, 'On the nature of Bata, the hero of the Papyrus d'Orbiney', *CdÉ* 59 (1984), pp. 248-257

Erik HORNUNG, *Les Dieux de l'Égypte: L'Un et le Multiple*, Flammarion, Paris, 1992

Erik HORNUNG, *L'Esprit du Temps des Pharaons*, Philippe Lebaud, Paris, 1996

Erik HORNUNG, *The Ancient Egyptian Books of the Afterlife*, Cornell University Press, Ithaca, London, 1999

Erik HORNUNG, 'Time in the Egyptian Netherworld', in *Cadmo* 11 (2001), pp. 7-14

Erik IVERSEN, 'The cosmogony of Shabaka Text', in Sarah Israelit-Groll (ed.) *Studies in Egyptology presented to Miriam Lichtheim*, vol. I, The Hebrew University, The Magnes Press, Jerusalém, 1990, pp. 485- 493

Gustave JÉQUIER, *Les frises d'Objects des Sarcophages du Moyen Empire*, col. MIFAO, vol. 47, IFAO, Cairo, 1921

Hermann KEES, ‚Herz und Zunge als Schöpferorgane in der ägyptischen Gotteslehre', in *Studium Generale*, 2, Berlin, Heidelberg, 1966, pp. 124-126

Yvan KOENIG, ‚L'eau et magie', in A. Amenta (ed.) *L'Acqua nell'antico Egitto: vita rigenerazione, incantesimo, medicamento – Proceedings of the First International Conference for Young Egyptologists*, vol. III, L'Erma di Bretschneider, Roma, 2005, pp. 191-200

Jean-Marie KRUCHTEN, *Les Annales des Prêtres de Karnak (XXI-XXIII Dynasties) et Autres Textes Contemporains Relatifs à l'Initiation des Prêtres d'Amon* (avec un chapitre archéologique par Thierry Zimmer), Orientalia Lovaniensia Analecta, 32, Departement Oriëntalistiek, Lovaina, 1989

Gustave LEFEBVRE, 'L'Oeuf divin d'Hermopolis', *ASAE* 23 (1923), pp. 65-67

Gustave LEFEBVRE, 'Rouge et nuances voisines', *JEA* 35 (1949), pp. 72-76

Gustave LEFEBVRE, *Tableau des Parties du Corps Humain mentionées par les Égyptiens*, IFAO, Cairo, 1952

Georges LEGRAIN, 'Le mot *ibwy*, image, icone', *RT* 11 (1905), pp. 180-182

Miriam LICHTHEIM, *Maat in Egyptian Autobiographies and related studies*, Orbis Biblicus et Orientalis, 120, University Press, Vandenheck & Ruprecht, Friburg, Göttinger, 1992

Miriam LICHTHEIM, *Moral Values in ancient Egypt*, Orbis Biblicus et Orientalis -155, University Press, Vandenheck & Ruprecht, Friburg-Göttinger, 1997

Alan LLOYD, 'Psychology and society in the Ancient Egyptian cult of the dead', in W. Kelly Simpson (ed.), *Religion and Philosophy in Ancient Egypt*, Yale, New Haven, 1989, pp. 117-133

Bernard LONG, 'Le *ib* et le *h3ty* dans les textes medicaux de l'Egypte Ancienne', in *Hommages à François Daumas, II*, Université de Montpellier, Montpellier, 1986, pp. 483-494

David LORTON, 'The expression *šms-ib*', *JARCE* 7 (1968), pp. 41-54

Michel MALAISE, 'La signification des pendentifs cordiformes dans l'art égyptien', *CdÉ* 50 (1975), pp. 105-135

Michel MALAISE, *Les Scarabées de coeur dans l'Égypte Ancienne*, Monographies Reine Élizabeth, Bruxelles, 1978

Alexandre MORET, 'De l'expression "plonger le coeur"', *RT* 14 (1893), pp. 120-123

Dieter MÜLLER, ‚Die Zeugung durch das Herz in Religion und Medizin der Ägypter', in *Orientalia*, 35, Pontificium Institutum Biblicum, Roma, 1966, pp. 247-274

Claudia MÜLLER-WINKLER, *Die Ägyptischen Objekt-Amulette*, Orbis Biblicus et Orientalis, Series Archaeologica, 5, Fribourg, 1987

Andrzej NIWINSKI, *XXI dynasty Coffins from Thebes: Chronological and Typological Studies*, Verlag Philipp von Zabern, Mainz am Reihn, 1988

Andrzej NIWINSKI, 'The solar-Osirian unity as principle of the theology of the "State of Amun" in Thebes in the XXI dynasty', *JEOL* 30 (1987-1988), pp. 87-106

Andrzej NIWINSKI, 'Relativity in iconography: Changes the shape and value of some Egyptian funerary symbols dependent upon their date and authorship', in J. Kamstra, H. Milde, K. Wagtendonk (ed.), *Funerary symbols and Religion. Essays dedicated to Professor M. Heerma van Voss on the occasion of his retirement from the Chair of the History of Ancient Religions at the University of Amsterdam*, J. H. Kok, Kampen, 1988, pp. 96-104

Andrzej NIWINSKI, *Studies on the Illustrated Theban Funerary Papyri of the 11th and 10th Centuries BC*, OBO, Academic Press, Fribourg, 1989

Andrzej NIWINSKI, '*Iconography of the 21st dynasty*', in Christoph Uehlinger (dir), *Images as Media: Sources for the cultural history of the Near East and the Eastern Mediterranean (Ist millennium BCE)*, Orbis Biblicus et Orientalis, University Press Fribourg, Vandenhoeck & Ruprecht, Götingen, 2000, pp. 21-43.

Andrzej NIWINSKI, '*The Book of the Dead on the Coffins of the 21st Dynasty*', in H. Backes, I. Munro, S. Stöhr, *Totenbuch-Forschungen: Gesammelte Beïtrage des 2. Internationalen Totenbuch-Symposiums*, Harrassowitz Verlag, Wiesbaden, 2006, pp. 245-264.

Rune NYORD, *Breathing Flesh: Conceptions of the Body in the Ancient Egyptian Coffin Texts*, CNI Publications 37, Copenhagen, 2009

Boyo OCKINGA, 'Hatschepsut's election to Kingship: the *ba* and the *ka* in Egyptian Royal Ideology', *BACE* 6 (1995), pp. 89-102

William Flinders PETRIE, *Amulets*, London, 1914

Olivier PERDU, 'Des pendentifs en guise d'ex-voto', *Rd'E* 54 (2003), p. 155-166

Alexandre PIANKOFF, *Le 'Coeur' dans les Textes Égyptiens depuis l'Ancien jusqu'à la fin du Nouvel Empire*, Librairie Orientaliste Paul Geuthner, Paris, 1930

Georges POSENER, 'L'expression *bj3.t '3.t* "Mauvais Caractére"', *RdÉ* 16 (1964), pp. 37-43

Georges POSENER, 'La piété personelle avant 1 âge amarnian', *RdÉ* 27 (1975), pp. 195-210

Stephen QUIRKE, 'Two Thirteenth Dynasty Heart Scarabs', *JEOL* 37 (2001-2002), pp. 31-40

Suzanne RATIÉ, 'Le scarabée de coeur du Musée d'Annecy', *BIFAO* 62 (1964), pp. 109-114

Heinrich SCHÄFER, ‚Die Entstehung einiger Mumienamulette', *ZÄS* 43 (1906), pp. 66-70

Heinrich SCHÄFER, ‚Altägyptische Geldgewichte', *ZÄS* 43 (1906), pp. 70-111

Alexander SCHARFF, ‚Ein Denkstein der römischen Kaiserzeitaus Achmim', *ZÄS* 62 (1927), pp. 86-89

Allan SHORTER, 'The study of Egyptian funerary amulets', *Cd'É* 11 (1931), pp. 312-314

Allan SHORTER, 'Notes on some funerary amulets', *JEA* 21 (1935), pp. 171-176

Christine SEEBER, *Untersuchungen zur Darstellung des Totengerichts im Alten Ägypten*, Deutscher Kunstverlag, Munich, 1976

Rogério SOUSA, *O Coração e o Homem no antigo Egipto: Contributos para a compreensão de uma 'Psicologia' antiga*, Faculdade de Letras da Universidade de Lisboa, Lisboa, 1998 (tese policopiada)

Rogério SOUSA, 'Os médicos no antigo Egipto', *Arquivos da Medicina* 17 (2003), pp. 64-67

Rogério SOUSA, 'A noção de coração no Egipto faraónico: uma síntese evolutiva', in *Percursos do Oriente Antigo-Homenagem a José Nunes Carreira*, Instituto Oriental da Faculdade de Letras da Universidade de Lisboa, Lisboa, 2004, pp. 529-554.

Rogério SOUSA, 'Heart and Water in the Religious Anthropology of Ancient Egypt', in A. Amenta (ed.) *L'Acqua nell'antico Egitto: vita rigenerazione, incantesimo, medicamento – Proceedings of the First International Conference for Young Egyptologists*, vol. III, L'Erma di Bretschneider, Roma, 2005, pp. 375-380

Rogério SOUSA, 'Os amuletos do coração no antigo Egipto: Tipologia e caracterização', *Cadmo* 15 (2005), pp. 105-130.

Rogério SOUSA, *Simbólica do coração no Antigo Egipto: estudo de antropologia religiosa sobre a representação da consciência*, dissertação de doutoramento em

História, Faculdade de Letras da Universidade do Porto, 2006

Rogério SOUSA, '*The Meaning of the Heart Amulets in Egyptian Art*', *JARCE* 43 (2007), pp. 59-70.

Rogério SOUSA, '*The cardiac vignettes of the Book of the Dead (Late Period)*', *in BAEDE* 17 (2007), pp. 39-53

Rogério SOUSA, '*The heart amulet in Ancient Egypt: A typological study*', in Goyon, J.-C., Cardin, C., *Proceedings of the Ninth International Congress of Egyptologists*, Vol. I, Peeters Publishers & Department of Oriental Studies, Leuvein, Paris, Dudley, 2007, pp. 713-721

Rogério SOUSA, 'Symbolism and meaning of pendulum heart amulets', *GM* 221 (2009), pp. 69-74

Rogério SOUSA, *Iniciação e Mistério no Antigo Egipto*, Ésquilo, Lisboa, 2009

Nili SHUPAK, *Where wisdom can be found? The Sage's Language in the Bible and in Ancient Egyptian Literature*, Orbis Biblicus et Orientalis, 130, University Press, Vandenhoeck & Ruprecht, Fribourg, Göttingen, 1993

Jorgen SORENSEN, '*Divine Access: The so-called democratisation of Egyptian funerary literature as a socio-cultural process*', in Gertie Englund (ed) *The religion of ancient Egyptians: Cognitive structures and popular expressions. Proceedings of Symposia in Uppsala and Bergen 1987 and 1988*, Acta Universitatis Upsaliensis, Boreas, Uppsala Studies in Ancient Mediterranean and Near Eastern Civilizations, 20, Uppsala, 1987, pp. 109-123

Maurice STRACMANS, 'Les termes *ib* et *haty* considérés sous l'angle métaphorique dans la langue de l'Ancien Empire', *Mélanges Mariette*, Col. Bibliothéque d'Étude, IFAO, Cairo, 1961, pp. 125-132

Maurice STRACMANS, 'Les fêtes de la circoncision chez les anciens Égyptiens', *CdÉ* 60 (1985), pp. 292-297

Florence THILL, 'Un nouveau pectoral-scarabée de coeur a Sai (Soudan)', in *Mélanges Offerts a Jean Vercoutter*, Éditions Recherches sur les Civilisations, Paris, 1985, pp. 331-341

Vincent Arieh TOBIN, 'The Secret of Sinuhe', *JARCE* 32 (1995), pp. 161-178

Elena TOLMATCHEVA, 'A reconsideration of the Benu-bird in Egyptian Cosmogony', in Zahi Hawass, *Egyptology at the Down of the Twenty-first Century: Proceedings of the Eighth International Congress of Egyptologists*, vol. 3, American University in Cairo Press, Cairo, New York, 2000, pp. 522-526

Lana TROY, 'Creating a god: the mumification ritual', *BACE* 4 (1993), pp. 55-81

Dominique VALBELLE, 'La notion d'identité dans l'Égypte Pharaonique', in *Sesto Congresso Internazionale di Egittologia, Atti, I*, Turim, 1992, pp. 551-556

Marie-Paule VANLATHEM, 'Scarabées de coeur *in situ*', *Cd'É* 76 (2001), pp. 48-56

Alexandre VARILLE, 'La grande porte du temple d'Apet à Karnak', *ASAE* 53 (1956), pp. 79-118

Pascal VERNUS, 'La formule du bon comportement (*bit nfrt*)', *RdÉ* 39 (1988), pp. 147-154

Pascal VERNUS, ‚Name', in Wolfgang Helck, Wolfhart Westendorf (ed.), *Lexikon der Ägyptologie*, IV, Otto Harrasowitz, Wiesbaden, 1982, cols. 320-326

Pascal VERNUS, ‚Namengebung', in Wolfgang Helck, Wolfhart Westendorf (ed.), *Lexikon der Ägyptologie*, IV, Otto Harrassowitz, Wiesbaden, 1982, cols. 326-337

James WALKER, 'Egyptian medicine and the gods', *BACE* 4 (1993), pp. 83-101

James WALKER, *Studies in Ancient Egyptian Anatomical Terminology*, The Australian Centre for Egyptology, Studies 4, Aris & Phillips Ltd., Warstminster, 1996

Vilmos WESSETZKY, 'Amulettes de coeur au Musée des Beaux-Arts', *BMH* 54 (1980), pp. 5-11

Wolfgang WETTENGEL, ‚Zur Rubrengliederung der Erzählung von den zwei Brü-dern', *GM* 126 (1992), 97-106

Alix WILKINSON, 'Jewellery for a procession in the bed-chamber in the tomb of Tutankhamun', *BIFAO* 84 (1984), pp., 335-345

Constant de WIT, 'Inscriptions des lions-gargouilles du temple d'Edfou', *CdE* 57 (1954), pp. 35-40

Jean YOYOTTE, 'Le jugement des morts dans l'Égypte ancienne', *Sources Orientales*, IV: Le jugement des Morts, Seuil, Paris, 1961

Jean YOYOTTE, 'Les os et la semence masculine à propos d'une théorie physiologique égyptienne', *BIFAO* 61 (1962), pp. 139-146

Louis ZABKAR, 'Herodutus and the egyptian idea of immortality', *JNES* 23 (1963), pp. 62-70

Louis ZABKAR, 'Some observations on T.G. Allen's edition of the Book of the Dead', *JNES* 24 (1965), pp. 75-85

Louis ZAKBAR, *A study of the Ba concept in Egyptian texts, SAOC*, 34, 1968

Louis ZABKAR, 'Ba', in Wolfgang Helck, Eberhard Otto (ed.), *Lexikon der Ägyptologie*, I, Otto Harrassowitz, Wiesbaden, 1972, cols. 558-590

Louis ZABKAR, 'A hymn to Osiris Pantocrator at Philae', *ZÄS* 108 (1981), pp. 141-171

Louis ZAKBAR, 'Six Hymns to Isis in the Sanctuary of her Temple at Philae and their Theological Significance', *JEA* 69 (1983), pp. 115-137

Louis ZAKBAR, 'Correlation of the transformation Spells of the Book of the Dead and the Amulets of Tutankhamun's mummy', in *Mélanges Offerts a Jean Vercoutter*, Éditions Recherches sur les Civilisations, Paris, 1985, pp. 335-383

Jan ZANDEE, *Death as an enemy according to ancient Egyptian conception*, Ed. Brill, Leiden, 1969

6. General bibliography

Cyril ALDRED, *Akhenaten: King of Egypt*, Thames & Hudson, London, 1988

James ALLEN, 'The Pyramid Texts of queens *Ipwt* and *Wḏbt-n.(i)*' *JARCE* 23 (1986), pp. 1-25

Luís Manuel de ARAÚJO, *Estudos sobre Erotismo no Antigo Egipto*, Edições Colibri, Lisboa, 1995

Luís Manuel de ARAÚJO, *O clero do deus Amon no Antigo Egipto: O clero amoniano no Império Novo e no pontificado tebano da XXI dinastia*, Edições Cosmos, Lisboa, 1999

Luís Manuel de ARAÚJO, *Egipto: As Pirâmides do Império Antigo*, Edições Colibri, Lisboa, 2003

Luís Manuel de ARAÚJO, 'Mumificação', in Idem (dir), *Dicionário do Antigo Egipto*, Editorial Caminho, Lisboa, 2001, pp. 594-595

Luís Manuel de ARAÚJO, 'Duat', in Idem (dir), *Dicionário do Antigo Egipto*, Editorial Caminho, Lisboa, 2001, pp. 285-286

D. ASTON, 'The Shabti box: A typological study', *OMRO* 74 (1994), pp. 21-54

Jan ASSMANN, 'Death and initiation in the funerary religion of Ancient Egypt', in W. Simpson (ed.), *Religion and Philosophy in Ancient Egypt*, Yale & New Haven, 1989, pp. 135-159

Jan ASSMANN, *Egyptian Solar Religion in the New Kingdom: Re, Amun and the crisis of polytheism*, Kegan Paul International, London, New York, 1995

Jan ASSMANN, *Images et Rites de la Mort dans l'Égypte Ancienne: L'apport des liturgies funéraires*, Cybele, Paris, 2000

Jan ASSMANN, *The Search for God in Ancient Egypt*, Cornell University Press, Ithaca, London, 2001

Jan ASSMANN, *Potere e salvezza: Teologia politica nell'antico Egitto, in Israele e in Europa*, Einaudi, Turim, 2002

Jan ASSMANN, *The Mind of Egypt: History and meaning in the time of the pharaohs*, Harvard University Press, Cambdrige, Massachusetts, London, 2002

Jan ASSMANN, *Maât, l'Égypte pharaonique et l'idée de justice social*, La Maison de Vie, Paris, 2003

Jan ASSMANN, *Mort et au-delà dans l'Égypte ancienne*, Éditions du Rocher, Monaco, 2003

Sydney AUFRÉRE, *L'Univers Minéral dans la pensée Égyptienne*, dois volumes, Institut Français d'Archaeologie Oriental, Cairo, 1991

Emoke BAILEY, 'Circumcision in ancient Egypt', *BACE* 7 (1996), pp. 15-28

Jean Christophe BAILLY, *La Llamada Muda: Los retratos de El Fayum*, Ediciones Akal, Madrid, 2001

John BAINES, 'Interpreting Sinuhe', *JEA 68 (1982)*, 31-44

John BAINES, Jaromír MÁLEK, *Egipto: Deuses, Templos e Faraós*, Círculo de Leitores, Lisboa, 1991

Paul BARGUET, 'Les chapitres 313-321 des Textes des Pyramides et la naissance de la lumière', *RdÉ* 22 (1970), pp. 7-14

Paul BARGUET, *Aspects de la pensée religieuse de l'Égypte ancienne*, La Maison de Vie, Paris, 2001

Nathalie BEAUX, 'La Douat dans les Textes des Pyramides: Espace et temps de gestation', *BIFAO* 94 (1994), pp. 1-6

Olivier BEIGBEDER, *La Symbolique*, col. Que sais je?, Presses Universitaires de France, Paris, 1957

Jocelyne BERLANDINI, 'Ptah-demiurge et l'exaltation du ciel', *RdÉ* 46 (1995), pp. 9-41

Edwin BEVAN, *Symbolism and Belief*, Beacon Press, Boston, 1957

Susanne BICKEL, 'Creative and destructive waters', in A. Amenta (ed.) *L'Acqua nell'antico Egitto: vita rigenerazione, incantesimo, medicamento – Proceedings of the First International Conference for Young Egyptologists*, vol. III, L'Erma di Bretschneider, Roma, 2005, pp. 191-200

Susanne BINDER, 'The hereafter: Ancient Egyptian beliefs with special reference to the *Amduat*', *BACE* 6 (1995), pp. 7-30

Aylward BLACKMAN, 'The funerary papyrus of Enkhfenkhons', *JEA* 4 (1917), pp. 122-129

Aylward BLACKMAN, 'The significance of incense and libations in funerary and temple ritual', *ZÄS* 50 (1912), pp. 69-75

Aylward BLACKMAN, 'Some notes on the Ancient Egyptian practice of washing the dead', *JEA* 5 (1918), pp. 117-123

Aylward BLACKMAN, 'Sacramental ideas and usages in ancient Egypt', *RT* 39 (1920), pp. 44-78

Rachel BLANCHARD, *Handbook of Egyptian Gods and Mummy Amulets*, Cairo, 1909

Martin BOMMAS, 'Situlae and the offering of water in the divine funerary cult: a new approach to the ritual of Djeme', in A. Amenta (ed.) *L'Acqua nell'antico Egitto: vita rigenerazione, incantesimo, medicamento – Proceedings of the First International Conference for Young Egyptologists*, vol. III, L'Erma di Bretschneider, Roma, 2005, pp. 257-272

Marie-Ange BONHÊME, *L'Art Égyptien*, Presses Universitaires de France, Paris, 1992

Marie-Ange BONHÊME, Annie FORGEAU, *Pharaon: Les Secrets du Pouvoir*, Armand Colin, Paris, 1988

R. van der BROEK, *The Myth of the Phoenix according to Classical and early Christian Traditions*, E. J. Brill, Leiden, 1972

Michèle BROZE, 'La création du monde et l'opposition *sḏm.f* - *sḏm.n.f* dans le temple d'Esna', *RdÉ* 44 (1993), pp. 3-9

Wallis BUDGE, *The Mummy: The Handbook of Egyptian Funerary Archaeology*, University Press, Cambridge, 1893

Benoit CLAUS, 'Osiris et Hapi: crue et regeneration en Égypte ancienne', in A. Amenta (ed.) *L'Acqua nell'antico Egitto: vita rigenerazione, incantesimo, medicamento* – Proceedings of the First International Conference for Young Egyptologists, *vol. III, L'Erma di Bretschneider, Roma, 2005, pp. 201-210*

Marc COENEN, 'The funerary papyri of the Bodleian Library at Oxford', *JEA* 86 (2000), pp. 81-98

Eugene CRUZ-URIBE, 'The Khonsu Cosmogony', *JARCE* 31 (1994), pp. 169-189

François DAUMAS, *La Civilisation de l'Égypte Pharaonique*, Éditions Arthaud, Paris, 1987

Georges DARESSY, 'Rituel des offrandes à Amenhotep I', *ASAE* 17 (1917), pp. 97-122

John DARNELL, *The Enigmatic Netherworld Books of the Solar-Osirian Unity: Cryptographic Compositions in the Tombs of Tutankhamun, Ramesses VI and Ramesses IX*, Academic Press, Fribourg, 2004

Diana DELLA, 'The Refreshing Water of Osiris', *JARCE* 29 (1992), pp. 181-190

Jean DELPECH-LABORIE, 'L'aura humaine et le *ka* égyptien', *CdÉ* 37 (1944), pp. 62-67

Philippe DERCHAIN, 'Sur le nom de Chou et sa fonction', *RdÉ* 27 (1975), pp. 110-116

Philippe DERCHAIN, 'L'auteur du Papyrus Jumilhac', *RdÉ* 41 (1990), pp. 9-30

Christiane DESROCHES-NOBLECOURT, *Le Secret des Temples de la Nubie*, Éditions Stock/Pernoud, Paris, 1999

Anthony DONOHUE, 'The vizier Paser', *JEA* 74 (1988), pp. 103-123

Rosemarie DRENKHAHN, Renate GERMER, *Mumie und Computer: ein multi-disziplinares Forchunger project in Hannover*, Kestner Museum, Hannover, 1991

Ramadan EL-SAYED, 'Les Kas de rayonnemet et de brillance', *ASAE* 70 (1970), pp. 409-413

Raymond FAULKNER, 'King and star religion in the Pyramid Texts', *JNES* 25 (1966), pp. 153-159

Walter FEDERN, 'The Transformations in the Coffin Texts: A new approach', *JNES* 19 (1960), pp. 241-257

Ragnhild FINNESTAD, 'Egyptian tought about life as a problem os translation', in Gertie Englund (ed.) *The religion of ancient Egyptians: Cognitive structures and popular expressions. Proceedings of Symposia in Uppsala and Bergen 1987 and 1988*, Acta Universitatis Upsaliensis, Boreas, Uppsala Studies in Ancient Mediterranean and Near Eastern Civilizations, 20, Uppsala, 1987, pp. 29-40

Ragnhild FINNESTAD, 'The Pharaoh and the Democratization of post-mortem life', in Gertie Englund (ed.) *The religion of ancient Egyptians: Cognitive structures and popular expressions. Proceedings of Symposia in Uppsala and Bergen 1987 and 1988*, Acta Universitatis Upsaliensis, Boreas, Uppsala Studies in Ancient Mediterranean and Near Eastern Civilizations, 20, Uppsala, 1987, pp. 89-93

Isabelle FRANCO, *Rites et Croyances d'Éternité*, col. Rites et Croyances d'Éternité, Pygmalion, Paris, 1993

Henri FRANKFORT, *Kingship of the Gods: A study of Ancient Near Eastern Religion as the integration of society and nature*, University of Chicago Press, Chicago, London, 1978

Gabala A. GABALA, *Ancient Egyptian Jewelry: Best Selection from the Egyptian Museum*, Ministry of Culture, Supreme Council of Antiquities & Egyptian Museum, Cairo, 1999

Alan GARDINER, 'The baptism of pharaoh', *JEA* 36 (1950), pp. 3-12

Renate GERMER, *Mumies: Life after Death in Ancient Egypt*, Prestel Verlag, Munich, New York, 1997

Beatrice GOFF, *Symbols of Ancient Egypt in the Late Period: the Twenty-first Dynasty*, Mouton Publishers, Haia, Paris, New York, 1979

Andrew GORDON, 'The *ka* as an animating force', *JARCE* 33 (1996), pp. 31-35

Bernhard GRDSELOFF, 'L'insigne du grand juge égyptien', *ASAE* 40 (1940), pp. 199-202

Bernhard GRDSELOFF, 'Nouvelles données concernant la tente de purification', *ASAE* 51 (1951), pp. 129-140

Gwyn GRIFFITHS, *The Conflict of Horus and Seth: From Egyptian and Classical sources*, Liverpool University Press, Liverpool, 1960

Gwyn GRIFFITHS, 'The frase *ḥr mw.f* in the Memphite Theology', *ZÄS* 123 (1996), pp. 111-115

Nicolas GRIMAL, *Histoire de l'Égypte Ancienne*, Fayard, Paris, 1988

Battiscombe GUNN, 'Inscriptions from the Step Pyramid site', *ASAE* 28 (1928), pp. 151-174

Hedvig GYORY, 'Les amulettes de l'oeil *Oudjat* ailé et le mythe de l'oeil du soleil', *BSEG* 18 (1994), pp. 23-31

Ahmed HAMADA, 'A stela from Manshiyet es Sadr', *ASAE* 38 (1938), pp. 217-230

Tom HARE, *Remembering Osiris: Number, Gender and Word in Ancient Egyptian representational systems*, Stanford University Press, Stanford, 1999

Stephen HARVEY, Melinda HARTWIG, *Gods of Ancient Memphis*, Institute of Egyptian Art & Archaeology, University of Memphis, Memphis, 2001

François-René HERBIN, 'Un hymne à la lune croissante', *BIFAO* 82 (1982), pp. 237-282.

Patrick HOURIHAN, *The Birds of Ancient Egypt*, Aris & Phillips, Warstminster, 1986

Erik IVERSEN, 'Reflections on some royal names', in I. S. Edwards, *Pyramid Studies and other Essays*, Egypt Exploration Society, London, 1988, pp. 78-88

T. G. H. JAMES, *Egyptian Painting*, British Museum Press, London, 1985

László KÁKOSY, 'The Ptah-Shu-Tefnut triad and the gods of winds on a ptolemaic sarcophagus', in Jacobus van Dijk (ed), *Essays on Ancient Egypt in honour of Heerma Te Velde*, vol. I, Publications Groningen, 1997, pp. 219-229

László KÁKOSY, 'A Memphite triad', *JEA* 66 (1980), pp. 48-53

Joachim Selim KARIG, ‚Die Kultkammer des Amenhotep aus Deir Durunka', *ZÄS* 95 (1968), pp. 27-32

Barry KEMP, *El Antiguo Egipto: Anatomia de una civilization*, Crítica, Barcelona, 1996

Yvan KOENIG, 'L'eau et magie', in A. Amenta (ed.), *L'Acqua nell'antico Egitto: vita rigenerazione, incantesimo, medicamento – Proceedings of the First International Conference for Young Egyptologists*, vol. III, L'Erma di Bretschneider, Roma, 2005, pp. 91-105

Yvan KOENIG, *Magie et Magiciens dans l'Égypte Ancienne*, Pygmalion, Paris, 1994

Claire LALOUETTE, *L'Empire des Ramsès*, Collection Champs, Flammarion, Paris, 1995

Claire LALOUETTE, *Thèbes ou la naissance d'un empire*, Collection Champs, Flammarion, Paris, 1995

Jean LECLANT, 'Les Rites de Purification dans le cérémonial de pharaonique du couronnement', *Proceedings of the XI International Congress of the*

International Association for the History of Religions, Vol. II: *Guilt or pollution and rites of purification*, E. J. Brill, Leiden, 1968, pp. 48-51

Leonard LESKO, 'Some remarks on the *Book of the Dead* composed for the high priests Pinedjem I and II', *For his Ka: Essays offered in memory of Klaus Baer*, The Oriental Institute od University of Chicago, Chicago, Illinois, 1994

Antonio LOPRIENO, *La Pensée et l'Écriture: Pour une analyse sémiotieque de la culture Égyptienne*, Cybele, Paris, 2001

Victor LORET, 'Quelques notes sur l'arbre *âch*', *ASAE* 16 (1916), pp. 33-51

Manfred LURKER, *The Gods and Symbols of Ancient Egypt*, Thames and Hudson, London, 1974

Christine EL-MAHDY, *Mummies: Myth and Magic*, Thames and Hudson, London, 1991

Jaromír MALEK, *Egypt, 4000 Years of Art*, Phaidon Press, London, 2003

Bill MANLEY, *Atlas de l'Égypte ancienne*, Éditions Autrement, Paris, 1998

Tiziana MARTINELLI, 'Geb et Nout dans les *Textes des Pyramides*: Essai de compréhension du caractère masculin de Geb et de la Terre ainsi que du caractère féminin de Nout et du Ciel', *BSEG* 18 (1994), pp. 61-77

Charles MAYSTRE, *Les grands prêtres de Ptah de Memphis*, Orbis Biblicus et Orientalis, Universität Freiburg Schweiz, Vandenhoeck & Ruprecht, Göttingen, 1998

Dimitri MEEKS, 'Les quatre *ka* du démiurge memphite', *RdÉ* 15 (1963), pp. 35-47

Dimitri MEEKS, Christine FAVARD-MEEKS, *La Vie Quotidienne des Dieux Égyptiens*, Hachette, Paris, 1993

Bernadette MENU, 'Le tombeau de Pétosiris, Maât, Thot et le droit', *BIFAO* 95 (1995), pp. 281-295

Henk MILDE, *The Vignettes in the Book of the Dead of Neferrenpet*, Nederlands Instituut voor het Nabije Oosten, Leiden, 1991

Cláudia Monte FARIAS, 'O templo no antigo Egipto: simbolismo e iconografia', *Artis* 1 (2002), pp. 17-30

Pierre MONTET, 'Le fruit défendu', *Kêmi* 2 (1950), pp. 85-116

Pierre MONTET, 'Ptah patèque et les orfèvres', *RA* 40 (1952), pp. 1-11

Siegfried MORENZ, *La Religion Égyptienne. Essay d'interprétation*, Ed. Payot, Paris, 1984

John NUNN, *Ancient Egyptian Medicine*, British Museum Press, London, 1991

Georges POSENER, 'Le conte de Neferkaré et du general Siséné', *RdÉ* 11 (1957), pp. 119-137

Stephen QUIRKE, *The Cult of Ra: Sun-worship in Ancient Egypt*, Thames & Hudson, London, 2001

Stephen QUIRKE, *Egyptian literature 1800 BC, questions and readings*, Golden House Publications, London, 2004

Hermann RANKE, *Die Ägyptischen Personennamen*, III, Verlag J. J. Augustin, Glückstadt, 1977

Maarten RAVEN, 'Corn-mummies', *OMRO* 63 (1982), pp. 7-34

Maarten RAVEN, 'A puzzling pataekos', *OMRO* 67 (1987), pp. 7-17

Carole REEVES, *Egyptian Medicine*, Shire Egyptology, London, 2001

Nicholas REEVES, *The complete Tutankhamun: The King, the Tomb, the Royal Treasure*, Thames and Hudson, London, 1990

Gay ROBINS, *The Art of Ancient Egypt*, British Museum Press, London, 1997

Ann ROTH, 'The *Pšs-kf* and the "Opening of the mouth" cerimony: A ritual of birth and rebirth', *JEA* 78 (1992), pp. 113-147

Ann ROTH, 'Fingers, Stars and the Opening of the mouth', *JEA* 79 (1993), pp. 57-79

José das Candeias SALES, *As Divindades Egípcias: Uma chave para a compreensão do Egipto antigo*, Editorial Estampa, Lisboa, 1999

Serge SAUNERON, *The Priests of Ancient Egypt*, Cornell University Press, Ithaca & London, 2000

Heinrich SCHÄFER, *Principles of Egyptian Art*, Grifith Institute, Oxford University Press, Oxford, 1980

Hans SCHNEIDER, 'Bringing the *ba* to the body: A glorification spell for Padinekhtnebef', *Hommages à Jean Leclant*, vol. 4, Bibliothèque d'Étude, IFAO, Cairo, 1994, pp. 355-362

Hans SCHNEIDER, 'Ptah in wings', in Jacobus van DIJK (ed), *Essays on Ancient Egypt in honour of Herman Te Velde*, Vol. I, Publications Groningen, 1997, pp. 293-297

Ian SHAW (dir.), *The Oxford History of Ancient Egypt*, Oxford University Press, Oxford, 2002

Jorgen SORENSEN, 'Ancient Egyptian religious thought and XVI Hermetic Tractate', in Gertie Englund (ed) *The religion of ancient Egyptians: Cognitive structures and popular expressions. Proceedings of Symposia in Uppsala and Bergen 1987 and 1988*, Acta Universitatis Upsaliensis, Boreas, Uppsala Studies in Ancient Mediterranean and Near Eastern Civilizations, 20, Uppsala, 1987, pp. 41-57

Jorgen SORENSEN, 'Divine Access: The so-called democratisation of Egyptian funerary literature as a socio-cultural process', in Gertie Englund (ed) *The religion of ancient Egyptians : Cognitive structures and popular expressions. Proceedings of Symposia in Uppsala and Bergen 1987 and 1988*, Acta Universitatis Upsaliensis, Boreas, Uppsala Studies in Ancient Mediterranean and Near Eastern Civilizations, 20, Uppsala, 1987, pp. 109-123

Anthony SPALINGER, 'Orientations on Sinuhe', *SAK* 25 (1998), pp. 311-339

Louis SPELLEERS, 'La résurrection et la toilette du mort selon les Textes des Pyramides', *RdÉ* 3 (1938), pp. 37-67

Cathie SPIESER, 'L'eau et la regeneration des morts d'après les représentations des tombes thébaines du Nouvel Empire', *CdÉ* 72 (1997), pp. 211-228

Aaron SMITH, 'Kingship, water and ritual: The ablution rite in the coronation ritual of the Pharaoh', in A. Amenta (ed.) *L'Acqua nell'antico Egitto: vita rigenerazione, incantesimo, medicamento – Proceedings of the First International Conference for Young Egyptologists*, vol. III, L'Erma di Bretschneider, Roma, 2005, pp. 329-336

Harry SMITH, 'Maet and Isfet', *BACE* 5 (1994), pp. 67-88

Stevenson SMITH, *The Art and the Architecture of Ancient Egypt*, Yale University Press, New Haven & London, 1998

Henri STIERLIN, *L'Or des Pharaons*, Terrail, Paris, 1993

John TAYLOR, *Death and the afterlife in ancient Egypt*, British Museum Press, London, 2001

Bruce TRIGGER, Barry KEMP, David O'CONNOR, Allan LLOYD, *Ancient Egypt: A social history*, Cambridge University Press, Cambridge, 2001

Vincent Arieh TOBIN, 'Mytho-Theology in Ancient Egypt', *JARCE* 25 (1988), pp. 169-183

Vincent Arieh TOBIN, 'Divine conflict in Pyramid Texts', *JARCE* 30 (1993), pp. 93-110

Kent WEEKS (ed.), *Egyptology and the Social Sciences: Five Studies*, The Amercican University in Cairo Press, Cairo, 1979

Alfred WIEDEMANN, *Religion of the Ancient Egyptians*, Dover Publications, Mineola, New York, 2003

Dietrich WILDUNG, *Egypt: From Prehistory to the Romans*, Taschen, Köhln, 1997

Richard WILKINSON, *Reading Egyptian Art*, Thames and Hudson, London, 1992

Richard WILKINSON, *Symbol and Magic in Egyptian Art*, Thames & Hudson, London, 1994

Richard WILKINSON, *The Complete Valley of the Kings*, Thames & Hudson, London, 1996

Richard WILKINSON, *The Complete Temples of Ancient Egypt*, Thames & Hudson, London, 2000

Richard WILKINSON, *The Complete God and Goddesses of Ancient Egypt*, American University in Cairo Press, Thames & Hudson, Cairo, 2003

Pascal VERNUS, *Athribis: Textes et documents relatifs à la Geographie, aux cultes, et à l'Histoire d'une ville du delta égyptien à l'Époque Pharaonique*, Bibliothéque d'Étude, 74, IFAO, Cairo, 1978

Jacobus VAN DIJK, 'The symbolism of the Memphite Djed-pillar', *OMRO* 66 (1986), pp. 7-17

Jacobus VAN DIJK, 'The birth of Horus according to the Ebers Papyrus', *JEOL* 26 (1979-80), pp. 10-25

Herman te VELDE, 'Some aspects of the god Shu', *JEOL* 26 (1979-1980), pp. 23-28

Jean VERCOUTTER, *L'Égypte et la Valée du Nil*, vol. I: *Des origines à la fin de l'Ancien Empire (12.000-2000 a. C.)*, Presses Universitaires de France, Paris, 1992

Andrea Paula ZINGARELLI, 'Some considerations about the water offered (poured) by the tree-goddess at TT 79', in A. Amenta (ed.) *L'Acqua nell'antico Egitto: vita rigenerazione, incantesimo, medicamento – Proceedings of the First International Conference for Young Egyptologists*, vol. III, L'Erma di Bretschneider, Roma, 2005, pp. 381-388

www.ingramcontent.com/pod-product-compliance
Lightning Source LLC
LaVergne TN
LVHW071218210926
848482LV00015B/846
* 9 7 8 1 4 0 7 3 0 7 6 9 5 *